Edward L. Acree
45 S. Idlewild #1014
274-4193

Abraham E. Nizel, D.M.D., M.S.D.

ASSISTANT CLINICAL PROFESSOR IN ORAL
PATHOLOGY (NUTRITION), TUFTS UNIVERSITY,
SCHOOL OF DENTAL MEDICINE.
RESEARCH ASSOCIATE IN FOOD TECHNOLOGY,
MASSACHUSETTS INSTITUTE OF TECHNOLOGY

Nutrition in Clinical Dentistry

W. B. Saunders Company

PHILADELPHIA AND LONDON

Reprinted November, 1960 and July, 1964

Nutrition in Clinical Dentistry

Library of Congress Catalog Card Number; 60-7462

Dedicated

to my wife,

Jeannette,

and my sons,

David and *Jonathan*

Preface

This textbook has been prepared to enable the general practitioner of dentistry to use nutrition as a practical objective discipline in his daily practice, and as a guide for teaching nutrition to the dental student and dental hygienist. It has been designed to conform to the recommendations on the teaching of nutrition in dental schools that were presented during the Conference Session on Nutrition and Dietetics at the 1956 meeting of the American Association of Dental Schools.

The dentist who appreciates the importance of nutrition in maintaining the integrity of the tissues of the oral cavity, the teeth, the periodontium and the adjacent oral structures, and can apply it in his daily practice, will be held in high esteem by the patient of today. The patient looks to the dentist for management of all types of problems that arise in the oral cavity, not only for individual tooth treatments. To solve some of these problems, local mechanical techniques do not always suffice; it requires an appreciation of the role and management of endogenous metabolic factors. Diet and nutrition are part of these systemic influences. As members of a health profession, it is our responsibility to use nutrition as one of our tools for the improvement of our patient's total oral health. Providing adequate diets during the periods of dental stress as well as utilizing proper diets for maintenance of tissue health postoperatively are as important adjuncts in the over-all management of a dental patient as are x-rays in diagnosis, anesthesia in surgery or oral physiotherapy in periodontology.

A knowledge of nutrition can help in the practice of dentistry in several ways:

1. It provides an understanding of some of the factors involved in the etiology, prevention and control of dental caries.

2. It explains some of the changes in the oral mucous membrane which reflect a systemic disease of nutritional origin.

3. It gives the dentist an answer to the inevitable question, "What can I eat, doctor?" after periodontal, prosthetic and oral surgery procedures.

The book is divided into two major parts, one on basic nutrition and one on applied nutrition.

In basic nutrition, the chemistry and physiology of each of the nutrients is discussed to give an understanding of its normal metabolism. This is followed by a consideration of the effects of abnormal metabolism of the nutrients on tissues and organs in general and on the mouth and its related structures in particular. In this section, subjects like intermediary metabolism and dietary interrelationships have been touched upon to give the reader a concept of how dynamic a subject nutrition really is. It is fully realized that a complete textbook could be written, and in many instances has already been written, on the subject matter included in each chapter. Therefore, no attempt has been made to deal in detail with any one nutrient; rather, the salient features of each are pointed out, particularly as they influence oral health.

In the section on applied nutrition, basic information on normal diets and the procedure for arriving at a nutritional diagnosis are presented as a preface to the specific dietetic management of the various dental problems that are encountered in daily practice. For the sake of convenience and simplicity the Daily Food Guide, which interprets adequacy of a diet in terms of servings of the 4 Food Groups, has been used throughout the text as the method of diet evaluation and diet teaching. The role of diet and nutrition in the control of rampant caries is probably the most important consideration in applied dental nutrition. For this reason detailed procedures, which include the "why" as well as the "what" of the diet, have been given for making a nutritional diagnosis and for prescribing diets to suit the patient's individual needs. For the patient whose dental conditions are classified as periodontal, prosthetic or surgical, specific dietary advice is suggested.

Several of my colleagues in the fields of nutrition and dentistry have motivated and inspired me to attempt the writing of this book. To my teacher and collaborator in research, Dr. Robert S. Harris, Professor of Biochemistry of Nutrition in the Department of Food Technology at Massachusetts Institute of Technology, I owe my special gratitude for his encouragement and continuous guidance. To Dr. Henry Sherman, who formerly was Assistant Professor of Biochemistry of Nutrition in the Department of Food Technology at Massachusetts Institute of Technology, I must express my thanks for his diligent and thorough editing as well as verification of the facts that pertained to the material on Basic Nutrition. Thanks also go to Dr. Sanford Miller, who is Assistant Professor in the same department as my other two colleagues and who has contributed two chapters, one on intermediary metabolism and the other on dietary interrelationships, as well as assisting with the chapter on calories and energy metabolism.

I am very appreciative and honored to have had the privilege of editorial advice on the chapter on the clinical assessment of nutritional status by Dr. Nevin S. Scrimshaw, Regional Advisor in Nutrition of the Pan-American Health Organization and Director of INCAP.

I also want to thank Miss Isabel Patterson, who is Assistant Professor of Nutrition at Boston University School of Nursing, for her counsel on dietetics and for the formulation of the several diets that are suggested in the text. She has also contributed two chapters, one dealing with interpreting nutritional needs and the other containing some practical suggestions for applying nutritional knowledge.

My dental colleagues who are or were associated with me at Tufts University School of Dental Medicine have been most helpful in making suggestions on several of the chapters that deal with nutrition in the various dental specialities—Dr. Irving Glickman in periodontology, Dr. Albert Yurkstas in prosthetics and Dr. Daniel Holland in oral surgery.

It was felt that rather than duplicate the numerous photographs and tables that describe so much of the review matter presented here, the purpose of the book would be better served if the original ones could be used. To the numerous authors and publishers who have given us permission for their use, many thanks. I also want to acknowledge the illustrations that Dr. G. Shklar, of Tufts University

School of Dental Medicine, and Dr. Jonathan Cohen, of the Children's Medical Center in Boston, have allowed me to use.

For the excellent typing services of Miss Rose Ann Roberto and Miss Patricia Rourke, my sincerest appreciation.

I am most grateful to my publishers, the W. B. Saunders Co., for their wonderful editorial help and meticulous attention to details.

Finally, to my beloved wife and children, I offer my everlasting gratitude for their understanding and patience in sparing me the many hours that were taken away from them and devoted to the writing of this book.

A. E. Nizel, D.M.D., M.S.D.

Contents

Section 1

Basic Nutrition and Its Effect on Oral Tissues in Health and Disease

Chapter I

Calories and Energy Metabolism

INTRODUCTION

"Behold, I have given you every herb bearing seed, which is upon the face of all the earth, and every tree, in which is the fruit of a tree yielding seed; to you it shall be for . . . (food)."

This is a quotation from the 29th verse of Chapter 1 of Genesis in the Old Testament and is probably the first reference to our source of food. But what is food?

To Adam, to many of our ancestors, and to some peoples even today, food connotes only one thing, satisfaction of hunger. But if we read the writings of the Hebrews, the Egyptians, the Greeks and the Romans, we find that there were some very learned and wise men who realized that food was more than a means of satisfying hunger; it meant edible substances that could nourish and give vigor to the body.

When scientists became interested in trying to determine how food functions to give strength to the body, how it yields energy, how it builds and repairs tissues and how it regulates body processes, then nutrition became, like anatomy, histology and biochemistry, a science unto itself. In fact, nutrition may be defined as a science which deals with the assimilation and effect of food on total health.

The science of nutrition actually originated at the end of the eighteenth century in the study of energy. This was the time when physicists were dealing with steam, power and energy. Men like

Priestley, Lavoisier, Liebig and others were intrigued with the thought that perhaps the basic concepts about energy that worked for inanimate objects could also be applied to the animate. They wanted to know how an animal functioned and what was the source of its energy.

Just as nutrition had its beginning as a science with the study of energy, so does this book. The most fundamental of all the requirements for life is energy. An animal can survive for relatively long periods of time without vitamins, minerals or other nutrients, but without the fuel to keep the "engine running," life soon ceases. Actually, an animal tends to select food instinctively, primarily for its caloric content and, secondarily, for any other benefit that his body can derive from it.

Another reason that calories are considered first is that the most prevalent clinical nutritional problems in the world in the last decade, and even today, stem not from vitamin deficiencies but rather from caloric undernutrition and caloric overnutrition. In fact, the rise in degenerative diseases in general has been attributed more to this latter factor than to any other.

EVOLUTION OF PRINCIPLES OF ENERGY METABOLISM[5]

Stahl, a German physician, proposed the imaginative hypothesis that there was an invisible, weightless substance called phlogiston which escaped from combustible material. He theorized that materials were made of calx (or ash) and phlogiston and that when a material burned, the calx remained and the phlogiston escaped. Attempts were made to identify phlogiston with some definite substance, but to no avail. Finally, in 1774, Priestley isolated and described a gas that escaped from mercuric oxide, which he called "dephlogisticated air." He also demonstrated that this same gas was present in the atmosphere.

On the basis of Priestley's discovery, Lavoisier began his numerous investigations in respiration and energy metabolism. He called "dephlogisticated air" by an alternate name, "oxygine principle," and was able to show that there were two factors involved in respiration: (a) the disappearance of oxygen, and (b) the appearance of "fixed air" (carbon dioxide). Later he was able to measure the quantity of heat produced during a chemical reaction by measuring the amount of ice that it melted in an ice calorimeter. Using both of these principles Lavoisier was then able to show that muscular work increased respiration and simultaneously increased the amount of heat liberated. The amount of carbon dioxide produced from respiration could be correlated to the amount of heat yielded. In short, through numerous experiments he related work, heat, respiration, transpiration and digestion.

Von Voit made one of the outstanding contributions to the study of metabolism when he built a respiratory chamber sufficiently large so that a man could sleep, work and eat within it. The in-going and out-going air could be sampled and analyzed. Rubner, von Voit's student and assistant, proved that the principle of conservation of energy was applicable to man as well as to matter. A second important contribution by von Voit was his development of a very accurate chemical calorimeter. Using similar principles, Bertholet, and later Atwater, developed a bomb calorimeter in which the amount of heat produced from food could be measured.

It is interesting that all these basic principles laid down at the end of eighteenth century and during the nineteenth century are still generally accepted today. Of course, the techniques have been refined and extended, and greater knowledge of metabolic events has supplied better explanations for the rationale of energy metabolism.

ENERGY VALUE OF FOOD[2,3,4,6]

All the energy required for growth, maintenance and work is derived from the oxidation of carbohydrates, fats and proteins. Proteins are used only if the other two nutrients are unavailable. Approximately 20 per cent of the potential energy of food is transformed into mechanical energy, the remainder being liberated as heat. The energy value of food depends upon the number of Calories that are produced when foodstuff is metabolized in the body.

Units of energy are calories; a calorie being defined as the amount of heat required to raise the temperature of one gram of water 1°C. The large Calorie or kilogram calorie is the term used in nutritional work and is 1,000 times the small calorie; it is defined as the amount of heat required to raise one kilogram of water from 15°C. to 16°C.

The amount of energy in a food can be determined by direct and indirect chemical calorimetric techniques as well as by nutrient analysis through predetermined Calorie equivalents. Direct calorimetry is the technique which involves the measurement of the amount of energy that is released as heat, whereas indirect calorimetry measures the energy content of the substance by determining the amount of oxygen utilized or carbon dioxide produced in the release of this heat.

Direct Chemical Calorimetry

As originally described by Atwater and Blakeslee, the direct chemical calorimetric method involves measuring the temperature

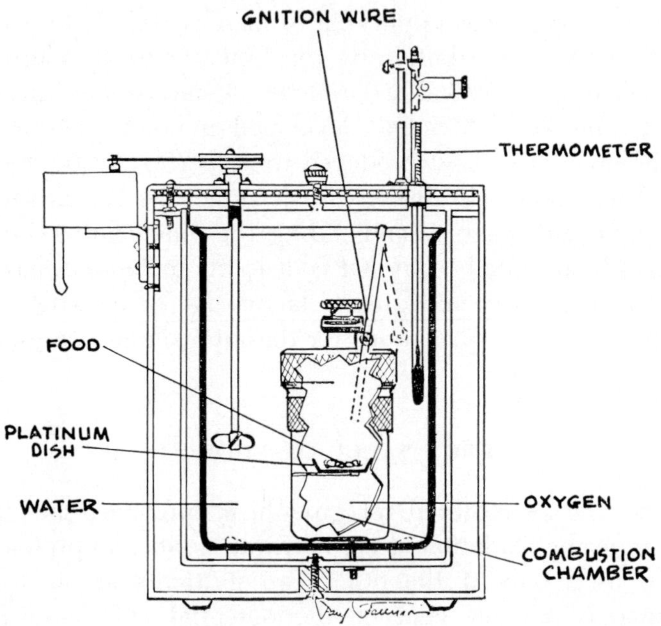

FIGURE 1. The bomb calorimeter. (Langley, L. L., and Cheraskin, E.: Physiology of Man. McGraw-Hill Book Company, Inc., 1954. Used by permission.)

rise of water that has been heated as a result of the combustion of a nutrient or nutrients. This technique is briefly described as follows:

A weighed amount of food is placed in a specially constructed steel bomb which is charged with oxygen (Fig. 1). This steel bomb is then immersed in a weighed amount of water (1 kg.). The sample of food is ignited by an electric fuse; in the presence of the oxygen, it is rapidly and completely burned. The heat liberated from this combustion is transferred to the water in which the bomb was immersed and the resulting rise in temperature of the water is measured. This temperature rise is corrected for losses due to radiation effects. The corrected rise multiplied by the amount of water gives a value for the amount of heat liberated in the bomb. Since the oxidation of the iron fuse wire produces a certain amount of heat, these Calories must be subtracted from the total amount of heat produced to arrive at a final figure. This value represents the number of Calories present in the sample of food tested.

Indirect Chemical Calorimetry

In the indirect chemical calorimetric method, the volume of oxygen required to combust the food is measured. This is done with an instrument called an oxycalorimeter.[1] The changes in the volume of oxygen are measured with a spirometer gauge. On the assumption that the same amount of oxygen is needed to release a Calorie of energy from any compound, a predetermined figure for the number of Calories released per liter of oxygen utilized can be computed. With the aid of this predetermined figure the calorie value of the test food can be calculated.

Nutrient Analysis Techniques

Predetermined Calorie Equivalents. Predetermined Calorie equivalents were established as a result of Atwater's measurements of the energy value of carbohydrates, fats and proteins. He found that carbohydrates yielded 4.1 Calories per gram, fats 9.45 Calories per gram, and protein 5.65 Calories per gram.

These values, which were obtained in a bomb calorimeter, he then corrected for each of the nutrients to take into account their respective coefficients of digestibility in man. In a mixed diet, the average per cent absorption for protein is 92 per cent, for fat, 95 per cent and for carbohydrates, 98 per cent.

Proteins are not oxidized completely to carbon dioxide and water; some carbon is eliminated in the urine as urea. Therefore, the conversion of "in vitro" to "in vivo" values must be accompanied by a correction factor (1.30 Calories) to account for this incomplete oxidation in the animal body. The calculations giving rise to the approximate physiological fuel values are as follows:

$$4.10 \times .98 = 4 \text{ Cal. per gm. of carbohydrate}$$
$$9.45 \times .95 = 9 \text{ Cal. per gm. of fat}$$
$$(5.65 - 1.30) \times .92 = 4 \text{ Cal. per gm. of protein}$$

These factors, 4, 9, 4, representing the Calorie equivalents per gram of carbohydrate, fat and protein, respectively, are quite adequate for practical purposes. However, it must be recognized that these are general factors and that specific Calorie factors are more desirable when individual foods are considered.

Technique for Calculating Nutrient Content of Foodstuffs. The method for determining the percentages of each of the nutrients in a foodstuff is as follows:

1. The protein concentration of a food is determined by measuring its total nitrogen content. A total nitrogen analysis measures nitrates, nitrites and other nitrogenous substances that are not necessarily part of the protein molecule. The assumption that the total nitrogen value measures protein alone is not completely valid, but it is sufficiently accurate for this type of calculation. Based on the assumption that the protein of the food contains 16 per cent nitrogen, a factor of 6.25 grams of protein per gram of nitrogen can be used to calculate the protein content of the food from its nitrogen value. Merely multiply the nitrogen value by 6.25. (If the protein in food contains an amount of nitrogen different from this percentage, the factor for converting nitrogen to protein is different.)

2. The amount of fat in a food is obtained by determining the amount of material that is extracted from it, after it has been dried, by ether or other fat solvents. The solvent extractable material is considered crude fat.

3. The moisture content and ash content of a food are determined by measuring weight losses following heating and ashing procedures respectively.

4. The carbohydrate content is often determined by calculation rather than by actual analysis. The difference between 100 and the sum of the percentages of crude protein, crude fat, moisture and ash content is called "total carbohydrate" or "carbohydrate by difference."

Using this technique of nutrient analysis, a sample calculation of the calorie content of a food such as bread is presented below. Bread contains, by analysis, the following:

51.8% carbohydrate
3.2% fat
8.5% protein
34.7% moisture
1.8% ash

If the percentages (grams per 100 grams) of carbohydrate, fat and protein are multiplied by the physiological fuel factors—4, 9, 4, respectively—the number of Calories contributed by each of these nutrients, in order, is 207, 29 and 34. Therefore, 100 grams of bread contains the sum of these, or 270 Calories. An average one-half inch slice of bread weighing 23 grams contains approximately 63 Calories.

ENERGY NEEDS OF THE BODY[2,3,4,6]

For what purposes must energy be supplied to the body? Power must be supplied to make a hand move, an eye blink or a jaw open and close. Heat is needed to maintain a constant body temperature. These two factors, power and heat, in addition to other body processes such as reproduction, respiration, circulatory activities, absorption, the conversion of food materials to their simpler components and the excretion of end products of metabolism, require energy.

The energy requirement for each of these metabolic processes is subject to great variation, depending on a number of factors. For example, the maintenance of body temperature is dependent upon the environment. In the tropics, the problem is to dissipate excess heat; in the arctic regions, heat must be supplied to maintain body temperature. Stress is another factor which influences the energy requirements of the body. Tissue synthesis, which occurs in growth and development as well as in the healing of wounds, is a third factor which requires large amounts of energy for its normal progress. A fourth factor may be the hormones like thyroxin which regulate body metabolism and, therefore, influence energy requirements. An imbalance in the functioning of the thyroid, of growth or gonadotrophic hormones or, in fact, of most of the endocrines, can directly or indirectly influence the basic activities of the body and, therefore, the body needs for energy.

Methods of Measurement

All of the preceding factors must be considered when energy requirements are being evaluated. But even though they cannot be quantitated individually, their total effect on the organism can be measured by two techniques, the direct and the indirect methods of animal calorimetry.

Direct Animal Calorimetry. This method is perhaps the more accurate, yet more complex, of the techniques. In practice, the test subject is placed in an insulated box and the total amount of heat radiated or transferred from the body is measured by two general methods: (1) by measuring the temperature change of a known amount of cold water flowing through tubing in the chamber, or (2) by measuring the temperature difference between the outer and inner walls of the calorimeter (Fig. 2). In each case, the corrections must be made for the amount of heat lost by evaporation of expired water and that evaporated from the skin. The amount of heat absorbed by the ventilation stream of air must also be considered.

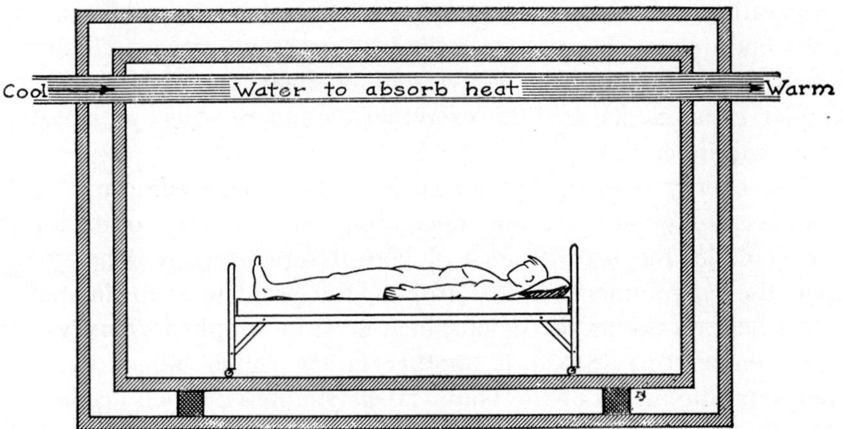

FIGURE 2. Method of determining basal metabolic rate by direct calorimetry. (From Amberson, W. R., and Smith, D. C.: Outline of Physiology. The Williams & Wilkins Company. Used by permission.)

The difficulties inherent in these measurements are numerous. For this reason this procedure has been used only when extreme accuracy and sensitivity are required.

Indirect Animal Calorimetry. The indirect or respiration exchange method of calorimetry is essentially a chemical method, in contrast to the physical techniques of direct calorimetry. It is generally simpler, less time consuming and less expensive than the direct method, but it is not quite so sensitive and is subject to a number of influences not inherent in the direct method.

The indirect method is based on the fact that during the oxidation of various nutrients oxygen is consumed and carbon dioxide is produced. Each type of nutrient requires a different amount of oxygen and, in turn, produces a different quantity of CO_2. The amount of oxygen consumed or carbon dioxide produced during the oxidation of a particular nutrient can be related to the energy produced by this oxidation. Therefore, a caloric equivalent of oxygen or carbon dioxide can be calculated for carbohydrate, protein and fat.

Respiratory Quotient. In addition to determining the energy released from a nutrient using caloric equivalents of O_2 and CO_2, a third measurement can be made. Since each type of nutrient consumes a specific amount of oxygen and produces a known amount of carbon dioxide during metabolism, the ratio of carbon dioxide produced to oxygen consumed is specific for each nutrient and is called the R.Q., meaning respiratory quotient. For example, when glucose is oxidized ($C_6H_{12}O_6 + 6\ O_2$) the number of carbon dioxide molecules produced ($6\ CO_2 + 6\ H_2O$) is equal to the number of oxygen molecules used. Therefore, its respiratory quotient is

$$\frac{6\ (CO_2)}{6\ (O_2)} = 1.$$

In the case of a glyceride like triolein ($C_{57}H_{104}O_6$), 80 molecules of oxygen are required to oxidize it. This reaction will produce 57 molecules of carbon dioxide and 52 molecules of water. Therefore, its respiratory quotient is

$$\frac{57\ (CO_2)}{80\ (O_2)} = 0.71.$$

The respiratory quotient is 1.0 for carbohydrate, 0.7 for fat, 0.8 for protein. Most R.Q. measurements are corrected for protein catabolism and, therefore, are the result of only fat and carbohydrate oxidations. Values between 0.7 and 1.0 are due to the oxidation of mixtures of fats and carbohydrates and can be related to the proportion of each.

The R.Q. is subject to a number of fluctuations. Hyperventilation, stress and severe exercise can interfere with the proper interpretation of R.Q. measurements. If it is measured shortly after a meal, the respiratory quotient will be about 1.0 because carbohydrates are the first to be metabolized. If it is measured 8 to 10 hours after a meal, the respiratory quotient will be closer to fat because this nutrient is last to be metabolized. A number of diseases can also influence the significance of the R.Q. For example, in acidosis excess carbon dioxide is expired through the lungs and, thus, can increase the R.Q. incorrectly. In diabetes, where very little carbohydrate is utilized by the body, most of the energy is derived from fat. Therefore, the respiratory quotient in this disease is about 0.7.

Techniques. In practice, the indirect approach is executed in either of two ways: (1) The test subject is placed in a sealed chamber and the air entering and leaving is analyzed for carbon dioxide, oxygen and water. Thus the amount of oxygen consumed and the amount of carbon dioxide produced are obtained. Corrections are made for the amount of protein metabolized so that the final calculations involve only the heat produced from carbohydrate and fat oxidation. (2) The more common technique, which is used for the measurement of basal metabolism in hospitals and physicians' offices, involves the use of a specially designed face mask which enables air of known composition to be inspired and which allows the collection of expired air for analysis.

Energy Balance. The technique of energy balance is used to determine how the body utilizes the energy obtained from food, i.e., how much is used for tissue synthesis, how much is stored as fat and how much is dissipated as heat. Basically the technique is as follows:

1. Animals are fed measured quantities of food of known composition.
2. The quantity of this food that is absorbed is determined by the difference between the amount consumed and the amount excreted.
3. At the end of the experimental period the carcasses of the animals are analyzed for fat, protein, water and, occasionally, carbohydrate.
4. The difference in the amount of energy consumed and the quantity stored in the form of protein and fat represents the amount of energy utilized for heat production, power and other physiological activities.

Basal Metabolism

The heat production of the body, in a post-absorptive state, during a physical and mental resting period is termed *basal metabolism.* The basal metabolic rate approximates the Calorie requirements of an individual for the maintenance of his essential life processes, e.g., circulation, excretion and respiration. In order to determine an individual BMR (basal metabolic rate), the patient's oxygen consumption is measured in a closed circuit system. The expired air can be breathed over and over again because the CO_2 and H_2O which are produced by the respiratory activity of the patient are absorbed by soda lime as fast as they arise. Utilization of oxygen is measured by a spirometer gauge which rises and falls with each respiration and is recorded on a kymograph. As the amount of oxygen in the chamber decreases, the average slope of the "zigzag" spirometer line falls. The oxygen consumption, therefore, can be measured by the slope of this line. The amount of oxygen consumed during a 6 minute period is corrected for temperature and barometric pressure. Since a calorie equivalent for oxygen can be calculated as being 4.825 Cal. for an average diet, the Calories produced per hour can be determined (Fig. 3).

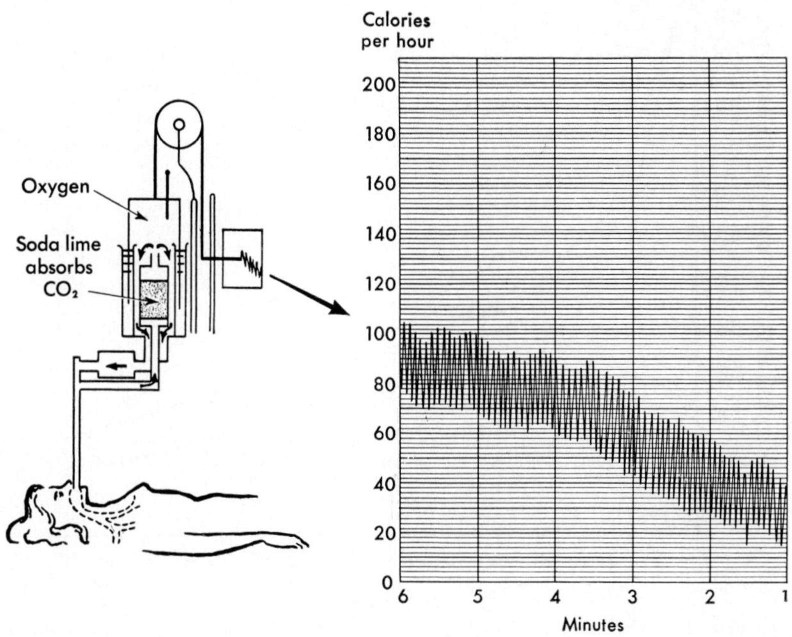

FIGURE 3. The Benedict-Roth apparatus for determining the metabolic rate. (Langley, L. L., and Cheraskin, E.: The Physiology of Man. 2nd ed. McGraw-Hill Book Company, Inc., 1958. Used by permission.)

Up to this point we have determined the amount of oxygen consumed in an hour under standard conditions, multiplied this determination by a factor, 4.825 Calories (the quantity of energy liberated for the average diet per liter of oxygen utilized in the body), and thus arrived at the number of Calories produced per hour.

Factors Influencing BMR. Size, age and sex must be evaluated and included in arriving at a figure for the basal metabolic rate of the individual. Size is related to surface area rather than weight because the amount of heat necessary to maintain a constant temperature depends on the area exposed to the environment. A nomogram is available for the estimating of surface area from weight and height data according to the Dubois formula. A straight line drawn from a point corresponding to the height of an individual on the left-hand scale to that of his weight on the right-hand scale crosses the surface area values in the middle scale at a particular point. This is the patient's surface area. (See Appendix I.)

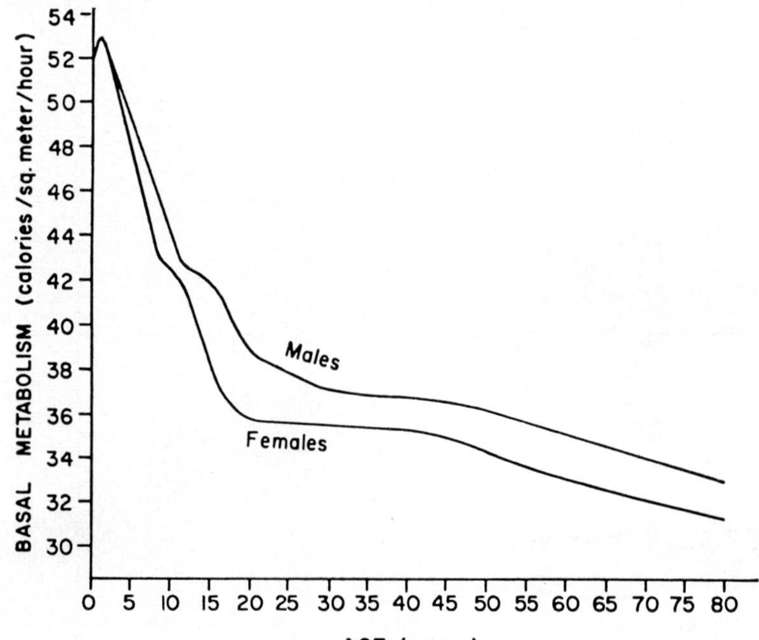

FIGURE 4. The normal basal metabolic rate at each age and for each sex. (Guyton, A. C.: Textbook of Medical Physiology.)

To correct for the variable of size, the BMR is expressed in Calories per square meter per hour. This value can be determined by dividing the number of Calories calculated from the closed circuit spirometer by the patient's surface area.

Interpretation of the BMR. The corrected BMR of the patient is compared to the average "normal" BMR for the age and sex of the individual (Fig. 4). The difference between the actual and normal values is the excess or deficit. To determine the per cent difference, merely divide the difference by the normal value and multiply by 100. Thus is derived the expression of the basal metabolic rate as plus or minus x per cent. For example, the actual

Calorie production per square meter per hour of a 20 year old male patient may be 40. The normal value for a 20 year old man derived from the reference chart is 38.5. The caloric excess is the difference, or 1.5.

$$\frac{1.5}{38.5} \times 100 = 3.9$$

Therefore, the patient's basal metabolic rate is +3.9 per cent or, in round figures, +4 per cent. A basal metabolic rate within the range of —10 per cent to +10 per cent is classified as being within normal limits.

Total Metabolism. Basal metabolism plus the heat that is produced by metabolism and physical activity represents the total heat production of the body or total metabolism. To determine the total energy expenditure and, therefore, the patient's requirements for maintaining metabolic balance, correction factors should be considered for specific dynamic action of food; for physiological conditions such as pregnancy, lactation and rate of growth, for environmental temperature and for physical activity.

Specific Dynamic Action of Food. Specific dynamic action is the term used to describe the extra heat production that occurs promptly after the ingestion of food. The specific dynamic action of proteins is the largest of the three major nutrients. It amounts to about 30 per cent, compared to 5 per cent for carbohydrates and 4 per cent for fat. However, these are not additive. The cause or explanation for this is not known. Approximately 6 per cent of the total caloric intake is usually regarded as sufficient to account for the specific dynamic action of the total diet. In balance studies, this amount of Calories must be added to the total intake.

Physiological Variables. During the latter half of pregnancy, an extra 300 Calories per day is recommended. During lactation, an extra 130 Calories should be taken in each day for every 100 cc. of milk produced; this may, on the average, amount to 1,000 Cal./day.

Environmental Factors. If the mean environmental temperature is 10°C. less than the normal 20°C., the caloric intake should be increased by 5 per cent; if the temperature is 10°C. higher than normal, it should be decreased 5 per cent.

Physical Activity. People who do heavy labor, such as carpenters and construction laborers, should ingest 25 per cent more Calories than the standard allowance.

TABLE 1. **DESIRABLE WEIGHTS FOR HEIGHT**

(Age disregarded because weight gains beyond ages of 25 to 30 years considered undesirable.)

Height, Inches	*Weight in Pounds* *Men*	*Women*
58	...	112 ± 11
60	125 ± 13	116 ± 12
62	130 ± 13	121 ± 12
64	135 ± 14	128 ± 13
66	142 ± 14	135 ± 14
68	150 ± 15	142 ± 14
70	158 ± 16	150 ± 15
72	167 ± 17	158 ± 16
74	178 ± 18	...

TABLE 2. **CALORIE ALLOWANCES AT VARIOUS BODY WEIGHTS AND AGES**

(20°C. mean external temperature, moderate activity.)

Desirable Weight		*Calorie Allowances*		
Kilograms	*Pounds*	*25 years*	*45 years*	*65 years*
Men				
50	110	2500	2350	1950
55	121	2700	2550	2150
60	132	2850	2700	2250
65	143	3000	2800	2350
*70	154	3200	3000	2550
75	165	3400	3200	2700
80	176	3550	3350	2800
85	187	3700	3500	2900
Women				
40	88	1750	1650	1400
45	99	1900	1800	1500
50	110	2050	1950	1600
55	121	2200	2050	1750
*58	128	2300	2200	1800
60	132	2350	2200	1850
65	143	2500	2350	2000
70	154	2600	2450	2050
75	165	2750	2600	2150

* "Reference" man and woman

(Table 1 and Table 2 modified from Metropolitan Life Insurance Company Statistical Bulletin 23, 1942; 24, 1943 and found in Recommended Dietary Allowance Revised 1958, Pub. 589, National Academy of Sciences-National Research Council, Washington, D.C.)

Estimation of Energy Requirements. The Calorie requirement for an individual is easily determined (1) by establishing from the patient's height the desirable weight in pounds or kilograms from Table 1; (2) by using this ideal weight figure and referring to Table 2, the Calorie allowance for different age groups and (3) by adding or deducting the Calories recommended for modification due to physical activity, age, stress or other factors, as suggested above.

If the individual consumes a greater number of Calories than those estimated as necessary, the excess Calories will be stored in the form of fat. The greater the excess, the more fat deposited and the more severe the obesity. On the other hand, if the individual consumes less Calories than are required, fat stores are utilized and the individual loses weight. It is obvious, therefore, that the problem of gaining or losing weight is a question of energy balance. This is presently one of the greatest nutritional problems.

REFERENCES

1. Benedict, F. G., and Fox, E. L.: The oxycalorimeter: principle and application to the determination of energy of fuel, foods, and excretory products. Ind. & Eng. Chem., *17*:912, 1925.
2. Fulton, J. F.: A Textbook of Physiology. 17th ed. Philadelphia, W. B. Saunders Co., 1955.
3. Guyton, A. C.: Textbook of Medical Physiology. Philadelphia, W. B. Saunders Co., 1956.
4. Langley, L. L., and Cheraskin, E.: The Physiological Foundation of Dental Practice. 2nd ed. St. Louis, The C. V. Mosby Co., 1956.
5. McCollum, E. V.: History of Nutrition. Boston, Houghton Mifflin Co., 1958.
6. Swift, R. W., and French, C. E.: Energy Metabolism and Nutrition. New York, Scarecrow Press, Inc., 1954.

Chapter II

Carbohydrates

Carbohydrate-rich foodstuffs such as rice, wheat, corn, potatoes, sugar cane and sugar beet comprise the major portion of everybody's daily food intake in our society.[27] Because they are so available and inexpensive, they are chosen in preference to the other major nutrients, the fats and the proteins. This excessive use of carbohydrates, particularly the refined fermentable type, is of major concern to us as dentists because of its high correlation with dental caries.

How are we to provide sufficient carbohydrates for caloric needs of the body and yet not jeopardize tooth integrity? Is fortifying our refined carbohydrates, sugar and flour, the answer? When and how much fat and protein can be substituted for carbohydrate? Is one type of carbohydrate less injurious to the tooth than another?

These and many other questions may, in part, be answered by a knowledge of the chemistry, physiology and pathology of carbohydrates.

CHEMISTRY

Definition

Carbohydrates are formed by the combination of carbon dioxide from the air and water from the soil in the presence of sunlight and chlorophyll. This process is called photosynthesis.[10] Chemically, this might be written,

$$6\ CO_2 + 6\ H_2O \xrightarrow[\text{sunlight}]{\text{chlorophyll}} C_6H_{12}O_6 + 6\ O_2$$

The definition of carbohydrates derived from this reaction might be that they are organic compounds consisting of carbon, hydrogen and oxygen in which the ratio of hydrogen to oxygen is two to one. However, because compounds like acetic acid and formaldehyde also have this proportional molecular constitution, this definition does not suffice. More accurately, carbohydrates should be defined as aldehyde or ketone derivatives of polyhydric alcohols or condensation products of such substances.

Classification

Carbohydrates are classified according to their chemical structure. The number of carbon atoms determines whether the carbohydrate is a mono-, di- or polysaccharide. The two end-carbon configurations determine whether it is an aldose, ketose or alcohol. For example, glucose is an aldohexose, and fructose is a ketohexose.

A classification of carbohydrates (see Table 3) suggested by Krehl[27] includes monosaccharides, disaccharides, polysaccharides, sugar alcohols and mucopolysaccharides.*

The most common saccharides in plants and animals are hexoses, of which glucose, fructose and galactose are the most important. When two of these monosaccharides combine by the loss of one molecule of water, they form a disaccharide. For example, two molecules of glucose combine to form maltose; one molecule of glucose and one molecule of fructose combine to form sucrose; and one molecule of glucose and one molecule of galactose combine to form lactose. Both starch, a vegetable type of polysaccharide, and glycogen, an animal type of polysaccharide, are formed by the polymerization of α-glucose molecules. The chain length of these α-glucose molecules contributes to the differentiation between glycogen and starch. When β-glucose molecules are polymerized, they form cellulose. The other classes of carbohydrates—pentoses, sugar alcohols and mucopolysaccharides—are not so important from a nutritional standpoint as the mono-, di- and polysaccharides and, therefore, they will not be discussed.

Monosaccharides. In general, the most common monosaccharides are readily soluble, diffusible and crystallizable. They are absorbed at different rates from the intestine, galactose $>$ glucose

* In carbohydrate nomenclature, the profile D- indicates that a substance belongs to the same configurational family as the reference substance, D-glyceraldehyde. Although this reference substance is dextrorotatory (rotates the plane of polarized light to the right) and its optical isomer, L-glyceraldehyde, is levorotatory, the optical activity of higher sugars whose names contain these symbols need not correspond with that of the parent glyceraldehyde.

TABLE 3. CLASSIFICATION OF CARBOHYDRATES

Monosaccharides	Polysaccharides
(a) *Hexoses*	Cellulose and hemicellulose
Glucose	Inulin
Fructose	Mannosans
Galactose	Pentosans
Mannose	Starch and dextrins
(b) *Pentoses*	Glycogen
Ribose	Galactogens
Xylose	
Arabinose	
Disaccharides	**Sugar Alcohols**
Sucrose	Sorbitol
Lactose	Mannitol
Maltose	

Mucopolysaccharides

Hyaluronic acid	*N*-acetyl-D-glucosamine; D-glucuronic acid
Chondroitin sulfuric acid	*N*-acetyl-S-galactosamine; D-glucuronic acid sulfate
Alpha-heparin	D-glucosamine; D-glucuronic acid sulfate
Beta-heparin	*N*-acetyl-D-galactosamine; D-glucuronic acid sulfate
Keratosulfate	*N*-acetyl-D-glucosamine; galactose sulfate

(Modified from Krehl, W. A.: Borden's Review of Nutrition Research, *16:*86 1955.)

> fructose.[9] None of these simple sugars ever comprises a major portion of a normal diet.

D-*Glucose** is an aldohexose and has the empirical formula, $C_6H_{12}O_6$, and the structural formula,

$$
\begin{array}{c}
\mathrm{CHO} \\
| \\
\mathrm{H{-}C{-}OH} \\
| \\
\mathrm{HO{-}C{-}H} \\
| \\
\mathrm{H{-}C{-}OH} \\
| \\
\mathrm{H{-}C{-}OH} \\
| \\
\mathrm{CH_2OH}
\end{array}
$$

Aldehyde form

There are also several cyclic forms of glucose known as "lactone pairs," or "lactals," which depend on the "oxygen bridge" for their specific structure. The two best established are 1-4 lactone (gluco-furanose) and 1-5 lactone (gluco-pyranose.)

* See footnote on p. 19.

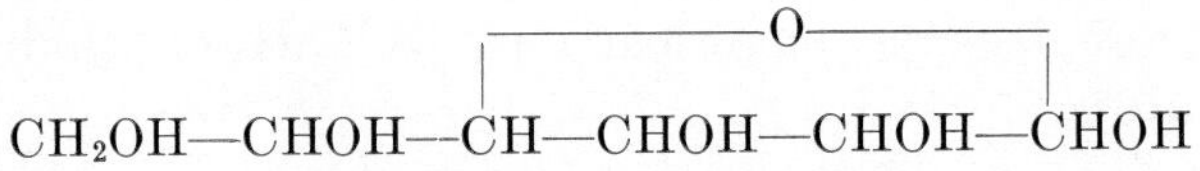

$$\overbrace{CH_2OH—CHOH—\underbrace{CH—CHOH—CHOH—CHOH}}^{O}$$

1-4 lactone (gluco-furanose)

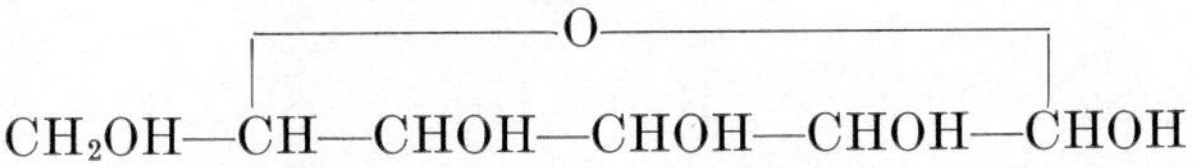

$$CH_2OH—\overbrace{CH—CHOH—CHOH—CHOH—CHOH}^{O}$$

1-5 lactone (gluco-pyranose)

The importance of these two cyclical forms is that the 1-5 lactone is the laboratory-made glucose, whereas the 1-4 lactone is the glucose that occurs in nature.

Glucose occurs in fruits and is sometimes called grape sugar; it is also called dextrose, because it rotates the plane of polarized light to the right. Hydrolysis of disaccharides and such polysaccharides as starch, glycogen and cellulose yields glucose as one of the hydrolytic products, and it is in the latter form that it can be utilized by tissues.

D-*Fructose* is a ketohexose with the empirical formula of $C_6H_{12}O_6$, and a structural formula of

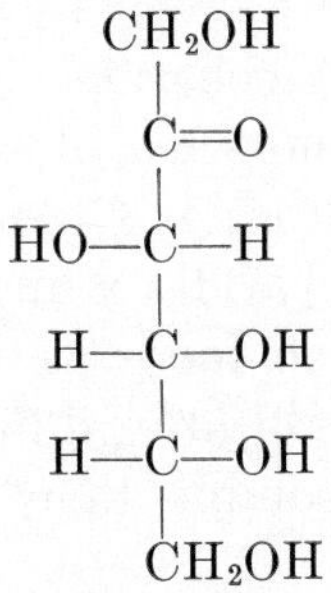

$$\begin{array}{c} CH_2OH \\ | \\ C{=}O \\ | \\ HO—C—H \\ | \\ H—C—OH \\ | \\ H—C—OH \\ | \\ CH_2OH \end{array}$$

It occurs in fruit and plant juices, particularly honey, and is often referred to as fruit sugar. Fructose is also obtained from inulin, which is found in the Jerusalem artichoke. It rotates the plane of polarized light to the left and, therefore, it is called levulose; but in the presence of dilute alkali, it is converted into the dextrorotatory type, glucose. It is the sweetest of all the sugars and its sweetness is graded in comparison with other sugars as follows:

fructose	173
sucrose	100
glucose	74
maltose	33
galactose	32
lactose	16

D-*Galactose* has the empirical formula $C_6H_{12}O_6$, and its structural formula is

$$
\begin{array}{c}
\mathrm{CHO} \\
| \\
\mathrm{H{-}C{-}OH} \\
| \\
\mathrm{HO{-}C{-}H} \\
| \\
\mathrm{HO{-}C{-}H} \\
| \\
\mathrm{H{-}C{-}OH} \\
| \\
\mathrm{CH_2OH}
\end{array}
$$

It is seldom found free in nature and usually results from the hydrolysis of lactose (galactose + glucose). It is found in nerve tissue as galactolipid. For the most part, galactose is formed from glucose in the mammary gland and, like glucose, it is converted into glycogen. In comparison to glucose it is less soluble in water, less sweet, and is fermentable much more slowly by yeasts.

Disaccharides. The disaccharides are a combination of two monosaccharides less one molecule of water, so their general empirical formula may be written as $C_{12}H_{22}O_{11}$. Sucrose, maltose and lactose are the three disaccharides which make up the bulk of the carbohydrate portion of such foods as sugar cane, malt and milk, respectively. They are crystallizable, diffusible and soluble in water, but lactose is much less soluble than sucrose or maltose. Their structural formulae are:

```
    H—C ———————————————————      CH₂OH
      |                   |  O—    |
    H—C—OH                |     —  C ————————
      |                   |          |       |
   HO—C—H                 |     HO—C—H       |
      |                   O          |       |
    H—C—OH                |      H—C—OH      O
      |                   |          |       |
    H—C ——————————————————       H—C ————————
      |                              |
     CH₂OH                          CH₂OH
  (D-glucose)                    (D-fructose)
```

Sucrose

```
                                     H
                                     |
        OH                      ┌────C────────┐
       /                        |    |        |
  H—C ──────────┐               |  H—C—OH     |
    |           |               |    |        |
  H—C—OH        |               |  HO—C—H     |
    |           O               O    |        O
  HO—C—H        |               |  HO—C—H     |
    |           |               |    |        |
  H—C ──────────┼───────────────┘  H—C ───────┘
    |           |                    |
  H—C ──────────┘                    CH2OH
    |
    CH2OH
```

(D-glucose (D-galactose)

Lactose

```
        OH                    ┌──────────┐
       /                      |         /
  H—C ──────────┐             |      H—C ────────┐
    |           |             O        |         |
  H—C—OH        |             |      H—C—OH      |
    |           |             |        |         |
  HO—C—H        O             |      HO—C—H      O
    |           |             |        |         |
  H—C ──────────┼─────────────┘      H—C—OH      |
    |           |                      |         |
  H—C ──────────┘                    H—C ────────┘
    |                                  |
    CH2OH                              CH2OH
```

(D-glucose) (D-glucose)

Maltose

Sucrose, or saccharose, which is ordinary table sugar, is consumed at the annual rate of about 100 lbs. per capita in the United States.[42] The primary sources of sucrose are the sugar beet, sugar cane and sugar maple. Because common table sugar is refined, many of the food faddists have suggested that natural sugars like honey and blackstrap molasses be used for sweetening agents. However, an actual analysis of the vitamin and mineral content of raw sugars has revealed that these protective nutrients are present in insignificant amounts.[21]

Sucrose is hydrolyzed by hydrochloric acid of the stomach and invertase of the intestine into one molecule of glucose and one molecule of fructose, which are the only forms that are utilizable. In fact, sucrose is never given intravenously or parenterally for the very reason that it is not hydrolyzed well if it by-passes the stomach. Therefore, only glucose should be given intravenously.

Invert sugar is a mixture of glucose and fructose obtained from hydrolyzed sucrose. This hydrolytic process is called inversion because the resulting fructose rotates the plane of polarized light more strongly to the left than the resulting glucose does to the right.

Maltose or malt sugar occurs in malt and malt products and it is most commonly derived from the digestive action of salivary and pancreatic amylases on starch. It is readily hydrolyzed by dilute mineral acids, yielding two molecules of glucose. Maltose is a sweet sugar, soluble in water and easily digested. In combination with dextrin it is usually the carbohydrate provided to infants in their formula feedings.

Lactose is the least soluble and least sweet of all the sugars and, consequently, it has the least commercial appeal. Lactose is formed in the mammary glands and is known as milk sugar. On hydrolysis it splits into one molecule of glucose and one molecule of galactose. Lactose is especially favorable to the development of desirable types of intestinal bacteria such as *Lactobacillus acidophilus.* It is also involved in the synthesis of galactosides in the central nervous system of growing young mammals.

Polysaccharides. As the name implies, polysaccharides are combinations of many sugars, and the size of the molecule may be very large. The molecular weight ranges from 10,000 to 1,000,000. This group, which makes up the major part of the daily food intake, consists of dextrins, cellulose, hemicellulose, glycogen and starch.

Starch, $(C_6H_{10}O_5)x$, is found in roots, stems and leaves of plants and makes up three-quarters of the solid matter of cereal grains such as wheat, rye, corn and barley. It also is found in potatoes, legumes and nuts. It is a high molecular weight polymer of glucose and insoluble, but dispersible, in water.

The carbohydrate material of the starch granule consists of two hexosans, amylopectin and amylose. Amylopectin, also called α-amylose, is the outer, almost insoluble phosphorus-containing portion of the granule which forms a viscous opalescent paste when heated in water. Amylose, also called β-amylose, is the inner relatively soluble portion of the granule and gives a blue color with iodine.

Dextrin, $(C_6H_{10}O_5)x$, is a mixture of low molecular weight polysaccharides which are derived from the hydrolysis of starch. "Soluble starch" is a dextrin which is a clear, colorless solution and forms a blue color with iodine. Dextrin is easily digested and in milk prevents the formation of large heavy curds. Dextrin provides a favorable medium for growth of *Lactobacillus acidophilus* in the intestine and promotes intestinal hygiene.

Glycogen, $(C_6H_{10}O_5)x$, is sometimes called animal starch. It reaches its highest concentration in the liver. However, it is also stored in muscles, bones and other tissues of the body. With iodine, glycogen gives a deep red color and it is opalescent in solution. On hydrolysis it yields D-glucose. During rest, glucose and other monosaccharides are stored in the body as glycogen. However, it is called upon, during active muscular work, to yield D-glucose for energy purposes.

Cellulose is the least soluble of the polysaccharides and is less readily hydrolyzable than those described above. It makes up a large part of the framework of plants. Cellulose does not have any nutritional value; it provides "roughage" for stimulating intestinal peristalsis and bulk for the formation of normal stools.

Methyl cellulose absorbs large quantities of water and is helpful in overcoming constipation. Oxidized cellulose retains its fibrous structure and serves as a matrix for clot formation. It is eventually dissolved by alkaline body fluids and then absorbed.

Hemicelluloses consist of pentosans, hexosans and hexopentosans; they are smaller in molecular size than cellulose and are usually found together with the latter in fruits, vegetables and bran.

PHYSIOLOGY

In order for the major nutrients of foodstuffs to be available to body tissues, they must first undergo the processes of digestion, absorption and metabolism. Digestion is the process of breaking down the complex molecules of nutrients in the original foodstuffs into smaller assimilable products. Absorption is the passage of a substance through a surface into body fluids and tissues. Metabolism is the continuous process of changing the end products of digestion and absorption into chemicals that are utilized by the cells and tissues of the body and then excreted.

Digestion

Carbohydrates are digested by the hydrolytic action of ptyalin, amylase and carbohydrase, special enzyme systems in the saliva, pancreas and intestinal mucosa. Through these processes, the complex carbohydrate molecules are broken down into the simpler six-carbon monosaccharides and absorbed through the intestinal wall. From a practical standpoint, the digestion of carbohydrates is primarily concerned with the polysaccharide starch because that constitutes the major portion of our daily carbohydrate intake.

If a starchy food like potatoes is cooked before it is eaten, the starch granules will be disrupted, making available for digestion the more soluble amylose portion of the starch molecule. In the mouth, the action of the tongue and buccinator muscles helps form a bolus, which is chewed and divided into small particles. Since most people do not chew their food as much as Fletcher advocated (a chew for each tooth), the amount of enzymatic digestion of starch to maltose by salivary ptyalin in the mouth is very little, only 3 to 5 per cent. However, the salivary ptyalin passes down into the stomach and, until it is inactivated by hydrochloric acid, continues to act on the starch. At this point 30 to 40 per cent of the starch has been converted to maltose.[16] The percentages of digestion suggested here are certainly subject to wide variation. For example, it has been shown that, in digesting a meal of bread and potatoes, 60 per cent of the former and 75 per cent of the latter were converted into maltose in the stomach.

In the small intestine the alkaline enzyme, amylopsin, which is derived from the pancreatic juices, contributes three carbohydrases (maltase, lactase and sucrase) which further digest maltose, lactose and sucrose into their respective hexoses. Because each of these disaccharides yields glucose on hydrolysis, it is readily seen why glucose is the main carbohydrate component of blood.

In addition to diet, two biochemical processes contribute to glucose levels in the blood. The first is the process of gluconeogenesis, which involves the conversion of glycerol, certain amino acids and fatty acids to glucose; and, second, during periods of acute stress, glycogen of the liver is reconverted into glucose through the process of glycogenolysis.

Absorption, Metabolism and Storage

Glucose, as well as other monosaccharides, is absorbed mainly through the capillaries in the villi of the small intestine. A very small amount of absorption (less than 1 per cent) takes place in the stomach. The hexoses pass through the intestinal wall phosphorylated or unchanged.[49] For the most part, glucose is converted to glucose-6-phosphate by the transfer of the phosphate radical from adenosine triphosphate (ATP). After traversing the intestinal wall as phosphorylated glucose, it is dephosphorylated before it passes into general circulation.

Several hormones, such as insulin, epinephrine and anterior pituitary growth hormone, control the level of glucose in the blood. Even though a large amount of carbohydrate may be ingested at one time, as a result of the regulating process of the endocrine glands only the amount of sugar which can be utilized at the moment is made available. The level of sugar in the blood before eating (fasting blood sugar) is usually 80 mg. per 100 ml. of whole blood, and immediately after a meal it rises to 120 to 130 mg.

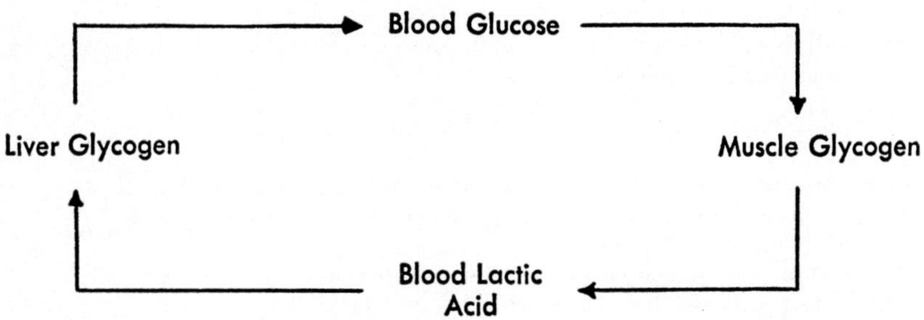

FIGURE 5. Cori cycle. (Krehl, W. A., in Borden's Review of Nutritional Research, Vol. XVI, No. 6, 1955.)

Most of the absorbed carbohydrate is transported from the intestine to the liver by way of the portal vein. In the liver the monosaccharides are converted into glycogen. When the body metabolism requires glucose, it calls on the liver to convert its stored glycogen into glucose, which can then serve as a source material for the formation of glycogen in muscle. Muscle glycogen, in contrast to the liver glycogen, is not broken down into glucose but rather to pyruvic acid and then to lactic acid. A cycle known as the Cori cycle is created in which lactic acid is converted to glycogen, which serves as a source of blood sugar from which muscle glycogen may again be formed (Fig. 5).

The main pathway of carbohydrate metabolism leads to the formation of lactic acid from glucose (Table 4). One of the intermediate products of this oxidation is pyruvic acid, which undergoes several changes. In the presence of oxygen, pyruvic acid is converted to carbon dioxide and water with the aid of the enzymes from the Krebs citric acid cycle.[34] By decarboxylation, pyruvic

TABLE 4. STEPS IN GLYCOLYSIS OF GLUCOSE TO LACTIC ACID

(1) glucose + adenosine triphosphate $\xrightarrow{\text{hexokinase}}$ glucose-6-phosphate + adenosine diphosphate

(2) glucose-6-phosphate $\overset{\text{isomerase}}{\leftrightarrows}$ fructose-6-phosphate

(3) fructose + adenosine triphosphate $\xrightarrow{\text{exokinase}}$ fructose-6-phosphate + adenosine diphosphate

(4) fructose-6-phosphate + adenosine triphosphate $\xrightarrow{\text{phosphohexokinase}}$ fructose-1, 6-diphosphate + adenosine diphosphate

(5) fructose-1,6-diphosphate $\overset{\text{zymohexase}}{\leftrightarrows}$ glyceraldehyde-3-phosphate + dihydroxyacetone phosphate

(6) dihydroxyacetone phosphate $\overset{\text{triose isomerase}}{\leftrightarrows}$ glyceraldehyde-3-phosphate

(7) glyceraldehyde-1,3-diphosphate + coenzym eI (ox.) $\rightleftarrows$ 1,3-diphosphoglyceric acid + coenzym eI (red)

(8) 1,3-diphosphoglyceric acid + adenosine diphosphate $\rightleftarrows$ 3-phosphoglyceric acid + adenosine triphosphate

(9) 3 phosphoglyceric acid $\overset{\text{triose mutase}}{\rightleftarrows}$ 2-phosphoglyceric acid

(10) 2-phosphoglyceric acid $\overset{\text{enolase}}{\leftrightarrows}$ phospho (enol) pyruvic acid + H_2O

(11) phosphopyruvic acid + adenosine diphosphate $\rightleftarrows$ pyruvic acid + adenosine triphosphate

(12) pyruvic acid + coenzyme I $\rightleftarrows$ lactic acid + coenzyme I (ox.)

(Adapted from Stetten, D.: Carbohydrate Metabolism. A symposium as prepared under the auspices of the Councils on Food and Nutrition of the American Medical Association. New York, Blakiston, 1951.)

acid is converted into acetic acid which, in turn, is converted into fatty acids and cholesterol through the acetyl–coenzyme A system. Pyruvic acid can also participate in the transamination reaction of certain amino acids. A more detailed discussion of the intermediary metabolism of carbohydrates is given in Chapter V.

TABLE 5. CONVERSION OF CARBOHYDRATES TO FAT

glucose $\xrightarrow{\text{glycolysis}}$ 2 molecules of pyruvic acid

pyruvic acid $\xrightarrow[\text{decarboxylation}]{\text{oxidation and}}$ acetic acid

2 acetic acid molecules $\xrightarrow{\text{condensation}}$ acetoacetic acid

acetic acid + acetoacetic acid $\xrightarrow{\text{condensation}}$ long-chain keto acids

long-chain keto acids $\xrightarrow{\text{reduction}}$ long-chain fatty acids

fatty acids + glycerol $\xrightarrow{\text{esterification}}$ neutral fat

The ingestion of amounts of sugar beyond energy needs is very easy because it does not impart the feeling of fullness that, for example, fats do. In view of the fact that the storage capacity for glycogen is limited, the remaining carbohydrate is converted into fat (Table 5) and stored as such in the subcutaneous tissue.

GENERAL SYSTEMIC PATHOLOGY OF ABNORMAL CARBOHYDRATE METABOLISM

Clinical evidence of abnormal carbohydrate metabolism may result from (1) improper dietary intake, (2) malfunctioning systemic regulatory processes, or (3) both. Improper intake implies the ingestion of amounts above or below that which is considered optimal for meeting the normal energy requirements. Conditions which may be aggravated by excesses of carbohydrates are diabetes, obesity and tooth decay. Clinical signs of vitamin B complex deficiency and negative nitrogen balance are also associated with excessive intake of carbohydrates. On the other hand, exceedingly low intake is associated with weight loss and ketosis. Storage of excess carbohydrate may lead to the condition known as von Gierke's disease.

Diabetes mellitus is a chronic disease due to an underutilization of glucose because of lack of insulin. Not only is pancreatic insulin production involved in this disease, but the hormones of the pituitary gland and the adrenals are also related to the development of diabetes. The prolonged inability to metabolize glucose will produce a hyperglycemic state and glucosuria. Therefore, the body will use fat as a source of energy which gives rise to excessive ketone body formation and acidosis. There is also a lipemia, largely cholesterol, which accompanies this disease and probably accounts for the propensity toward vascular disease. Clinically, diabetic patients have polyphagia, polydipsia and polyuria. In addition, there are weight loss, increased fatigability, susceptibility to infection, retinal changes and peripheral nerve degeneration.

Effects of Excess Carbohydrate Intake

Obesity is the result of ingesting more calories than are expended as energy. When both energy and storage needs for carbohydrates have been satisfied, any excess is converted into fat and stored as adipose tissue. As long as the regulating mechanisms are functioning normally, carbohydrates are never excreted or wasted. Therefore, to prevent obesity, it is imperative that calorie intake and output be in balance.

Tooth decay may be initiated and extended by fermentable carbohydrates. The present knowledge on the relation of carbohydrates to dental caries will be discussed in detail in the pages which follow this discussion of general pathology.

Vitamin B complex deficiencies are initiated when excess carbohydrates are ingested. The B complex vitamins, such as thiamine and pantothenic acid, act as coenzymes in the oxidation of the carbohydrate. If excess sugar is ingested, these vitamins may be diverted to this oxidative process so that little will be left to perform other necessary functions in the tissues, thus creating a deficiency. The classic signs of vitamin B complex deficiency are epithelial changes of the tongue papillae as well as general neurologic and dermatologic changes.

A *negative nitrogen balance* is the result of ingesting less protein than is normally required for cell metabolism and is usually due to excessive carbohydrate intake. Hypoproteinemia is manifest by general weakness and tissue breakdown; the total serum albumin falls below 4 Gm. per 100 cc. and the total serum protein below 6 Gm. per 100 cc.

Diseases Involving Deficiency of Carbohydrate Intake and Abnormal Storage

Von Gierke's disease is a condition in which there is storage of excess glycogen, particularly in the liver, kidney and, occasionally, in small amounts, in heart and voluntary muscles. This is a rare disease which occurs in infants and leads to death before adulthood. The children have enlarged livers which produce a characteristic protuberant abdomen. Usually they suffer from hypoglycemic convulsions and comas.

Weight loss is a result of excessive use of storage fat. When energy requirements are not met by dietary means, or when carbohydrate stores are depleted, the storage fats are utilized. This withdrawal of adipose tissue from the subcutaneous storage area results in emaciation.

Ketosis is the excessive formation of ketones in the body. When carbohydrate intake is inadequate, there is a tendency for the body to metabolize excessive amounts of fat to meet caloric requirements. When fatty acid breakdown becomes excessively rapid, the rate of ketone formation in the liver exceeds the rate of disposal; this produces ketosis and, eventually, acidosis.

EFFECTS OF CARBOHYDRATES ON THE TEETH, ORAL ENVIRONMENT AND PERIODONTIUM

Dental Caries and Carbohydrate Relationships

"The effect of sugar and other carbohydrates on the teeth remains one of the foremost dental problems. . . . The presence of carbohydrates—especially sugars—on the teeth is an essential in the production of dental decay." These excerpts quoted from an editorial in the Journal of the American Dental Association[1] express the commonly accepted clinical impression of the dental practitioner. To substantiate the impression there are numerous well controlled animal experiments, some epidemiologic data and controlled clinical studies which definitely point to carbohydrates as an important etiologic agent in dental caries.

Shaw[39] suggests that there are three main periods in the development of the tooth which should be related to nutrition and dental caries: (a) pre-eruptive, when calcification begins; (b) newly erupted, when maturation continues to take place; and (c) post-eruptive, when teeth are fully mature and calcified. The second or maturation period of the tooth, when composition of the saliva may have some effect, is the one about which we know least. Therefore, it will not be discussed here. However, there is much experimental data which indicates that susceptibility to caries initiation is influenced by carbohydrate ingestion during tooth formation and that the rate of caries progression is influenced by the extent of carbohydrate contact with the fully formed tooth.

Effects of Carbohydrate on the Unerupted Tooth

A fine-particle-size purified ration which contained 67 per cent granulated cane sugar, in addition to adequate amounts of recognized essential nutrients, was found to be very cariogenic when fed preweaning to the ordinary laboratory rat (*Mus norwegicus*).[44] In contrast, this same diet proved to be much less cariogenic when it was introduced after the complete eruption and maturation of the teeth. This proved that mechanical fracture because of coarse particle size was not necessary to initiate caries. In fact, the finding of extensive caries during the tooth formative period suggested that caries might be a systemic or nutritional effect.

In a subsequent experiment, Sognnaes[44] found that the teeth of the offspring of female hamsters fed a purified diet throughout pregnancy and lactation were 3 to 4 times as caries-susceptible to postweaning cariogenic diets as the teeth of the offspring of hamsters which were fed a natural diet through pregnancy and lactation (Fig. 6).

Mitchell and Shafer[33] reported a similar finding of high caries susceptibility in the offspring of dams which were transferred to a caries-producing ration early in pregnancy.

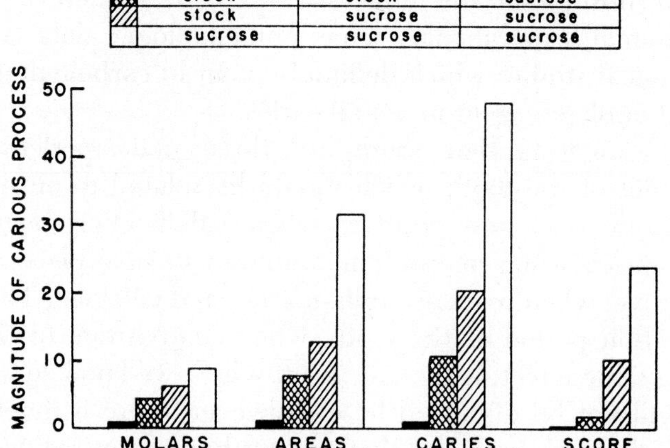

FIGURE 6. Pre-eruptive influence of the purified (sucrose) ration on the caries susceptibility of hamsters. (Sognnaes, R. F., in J.A.D.A., 37:676, 1948.)

Monkeys that were started on a purified ration when they were just under two years of age developed no caries in their second deciduous molars even though they were fed this ration for five and one-half years. In contrast, monkeys that were started on this purified ration when they were about nine months old developed over three carious second deciduous molars per animal at the end of only two and one-half years on the purified ration.[45]

Steinman et al.[47] produced in rats a 100 per cent increase in the incidence of molar tooth decay through the administration, by dropper, of a 20 per cent sucrose solution three times a day for at least seven days during the preweaning, calcifying period.

In addition, there is evidence from human epidemiologic studies[43,50] that tooth quality is influenced by the kinds of foodstuff eaten before the teeth erupt. The incidence of postwar dental caries and the consumption of sugar during the war showed a high degree of correlation. Molars of Scandinavian children were made caries resistant during the war period when less refined foods were available. Three to five years later when the tooth was exposed to a more cariogenic diet, the innate resistance was sufficient to ward off the local attacking forces of increased sweets. Likewise, the incidence of decay in first permanent molars was found lowest in German children who five years previously had been on a low sugar ration (Fig. 7).

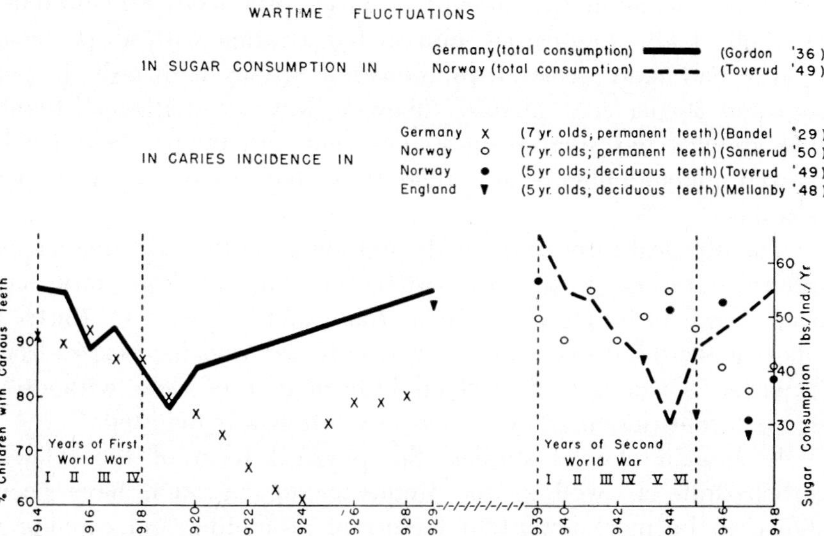

FIGURE 7. Sognnaes, R. F.: Is the susceptibility to dental caries influenced by factors operating during the period of tooth development? Sugar and Dental Caries Symposium, J. of Calif. Dent. Assoc., *26*:47, 1950.

In the majority of children ill with diabetes mellitus who ate more liberal amounts of milk, eggs, meat, vegetables and fruit than most children, there was little or no extension of caries for years.[5] The small number who failed to observe their dietary regime experienced a much higher rate of caries. The children who were put on this low sugar diet early had less caries than those who started the diet later.

Effects of Carbohydrate on the Erupted Tooth

It has been shown that animals must be fed refined carbohydrates to produce dental decay. Even after sialoadenectomy,[37] a most severe caries-promoting factor, experimental animals did not show any tooth decay when fed high protein-fat diets devoid of carbohydrate. However, the inclusion of sucrose in the animals' ration does not necessarily insure the production of dental caries.[20,24,28,31,35] This finding lends strength to the argument that dental caries is a disease of complex etiology and that it is dependent upon not one but several factors.

With regard to the type of carbohydrate that is most conducive to caries, it has been found that glucose and sucrose are the most cariogenic, while starch and dextrin are the least.[38]

The level of sucrose and glucose in the diet has also been found to be significant in the amount of caries produced. For example, Mitchell et al.[32] found that animals fed a ration with 45 per cent sucrose had more caries than those fed rations with only 15 per cent and 30 per cent sucrose. Likewise, Keyes and Likens[23] found that animals fed sucrose at 40 per cent and 60 per cent levels showed much higher scores than those fed sucrose at a 20 per cent level.

The physical form of the carbohydrate is another variable which influences the extent of caries production. Sugar in solid form has been shown to be more cariogenic than liquid sucrose. Of thirteen rats that were fed granulated sugar, only two remained caries free. However, seven out of thirteen litter-mate rats were without a single carious lesion when a sucrose solution was ingested.[17]

In human clinical studies, the physical form of the refined carbohydrate as well as the frequency of ingestion have been shown to be most important factors in promoting and extending dental decay in fully developed adult teeth.[15] Institutionalized adults were divided into ten groups. As a basis of comparison a caries index was established for each individual by observing his rate of dental decay increase over a period of one year while eating the regular ration. For the next four years the diet was supplemented with a sugar-containing foodstuff. Some subjects had liquefied sucrose, others bread and sugar, and others different candies, but the total amount of sugar was the same for each group. The results indicated that the caries incidence did not parallel the amount but rather the physical nature of the sugars consumed. The comparative cariogenicity of groups was as follows; liquid sucrose < bread < caramels < toffees. Furthermore, the frequent eating of sweets between meals contributed significantly to the increased caries experience (Fig. 8 and Table 6).

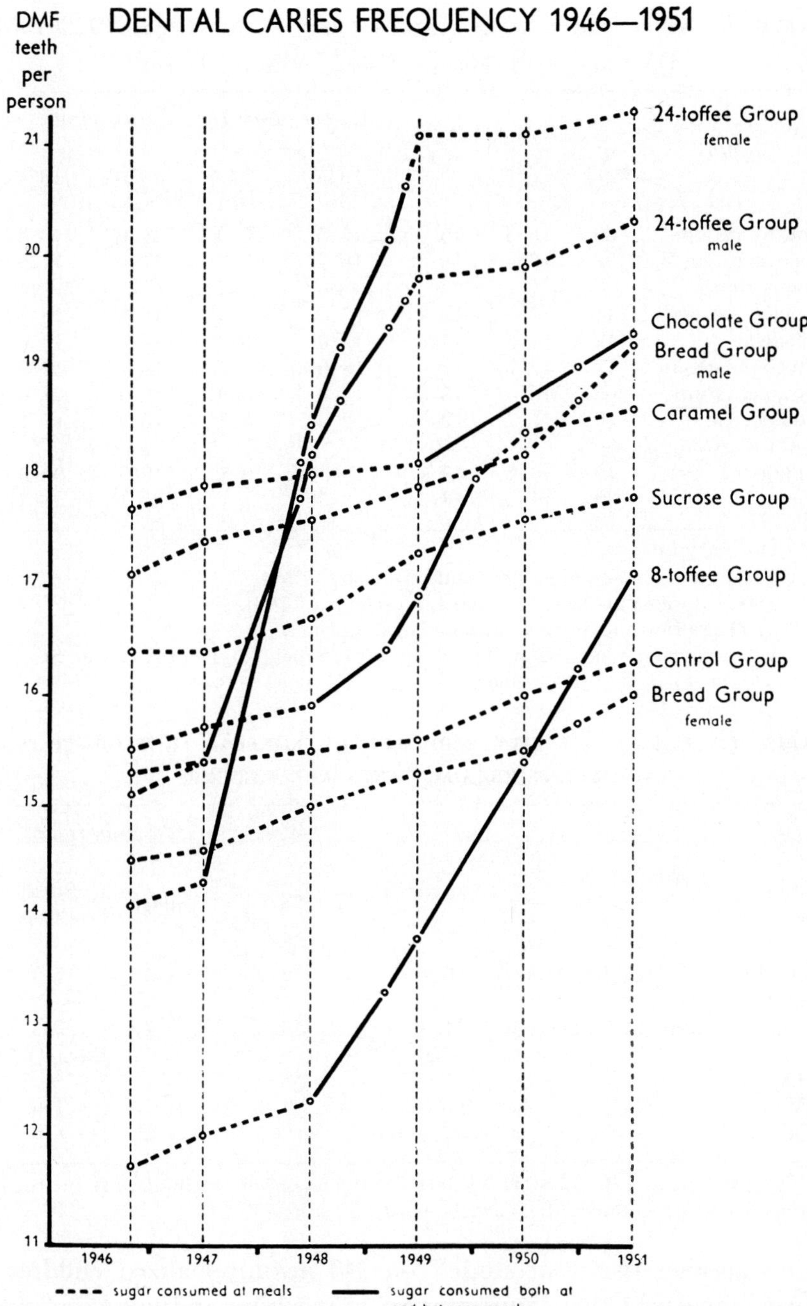

FIGURE 8. Gustafsson, B., Quensel, C., Lanke, L., Lundqvist, C., Grahnen, H., Bonow, B., Krasse, B.: The Vipeholm Dental Caries Study: The effect of different levels of carbohydrates intake on caries activity in 436 Individuals observed for five years, Acta Odont. Scand., *11*:232, 1954.

TABLE 6. VIPEHOLM DENTAL CARIES FREQUENCY STUDY, 1946–1951

DMF (Decayed, Missing, Filled) Teeth per Person

Group	*No. of Pers.*	*Basic*[1] 1946	*Vitamin*[2] 1947	*Carbohydrate I*[3]		*Carbohydrate II*[4]	
				1948	1949	1950	1951
Control group	60	15.3	15.4	15.5	15.6	16.0	16.3
Sucrose group	57	16.4	16.4	16.7	17.3	17.6	17.8
Bread group							
male	41	17.1	17.4	17.6	17.9	18.2	19.2
female	42	14.5	14.6	15.0	15.3	15.5	16.0
Chocolate group	47	17.7	17.9	18.0	18.1	18.7	19.3
Caramel group	62	15.5	15.5	15.9	16.9	18.4	18.6
8-toffee group	40	11.7	12.0	12.3	13.8	15.4	17.1
24-toffee group							
male	48	15.1	15.4	18.2	19.8	19.9	20.3
female	39	14.1	14.3	18.5	21.1	21.1	21.3

[1] Ordinary hospital diet.
[2] Vitamin and mineral supplements to hospital diet.
[3] 1800 calories plus twice normal sucrose consumption.
[4] 2700 calories plus normal sucrose consumption.

(Adapted from Gustafsson, B., et al.: The Vipeholm Dental Caries Study. Acta Odont. Scand. *11*:232, 1954.)

TABLE 7. CARIES ACTIVITY AND WEEKLY CONSUMPTION OF TOOTH-ADHERENT BREADS, CAKES AND PASTRIES

Region	*Caries Activity*	*Weekly Consumption in Lbs.*		
		Farms	Villages	Small Cities
New England, Middle Atlantic and North Central	High	7.2	8.4	7.8
Plains, Mountain and Pacific	Moderately high	4.3	6.7	7.3
Southeast:				
White farm operators	Low	1.4	4.1	4.9
Negroes	Very low	.4	1.2	1.6

Adapted from Bibby, B. G.: Effect of sugar content of foodstuffs on their caries-producing potentialities. J.A.D.A. *51*:302, 1955.

In another two year study[25] on 243 institutionalized children, it was found (1) that liquid sucrose at mealtime did not affect the caries rate and (2) that doubling the normal intake of sugar did not increase the caries incidence. The sugar was eaten with the meals.

The quantity of different kinds of sugar products, cakes and soft drinks ingested in various sections of the country has been related to caries prevalence.[4] New Englanders, compared to Texans, eat approximately twice the amount of pastries and cakes, which could contribute to the fact that the caries rate in New England is double that in Texas. On the other hand, doubling the intake of sucrose solution in the form of soda pop by Texans does not materially affect this comparatively low caries experience (Table 7 and Fig. 9). Evidently, the retention of the sweets in and around the teeth is more important from a caries-producing standpoint than the amount of sugar. (See Chapter XIV for further discussion.)

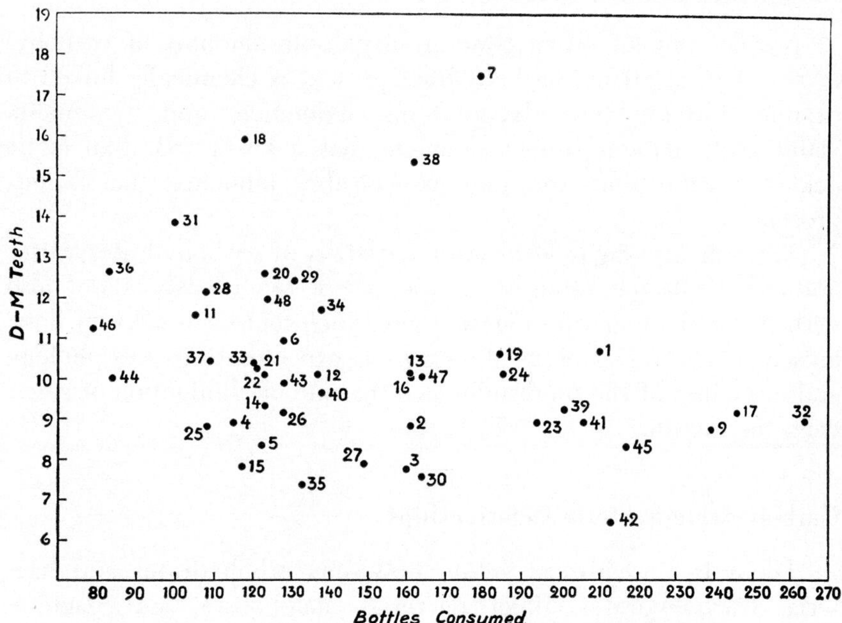

FIGURE 9. Relation between consumption of carbonated beverages and dental caries. Data for DM teeth from Nizel, A. E., and Bibby, B. G.: Geographic variations in caries prevalence in soldiers. J.A.D.A. *31:*1619, Dec. 1944. Data for beverage consumption based on 1947 information from U. S. Department of Commerce, Bureau of the Census. Points represent DM teeth and per capita consumption of carbonated beverages for states as follows:

1, Ala.	9, Fla.	17, La.	24, Mo.	31, N.Y.	38, R.I.	45, Va.
2, Ariz.	11, Idaho	18, Maine	25, Mont.	32, N.C.	39, S.C.	46, Wash.
3, Ark.	12, Ill.	19, Md.	26, Neb.	33, N.D.	40, S.D.	47, W. Va.
4, Calif.	13, Ind.	20, Mass.	27, Nev.	34, Ohio	41, Tenn.	48, Wis.
5, Colo.	14, Iowa	21, Mich.	28, N.H.	35, Okla.	42, Texas	49, Wyo.
6, Conn.	15, Kan.	22, Minn.	29, N.J.	36, Ore.	43, Utah	
7, Del.	16, Ky.	23, Miss.	30, N. Mex.	37, Pa.	44, Vt.	

(Bibby, B. G.: Effect of sugar content of food stuffs on their caries-producing potentialities. J.A.D.A., *51:*293, 1955.)

Studies have also been made on the comparative effects of refined sugar and natural sugars.[8] No evidence has been found in animals that natural cane sugar, as a syrup, is less cariogenic than refined sugar. However, the substitution of spray-dried blackstrap molasses for sucrose did produce a lower incidence of caries in rats.[41] Dental surveys[11,46] among the habitual sugar cane chewers on sugar plantations showed a high caries attack rate, suggesting that natural sugars were not necessarily less deleterious to teeth than refined sugar.

Carbohydrate-Saliva Relationships

Normal human saliva contains negligible amounts of carbohydrates. Almost all the carbohydrate present is chemically linked to protein, forming two glycoproteins, sialomucin and fucomucin. Sialic acid, derived from sialomucin, has a lower *p*H than lactic acid or acetic acid and may conceivably influence the carious process.[3]

The salivary sugar level after ingestion of carbohydrates varies not only with the retentive properties of the foodstuffs but also with the individual who ingests them. Such factors as salivary flow, muscular control over swallowing or expectorating, morphology and crowding of the teeth influence the rate of elimination of sugar from the mouth.

Carbohydrate-Bacteria Relationships

There is a reciprocal action between carbohydrates and bacteria. Carbohydrates affect bacterial metabolism, and bacteria ferment and degrade the simple sugars. Carbohydrates are absolutely essential for the nutrition of the oral bacteria because they (a) supply energy to the cells, and (b) supply carbon for cell synthesis.[52] Carbohydrates can promote either symbiosis or antagonism between organisms. Thus, a particular acidogenic bacteria might flourish or diminish, depending on the amount of carbohydrate present in the medium.

The effects of bacteria on carbohydrate metabolism depend on (a) the type of bacteria and (b) the type of carbohydrate. Homofermentative lactobacilli like *lactobacillus casei* are more effective in reducing pyruvate to lactic acid than the heterofermentative type.[48] As for the type of saccharide that will produce the most acid as a result of bacterial action, it has been found to follow this sequence: glucose $>$ fructose $>$ sucrose $>$ maltose $>$ lactose $>$ starch.[29,38]

The increased bacterial aggregation of the oral cavity after carbohydrate ingestion, according to Hellstrom and Ericsson,[18] is the source of salivary lactic acid. Neither the saliva nor the dental plaque contributes to the increased lactate content of the saliva.

A positive correlation has been shown to exist between lactobacillus counts and the presence of fermentable carbohydrates. High counts of lactobacilli definitely indicate an increased oral environment of sugar. Whether this is directly associated with present or future caries incidence is a moot question.[6,7,12,19,22,26,51] No clinician should feel that lactobacillus counts are the infallible yardstick for measuring caries activity. Miller, at the end of the nineteenth century, stated, "I do not, however, wish to be understood as saying that acids, or pathogenic bacteria, or putrefactive bacteria, or all together are the sole and only cause of decay of the human teeth."[30]

Periodontal Effects of Diabetes and Carbohydrate-free Diets

Faulty carbohydrate metabolism, as manifest by uncontrolled diabetes mellitus, does produce oral mucous membrane changes which are characterized by a dryness and erythema of the buccal mucosa as well as of the tongue. In uncontrolled diabetes of long

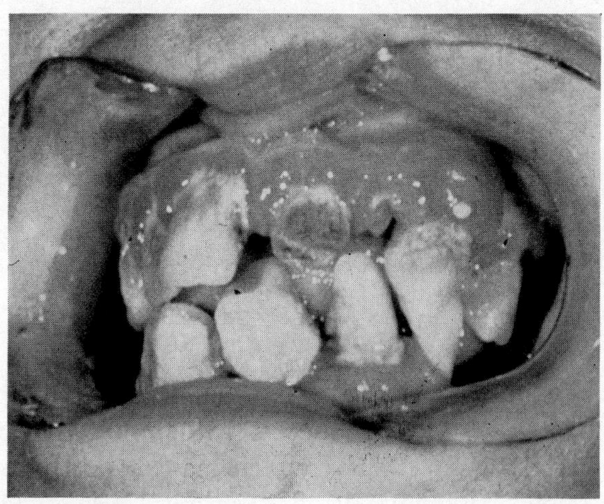

FIGURE 10. Gingival hyperplasia in patient with uncontrolled diabetes. (Courtesy Dr. G. Shklar.)

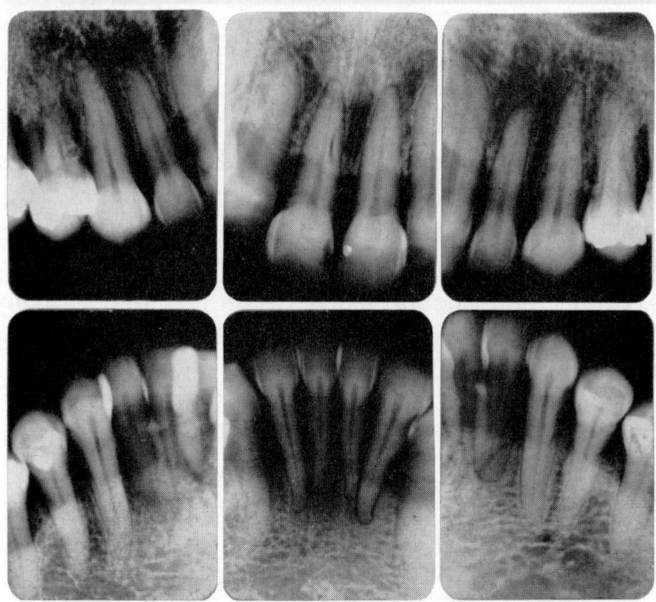

FIGURE 11. The dental radiographs of a patient showing marked alveolar bone loss. (Courtesy Dr. G. Shklar.)

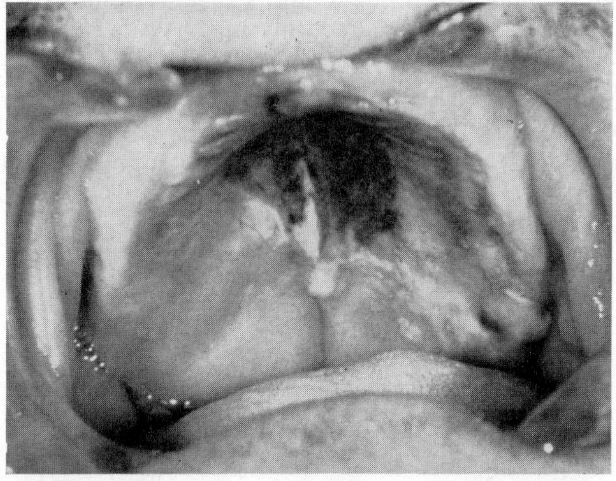

FIGURE 12. Ulcer of the palatal mucosa in patient with uncontrolled diabetes. (Courtesy Dr. I. Meyers.)

standing, acidosis and negative nitrogen balance will contribute significantly to lowered resistance to infection. This, in turn, will produce lowered tissue vitality, which may make the patient more susceptible to the development of periodontal disease (Figs. 10 and 11), as well as ulcerations of the oral mucous membrane (Fig. 12).

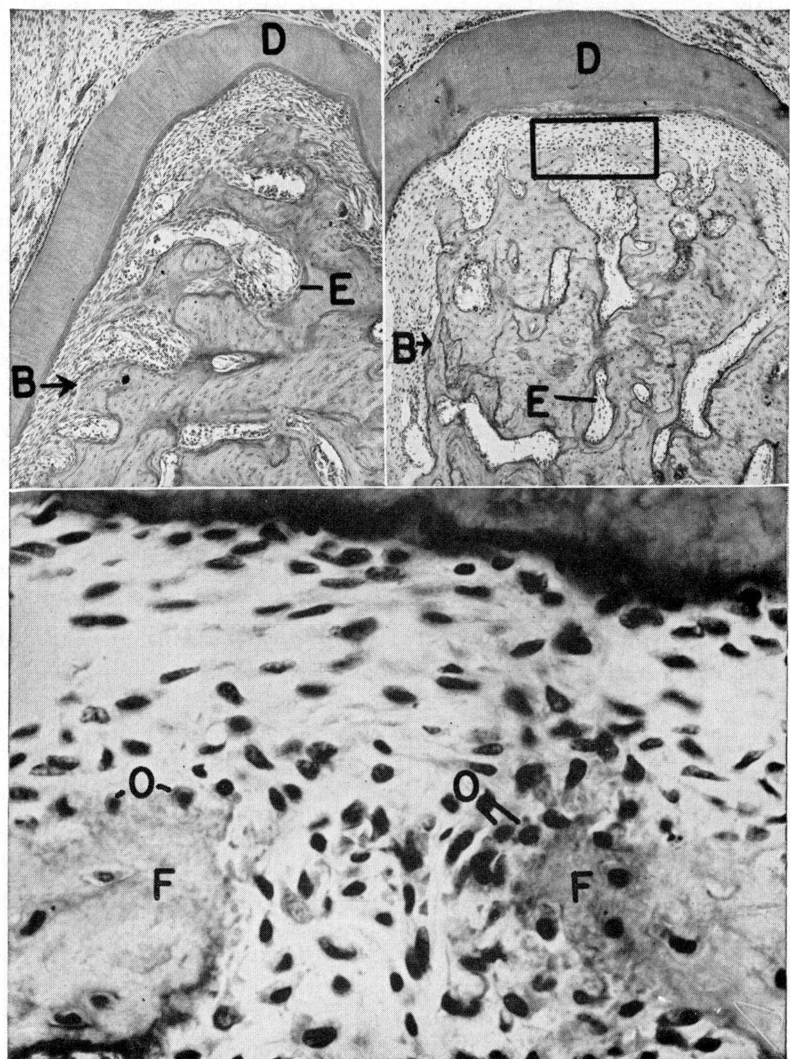

FIGURES 13–15. CHANGES IN THE PERIODONTIUM IN EXPERIMENTAL DIABETES.

FIGURE 13. *Control animal.* Bifurcation area of a mandibular molar (*D*) showing normal bone deposition adjacent to the periodontal membrane (*B*). The vessel channels and marrow spaces (*E*) are lined in part by newly formed bone and in part by resorption lacunae.

FIGURE 14. Diabetic animal. Bone in bifurcation of mandibular molar (*D*). Note absence of normal bone formation adjacent to the periodontal membrane (*B*) and along the vessel channels and marrow spaces (*E*). (Compare with Fig. 13.)

FIGURE 15. High power study of the area enclosed within the rectangle in Fig. 14 showing fragmentation of the bone matrix (*F*) and release of the osteocytes (*O*). (Glickman, I.: Clinical Periodontology. 2nd ed.)

Gingival abscesses, gingival proliferations and diffuse alveolar atrophy, found in diabetic patients, are probably not related to glycosuria or hyperglycemia, according to Rudy and Cohen,[36] but may be due to prolonged vitamin and mineral deficiencies as a result of restricted diets. From a clinical standpoint, Glickman[14] states that diabetic patients present a tendency toward loss of alveolar bone, but the assumption that the origin and progress of periodontal disease is related to diabetes has not been substantiated. In experiments conducted on alloxan-induced diabetes in albino rats, Glickman concluded that in these animals (1) there were no gingival, periodontal membrane or cementum changes peculiar to diabetes; and (2) there was a tendency toward varying degrees of nonspecific osteoporotic changes of alveolar bone (Figs. 13-15).

Recently the rice rat has been used as an experimental animal to study the effects of diet on the soft tissue of the periodontium.[2] A most dramatic and significant reduction in soft tissue lesions of the periodontium was noted in rats that were fed a diet completely free of carbohydrates. The experimental group fed a complete, though carbohydrate free, diet had 81 per cent less gingival disturbance than the group fed a nutritionally complete diet containing carbohydrate.

REFERENCES

1. Anon.: Recent reports cast new lights and new shadow on the etiology of dental decay. J.A.D.A., *51:*349, 1955.
2. Auskaps, A. M., Gupta, O. P., and Shaw, J. H.: Periodontal disease in the rice rat. III. Survey of dietary influences. J. of Nut., *63:*325, 1957.
3. Beggard, I., and Werner, I.: Carbohydrate constituents of human saliva. Acta Odont. Scand., *16:*43, 1958.
4. Bibby, B. G.: Effect of sugar content of foodstuffs on their caries producing potentialities. J.A.D.A., *51:*293, 1955.
5. Boyd, J. D.: Long term prevention of tooth decay among diabetic children. Am. J. Dis. of Children, *66:*349, 1943.
6. Boyd, J. D., Zentmire, Z., and Drain, C. L.: Bacteriological studies in dental caries. J. D. Res., *13:*443, 1933.
7. Bunting, R. W., and Palmerlee, F.: The role of *Bacillus acidophilus* in dental caries. J.A.D.A., *12:*381, 1925.
8. Constant, M. A., Phillips, P. H., and Elvehjem, C. A.: Dental caries in the cotton rat. XII. Natural versus refined sugars. J. of Nut., *43:*551, 1951.
9. Cori, C. F.: The fate of sugar in the animal body. I. The rate of absorption of hexoses and pentoses from the intestinal tract. J. Biol. Chem., *66:*691, 1925.
10. Daniel, F.: Photosynthesis. Borden's Rev. of Nut. Res., *15:*77, 1954.
11. Dreizen, S., and Spies, T. D.: The incidence of dental caries in habitual sugar cane chewers. J.A.D.A., *45:*193, 1952.

12. Glass, R. L.: Lack of relationship between salivary lactobacillus counts and dental caries activity. Oral Surg., Oral Med. and Oral Path., *5:*210, 1952.
13. Glickman, I.: The periodontal structures in experimental diabetes. New York J. Dent., *26:*226, 1946.
14. Glickman, I.: Clinical Periodontology. 2nd ed. Philadelphia, W. B. Saunders Co., 1958.
15. Gustafsson, B. E., Quensel, C., Lanke, L., Lundqvist, C., Grahnen, H., Bonow, B., and Krasse, B.: Vipeholm dental caries study: The effect of different levels of carbohydrate intake on caries activity in 436 individuals observed for five years. Acta Odont. Scand., *11:*232, 1954.
16. Guyton, A. C.: Textbook of Medical Physiology. Philadelphia, W. B. Saunders Co., 1956.
17. Haldi, J., Wynn, W., Shaw, J. H., and Sognnaes, R. F.: The relative cariogenicity of sucrose when ingested in the solid form and in solution by the albino rat. J. Nut., *49:*295, 1953.
18. Hellstrom, I., and Ericsson, Y.: Lactic acid content of the saliva after carbohydrate ingestion. II. Source of the salivary lactic acid and inhibition of its formation. Acta Odont. Scand., *10:*118, 1953.
19. Jay, P., and Voorhies, R. S., Jr.: *Bacillus acidophilus* and dental caries. Dent. Cosmos., *69:*977, 1927.
20. Jackson, C. M.: The effects of high sugar diets on the growth and structure of the rat. J. Nut., *3:*61, 1930.
21. Jackson, W. R., and Macek, T. J.: B complex vitamins in sugar cane and sugar cane juice. Ind. Eng. Chem. Anal. Ed., *36:*261, 1944.
22. Kesel, R. G.: Dental caries: Etiology, control, and activity tests. J.A.D.A., *30:*25, 1943.
23. Keyes, P. H., and Likens, R. C.: Plaque formation, periodontal disease and dental caries in Syrian hamsters. J. D. Res., *25:*166, 1946.
24. Keyes, P. H.: Minimal caries activity in Syrian hamsters. J. D. Res., *31:*477, 1952.
25. King, J. D., Mellanby, M., Stones, H. H., and Green, H. N.: Effect of Sugar Supplements on Dental Caries in Children. Medical Research Council Special Report Series No. 288. London, Her Majesty's Stationery Office, 1955.
26. King, J. D., and Croll, J. M.: Dental caries, carbohydrate and *B. acidophilus.* Brit. D. J., *66:*19, 1939.
27. Krehl, W. A.: The nutritional significance of the carbohydrates. Borden's Rev. of Nut. Res., *16:*85, 1955.
28. Lilly, C. A.: Failures to produce experimental dental caries in the white rat with high carbohydrate diet and *Bacillus acidophilus* or with vitamin D deficiency. J. Nut., *5:*175, 1932.
29. McClure, F. J.: Observations on induced caries in rats. V. Effects of excessive sugar in the diet. J. D. Res., *24:*239, 1945.
30. Miller, W. D.: Agency of micro-organisms in decay of human teeth. Dent. Cosmos, *25:*1, 1882.
31. Mitchell, D. F.: Caries resistance in hamsters. J. D. Res., *33:*676, 1954.
32. Mitchell, D. F., Chernausek, D. S., and Helman, E. Z.: Hamster caries. The effects of three different dietary sugar levels and an evaluation of scoring procedures. J. D. Res., *30:*778, 1951.
33. Mitchell, D. F., and Shafer, W. G.: The effects of caries producing diets initiated at various stages of pre- and post-natal development of the hamster. J. D. Res., *28:*464, 1949.

34. Ochoa, S.: Enzymic mechanisms in the citric acid cycle. Advances in Enzymology, *15:*183, 1954.
35. Rosebury, T., and Karshan, M.: Studies in the rat of susceptibility to dental caries. I. Bacteriological and nutritional factors. J. D. Res., *11:*121, 1931.
36. Rudy, A., and Cohen, M. M.: The oral aspects of diabetes mellitus. New England J. Med., *219:*503, 1938.
37. Schwartz, A., and Shaw, J. H.: Studies on the effect of selective desalivation on the dental caries incidence of albino rats. J. D. Res., *34:*239, 1955.
38. Shafer, W. G.: The caries-producing capacity of starch, glucose, and sucrose diets in the Syrian hamster. Science, *110:*143, 1949.
39. Shaw, J. H.: Nutritional relationships to dental caries. Borden's Rev. of Nut. Res. *16:*1, 1955.
40. Shaw, J. H.: Effect of carbohydrate-free and carbohydrate-low diets on the incidence of dental caries in white rats. J. Nut., *53:*151, 1954.
41. Shaw, J. H.: Caries-producing factors: A decade of dental research. Project No. 3 of the Sugar Research Foundation, Inc., J.A.D.A., *55:*785, 1957.
42. Sherman, H. C.: Chemistry of Food and Nutrition. 7th ed. New York, The Macmillan Co., 1946.
43. Sognnaes, R. F.: Analysis of wartime reduction of dental caries in European children with special regard to observation from Norway. Am. J. Dis. of Children, *75:*792, 1948.
44. Sognnaes, R. F.: Caries-conducive effect of a purified diet when fed to rodents during tooth development. J.A.D.A., *37:*676, 1948.
45. Sognnaes, R. F.: Is the susceptibility to dental caries influenced by factors operating during the period of tooth development? Sugar and Dental Caries Symposium. Supplemental issue, J. Calif. Dent. A. *26:*37, 1950.
46. Steggarda, M., and Hill, T. J.: Incidence of dental caries among Maya and Navajo Indians. J. D. Res., *15:*233, 1936.
47. Steinman, R. R., and Haley, M. I.: The biological effect of various carbohydrates ingested during the calcification of the teeth. J. Dent. Children, *24:*211, 1957.
48. Stephan, R. M., and Hemmens, E. S.: Studies of changes in *p*H produced by pure cultures of oral micro-organisms. J. D. Res., *26:*15, 1947.
49. Stetten, D.: Carbohydrate Metabolism, in Council on Foods and Nutrition of the American Medical Association's Handbook of Nutrition. 2nd ed. New York, Blakiston, 1951.
50. Toverud, G.: Dental caries in Norwegian children during and after the last World War: A preliminary report. Proc. Roy. Soc. Med., *42:*249, 1949.
51. Whyte, R.: A dietetic, dental and bacteriological study of fifty institutional inmates. Brit. Dent. J., *75:*247, 273, 301, 1943.
52. Williams, N. B.: Effect of sugars and other carbohydrates on the oral flora. J.A.D.A., *51:*278, 1955.

Chapter III

Fats

Fats were not only used as illuminants, cosmetics, medicines and lubricants in ancient times but also were considered an important foodstuff. Glycerol was obtained from olive oil by Schule in 1779, and in 1823 Chevreul determined chemically that animal and vegetable fats are combinations of glycerol and fatty acids.[4] Even though fats were discovered so early in history, it is only recently, with the newer methods of separation and purification (molecular distillation) and with newer identification procedures (infrared and ultraviolet absorption curves), that better knowledge has evolved concerning this group of substances.

It is estimated that the average American obtains about 33 per cent of his total calories from fats.[12] Furthermore, fats provide the maximum energy with the least amount of bulk. But, in addition to their caloric function, there are substances in the fat family which have vital biological activity; examples are essential unsaturated fatty acids, tocopherols, carotenoids and sterols.

CHEMISTRY

Definition

Fat and fatlike substances have been given by Bloor[2] a more comprehensive name, lipids. Deuel[4] defines lipids to "include all those substances which are insoluble in water but soluble in the so-called fat solvents (diethyl ether, petroleum ether, chloroform, hot alcohol, benzene, carbon tetrachloride, acetone, etc.), which are related either actually or potentially to fatty acid esters, and which at the same time are utilizable by the animal organism."

Classification

Bloor[2] has classified the lipids into three general groups, simple, compound and derived (see Table 8).

TABLE 8. CLASSIFICATION OF LIPIDS

I. Simple lipids—Esters of fatty acids with various alcohols
   1. Neutral fats: Triesters of fatty acids with glycerol
   2. Waxes: Esters of fatty acids with monohydroxy aliphatic alcohols higher than glycerol
      (a) True waxes: Products of both animal and vegetable origin in which the esters are composed of palmitic, stearic, oleic, or other higher fatty acid esters of cetyl alcohol ($CH_3[CH_2]_{14}CH_2OH$) or other higher straight chain alcohols
      (b) Cholesterol esters: Esters of fatty acids with cholesterol
      (c) Vitamin A esters: Palmitic or stearic acid esters of vitamin A
      (d) Vitamin D esters

II. Compound lipids—Esters of fatty acids with alcohols plus other radicals
   1. Phospholipids: Lipids containing phosphoric acid and a nitrogenous base
   2. Glycolipids or cerebrosides: Lipids containing a carbohydrate and also nitrogen but no phosphorus and no glycerol
   3. Sulfolipids: Lipids characterized by possessing sulfate groups

III. Derived lipids—Derivatives obtained by hydrolysis of those given in Groups I and II which still possess the general physical characteristics of lipids
   1. Saturated and unsaturated fatty acids
   2. Monoglycerides and diglycerides
   3. Alcohols
      (a) Straight chain alcohols: Water-insoluble alcohols of higher molecular weight obtained on hydrolysis of waxes
      (b) Sterols
      (c) Alcohols containing the β-ionone ring: Include vitamin A and certain carotenols
   4. Miscellaneous
      (a) Aliphatic hydrocarbons: Include iso-octadecane found in liver fat and certain hydrocarbons found in beeswax and plant waxes
      (b) Carotenoids
      (c) Squalene: A hydrocarbon found in shark and mammalian liver and in human sebum
      (d) Vitamins D, E, and K

(Adapted from Bloor by Kleiner, I., and Orten, J.: Human Biochemistry. 5th ed. St. Louis, The C. V. Mosby Co., 1958.)

Simple lipids are the visible and invisible fats of our diet. Butter, margarine, lard and edible oils, which are eaten to the extent of 43 to 46 pounds a year by the average American, are classified as visible fats. These provide about half the fat calories. The other half come from the invisible fats found in meats, eggs, dairy products, cereals, nuts and fruits.

Chemically, simple lipids are glyceryl esters of fatty acids which are structurally written:

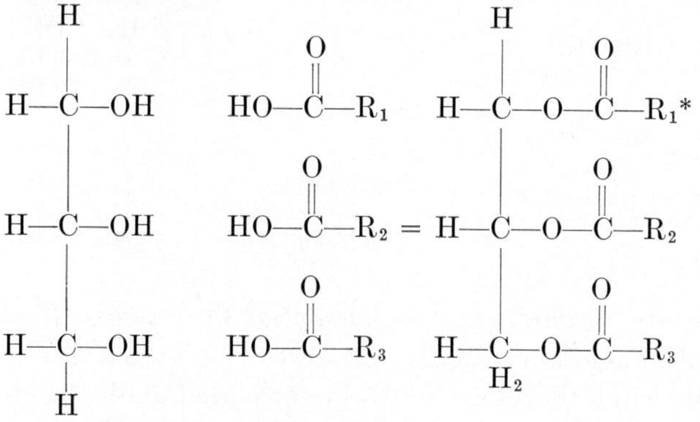

$$
\begin{array}{cccc}
\mathrm{H} & & & \mathrm{H} \\
| & \mathrm{O} & & |\quad\quad \mathrm{O} \\
| & \| & & |\quad\quad \| \\
\mathrm{H{-}C{-}OH} & \mathrm{HO{-}C{-}R_1} & & \mathrm{H{-}C{-}O{-}C{-}R_1}^{*} \\
| & \mathrm{O} & & |\quad\quad \mathrm{O} \\
| & \| & & |\quad\quad \| \\
\mathrm{H{-}C{-}OH} & \mathrm{HO{-}C{-}R_2} & = & \mathrm{H{-}C{-}O{-}C{-}R_2} \\
| & \mathrm{O} & & |\quad\quad \mathrm{O} \\
| & \| & & |\quad\quad \| \\
\mathrm{H{-}C{-}OH} & \mathrm{HO{-}C{-}R_3} & & \mathrm{H{-}C{-}O{-}C{-}R_3} \\
| & & & \mathrm{H_2} \\
\mathrm{H} & & & \\
\text{Glycerol} \quad + & \text{Fatty acids} & = & \text{Fat}
\end{array}
$$

* (R_1, R_2, R_3 represent fatty acid chains.)

Compound lipids are constituents of serum and of cells. They are glycerides in which one fatty acid molecule is replaced by a fraction containing organic nitrogen and orthophosphate. These are the phosphatides found in blood, bile and brain and nerve tissue.

Derived lipids are compounds which have the same solubility properties as fats but, in reality, are not chemically true fats. Chemically, they are derivatives of phenanthrene and include the sterols, the bile acids, the sex hormones, the adrenocortical hormones, vitamin D and certain carcinogens.

Chemical and Physical Properties

Solubility in fat solvents and insolubility in water are, according to Bloor's definition of lipids, the most characteristic properties of this group of nutrients.

To a large degree, the *melting* point determines the physical state of a fat. Those fats which have a predominance of unsaturated fatty acids are liquid at room temperature and are called oils, whereas those compounds which contain mostly saturated fatty acids are solid at room temperature. A saturated fatty acid is one that has no double bonds except the one in the carboxyl group.

Unsaturated fatty acids have one or more double bonds in the chain in addition to the carboxyl bond; a few even have triple bonds.

The most common fatty acids and their empirical formulae are:

Saturated	Butyric	C_3H_7COOH
	Caproic	$C_5H_{11}COOH$
	Palmitic	$C_{15}H_{31}COOH$
	Stearic	$C_{17}H_{35}COOH$
Unsaturated	Oleic	$C_{17}H_{33}COOH$
	Linolenic	$C_{17}H_{29}COOH$
	Linoleic	$C_{17}H_{31}COOH$
	Arachidonic	$C_{19}H_{31}COOH$

There are *essential* and *nonessential* fatty acids. Linoleic, linolenic and arachidonic acids are fatty acids that are considered "essential," and therefore must be provided daily in the dietary. All the others are the so-called "nonessential" fatty acids, i.e., they are synthesized by the body in amounts adequate to meet the needs of the body so that they need not be included in the daily menu. This does not mean that they are "nonessential" for body function.

The *specific gravity* of fats is less than 1.0, which is the reason they float on water.

There is no *color* to pure fat; human body fat is yellowish because it contains the pigments carotene and xanthophyll, acquired from the ingested food.

The degree of unsaturation in fats is expressed by the *iodine number.* Fats will generally combine with iodine in proportion to the number of double bonds in the constituent fatty acids; thus, usually, the higher the iodine number the more unsaturated is the fat.

Fats can be hydrolyzed (saponified) by bases, such as sodium hydroxide and potassium hydroxide, into glycerol and the alkaline salts of the fatty acids. The amount of alkali needed to saponify a given quantity of fat, the *saponification number,* will depend upon the average chain length of the constituent fatty acids. Butter has a higher saponification number than oleomargarine because it has more fatty acids and, owing to the presence of short-chained fatty acids, such as butyric and caproic acids, more carboxyl groups per gram of fat.

By a process known as *hydrogenation,* which basically involves the addition of hydrogen to double bonds, the soft fats or oils are converted into the harder, more saturated type. The popular shortenings used by the housewife in her cooking are hydrogenated fats.

The unsaturated fatty acids of fats and oils combine with oxygen very readily to produce auto-oxidized or *rancid fats,* which then impart their objectionable paintlike odor to the fat or oil. The amount and speed of rancidity is favored by (1) the degree of unsaturation, (2) the absence of natural antioxidants such as tocopherol (vitamin E), (3) poor storage conditions, and (4) the absence of added antioxidants such as butylated hydroxyanisole (BHA).

PHYSIOLOGY

Digestion

It is doubtful that any dietary fat is digested in the stomach by gastric lipase and hydrochloric acid. It is in the small intestine, where the bile comes in contact with the fat, that almost all the digestion takes place.

Because fats are insoluble in water, they must be emulsified by bile so that they may become miscible with the aqueous intestinal lipases. This emulsification is accomplished by the action of bile salts, which surround the fat globule and lower its surface tension. As a result of this action, the fat globules can be fragmented into smaller particles which then become miscible with the intestinal contents. Triglycerides are then hydrolyzed by the pancreatic lipase, steapsin, into mono- and diglycerides, fatty acids and glycerol. In addition to their emulsifying action, the bile acids (taurocholic and glycocholic) aid considerably in the absorption of fats and fatty acids.

Absorption

The end products of digestion are absorbed by the cells of the intestinal mucosa. In the mucosa there is a resynthesis and rearrangement of these products into triglycerides.

Less than half the absorbed fat is transported to the lymphatics via the lacteals; the rest is presumed to go directly to the liver via the portal blood. What is not utilized for caloric or biological functions is stored as neutral fat. However, depot fats are in a continuous state of dynamic equilibrium with the dietary fatty acids (Fig. 16).

There are two theories on the mechanism of fat absorption: (1) the lipolytic theory, and (2) the partition theory. The *lipolytic theory* suggests that all fat must be digested to fatty acid and glycerol and can be absorbed only as such. On the other hand, the *partition theory* states that fat can be absorbed as such after having been emulsified by monoglycerides and bile acids.

Phospholipids may be digested into their compounds, but they can be absorbed without hydrolysis.

The amount of cholesterol present in the body may often exceed the amount ingested because it is manufactured in the body.

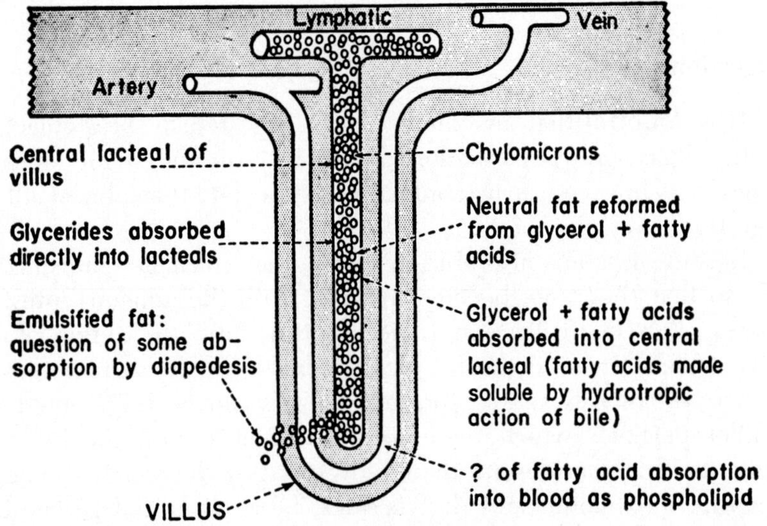

FIGURE 16. Absorption of fats. (Guyton, A. C.: Text of Medical Physiology.)

However, the absorption of cholesterol, like other fatty substances, is dependent upon the presence of bile in the intestine.

Oxidation

The digestion product glycerol may be oxidized into glyceric aldehyde or some related compound, which then may be metabolized like other three-carbon compounds. The other component of the digestive action, fatty acid, is first "activated" by conversion to coenzyme A derivatives and then oxidized, principally at the β-carbon atom, to form β-hydroxy and, subsequently, β-ketonic acids. Further oxidation will produce a fatty acid with two less carbon atoms. For example, stearic acid, with an empirical formula

$C_{17}H_{35}COOH$, loses two carbon atoms via β-oxidation; this results in the formation of palmitic acid, $C_{15}H_{31}COOH$.

As this process of β-oxidation continues, the palmitic acid is changed to myristic acid which, in turn, is oxidized to lauric acid, and so on, to butyric acid. Beta oxidation of butyric acid will yield β-hydroxybutyric acid and acetoacetic acid. From this, two molecules of acetic acid result which then may be oxidized via the Krebs citric acid cycle to the end products, carbon dioxide and water. At each one of the oxidation steps, small amounts of energy are usually released; these small packets of energy are more efficiently used than one complete evolution of energy.

Functions

The supplying of energy sources takes priority over all other body functions. If adequate amounts of fat are present in the diet to provide the body with fuel for energy, then it will spare protein from being diverted from tissue production to energy production. This is called the "protein-sparing" action of fat.

The layer of adipose tissue over the skeleton provides protection against mechanical injury by absorbing the shock of any trauma. Its thickness also prevents loss of body heat, thus serving as a thermal regulator.

Fats act as a source of, and as a vehicle for, the transport of the fat-soluble vitamins A, D, E and K as well as the essential fatty acids.

Fats delay hunger by slowing down stomach contractions and the rate of chyme production. This slows down the passage of food through the alimentary tract. A person who eats a high proportion of fat thus feels "full" for a relatively longer period of time. This feeling of satiety is commonly misinterpreted as indigestion.

Compound fats such as the phospholipids serve as integral components of cells and cell membranes.

Derived lipids play an important role in steroid metabolism.

GENERAL SYSTEMIC PATHOLOGY OF ABNORMAL FAT METABOLISM

Diseases Due to Low Fat Intake or Faulty Utilization

Vitamin Deficiency. If the ingestion of fats is low, the intake of fat-soluble vitamins is usually below normal. A vitamin D deficiency will contribute to defective mineralization of teeth and bones because proper calcification of bone matrix depends on having available an optimal ratio of calcium to phosphorus to vitamin D. Thus, a deficiency in fat intake can conceivably contribute to hypoplasia of enamel or dentin, or to the formation of a tooth of poor mineral quality.

If vitamin K is deficient due to low fat intake or faulty absorption, a condition of hypoprothrombinemia will result, in which hemorrhagic or bleeding tendencies can be expected in the patient.

Underweight. Without an adequate fat intake, dietary and tissue proteins and carbohydrates may be called upon to satisfy the body's need for energy. The excessive withdrawal of these two nutrients from the body will result in the catabolism of muscle and adipose tissue. This may contribute to underweight and emaciation.

Celiac Disease and Sprue. Steatorrhea, which is characterized by loose, frothy and whitish stools, is a symptom of faulty fat digestion and absorption.

Diseases Due to High Fat Intake

Obesity. Obesity will result from an intake of fat that is higher than necessary to meet the energy needs of the body; it will also result from excess carbohydrate intake. This is probably the most prevalent nutritional disease in the overfed population of the United States. Not only does obesity produce unsightly body disfigurement, it is also an important contributing factor to the incidence of diabetes and coronary heart disease.

Atherosclerosis. Atheromas are plaques created by the deposition of lipids, particularly cholesterol and its esters, in the subendothelial connective tissue of the intima—the inner lining of an artery. There appears to be a high correlation between the incidence of atheromas and the presence of lipoprotein with a low flotation rate* (S_f 10–20). An accumulation of atheromas causes a thickening and loss of elasticity of the arterial wall, or arteriosclerosis (hardening of the arteries). Atherosclerosis is, directly or indirectly, the cause of 25 per cent of all deaths in the United States.

* The rate at which particular lipoproteins can be made to travel, under proper experimental conditions, toward the axis of an ultracentrifuge instead of toward the periphery as ordinary proteins do.

The normal daily intake of cholesterol-containing foods such as eggs, fatty meats and dairy products is 250 to 800 mg.[10] On the basis of results from animal experimentation and the projection of these results to human beings on a weight basis, this intake is theoretically not high enough to produce atherosclerosis.

To control or prevent atherosclerosis, diets that are low in saturated fats and cholesterol have been recommended. However, because there is an innate individual ability to synthesize cholesterol, it is questionable whether diet alone can exert sufficient influence to reduce serum lipids. While the ingestion of corn oil, sunflower seed oil and other oils containing unsaturated fatty acids has been suggested[11] as a means of lowering serum cholesterol, there are other means which are also efficacious, e.g., moderate exercise, a low calorie diet, adequate protein and adequate vitamin B_6 intake.

Ketosis. When too much fat is ingested or when there is a disturbance in carbohydrate metabolism (diabetes), the oxidation of fatty acids beyond the acetoacetic acid stage is retarded. Thus, β-hydroxybutyric and acetoacetic acid accumulate and cause a condition known as ketosis, or acidosis.

Diseases Due to Disturbances in Lipid Metabolism

Xanthoma is characterized by excessive accumulation of lipid, especially cholesterol esters, in the skin around the eye, on the tendons or in the blood vessels. It may appear as a yellow macular discoloration or on the eyelids as slightly elevated, soft, rounded yellow nodules.

An accumulation of lipid in the spleen, liver, lymph nodes and bones is seen in three diseases, Hand-Schüller-Christian complex, Niemann-Pick disease and Gaucher's disease.

Xanthomatoses. Hand-Schüller-Christian disease is not a single entity but actually a complex of three morphologically related variants, namely Letterer-Siwe disease, Hand-Schüller-Christian disease and eosinophilic granuloma. These three differ clinically in the age group they affect, the rapidity of the clinical course and the duration of the inflammatory change. When Hand-Schüller-Christian disease was first described, it was thought to be due to accumulation of cholesterol and, therefore, was considered a disease of lipid metabolism. However, it now appears that the chronic inflammatory condition is the primary pathology and the foamy macrophages containing cholesterol are secondary invaders.

Letterer-Siwe disease, which occurs in infants, usually terminates in death within a few months after its onset. It is a nonlipid reticuloendotheliosis which produces marked enlargement of the spleen, liver, lymph nodes and bone marrow. The infants develop an anemia and a leukocytosis or leukopenia.

Hand-Schüller-Christian disease, which affects children, is characterized by three clinical features: (1) defects in the membranous bones of the skull (Fig. 17), (2) diabetes insipidus, and (3) exophthalmos.

Because of the expansive characteristics of the inflammatory tissues in the skull there may be pressure on the hypothalamus

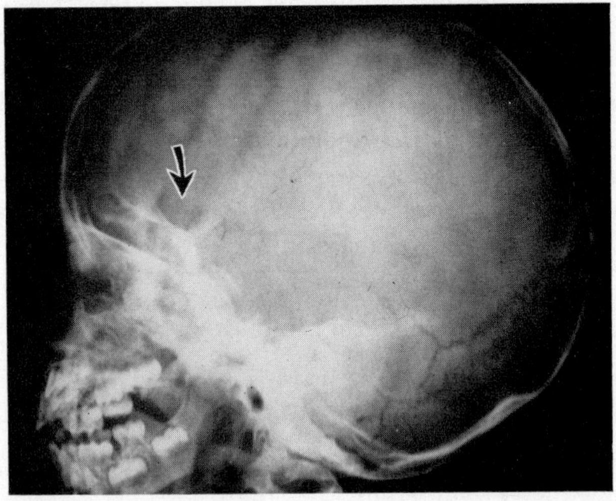

FIGURE 17. Skull plate of Hand-Schüller-Christian disease. Arrow points to lesion. (Courtesy Dr. G. Shklar.)

which causes it to bulge into the posterior orbit, producing exophthalmos. The pressure on the pituitary from the excessive inflammatory tissue causes diabetes insipidus.

Eosinophilic granuloma, which occurs in older children and young adults, is a granulomatous tumor in bone, producing pain from the pressure of its expansion. Occasionally eosinophils are seen in the tumor.

Non-xanthomatoses. *Gaucher's disease* is a rare familial disease in which cerebrosides or galactolipids are found in the foamy phagocytes which accumulate in the spleen, liver and lymph nodes. Enlargement of these organs and skeletal defects result. Histologically, there is found a characteristic ovoid cell having a large cytoplasm with an eccentrically placed nucleus.

Niemann-Pick disease is a congenital familial disease, predominantly affecting children of Jewish extraction. There is a rapid increase in the size of the abdomen. The skin assumes a pale yellow-brown discoloration and it becomes edematous. Bronchitis may appear. The cells of the spleen and bone marrow are filled with deposits of the phosphatide, sphingomyelin. Every tissue and organ of the body, especially the brain, is affected by this disease. This is in contrast to Gaucher's disease, in which only the reticulo-endothelial system is affected.

EFFECTS OF FATS ON TEETH AND ORAL STRUCTURES

Teeth

A very small percentage of lipid, primarily phospholipid and cholesterol, has been found in the organic portion of dentin and enamel.[9] The enamel contains more phospholipid but less cholesterol than dentin. Fats containing highly unsaturated fatty acids fed to vitamin E-deficient rats produce white opaque incisor teeth and histologic changes in the enamel organs.[5]

Dental Caries. In a human clinical study[3] that attempted to correlate dietary fat intake with dental caries incidence, significant reductions in caries were not found in association with a high fat diet. Boyd fed a group of children a high fat diet consisting of a protein:carbohydrate:fat ratio of 7:9:21. Later to the same group a lower fat diet was fed, in which the protein:carbohydrate:fat ratio was 7:15:11. Even though the caries experience was found to be slightly lower while they were on the high fat diet, Boyd concluded that this result was not due to the high fat:low carbohydrate intake but rather to better supervision during the period when the high fat diets were given.

In feeding experiments with cotton rats[16,17] and hamsters[6] replacement of a portion of the carbohydrate component of the cariogenic diet with lard seemed to produce a trend toward lower caries incidence.

Rosebury[15] found that if he added corn oil to a cariogenic diet, the food particles became coated with a fatty film. Thus bacterial enzymes could not penetrate the food to degrade it to acid, and decalcification of the teeth was prevented.

Gustafson[7,8] fed three groups of common laboratory rats purified isocaloric diets containing 4.8 per cent, 13.8 per cent and 25 per cent fat, respectively. There was an inverse relationship among the groups with respect to the number and extent of carious lesions and the percentage of fat in the diet. The group receiving 25 per cent fat had two-thirds less caries than the control (Fig. 18). Furthermore, all fats, regardless of their melting points and degree

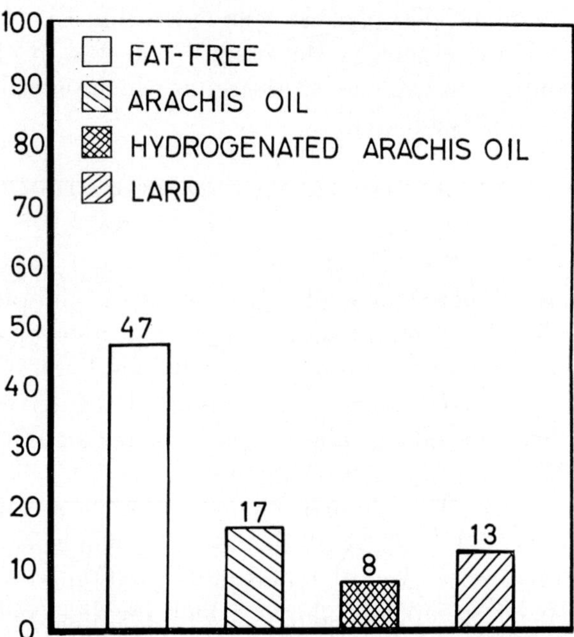

FIGURE 18. Number of carious units for males and females. (Gustafson, G., et al. Acta Odontologica Scandinavica, Vol. 13, 1956.)

of unsaturation, were associated with an almost equally significant reduction in caries incidence.

Oral Mucous Membranes and Alveolar Bone

In general, disturbed lipid metabolism produces a characteristic yellowing of the oral mucous membrane and gingiva and also halitosis.[18]

Hand-Schüller-Christian disease may manifest itself orally by hyperplastic and bleeding gingiva.[19] The teeth become sore and extremely mobile to the point of exfoliation. This periodontitis is due to the infiltration of the supporting bone by chronic inflammatory tissue and secondary fatty infiltration. Roentgenograms of the jaws show radiolucent areas which are indicative of osteolytic action (Fig. 19).

Letterer-Siwe disease and eosinophilic granuloma also show tumorlike destructive lesions in the mandible. Bernier[1] describes eosinophilic granuloma as granulomatous lesions accompanied by "foamy" macrophages. Eosinophils are predominantly present, but

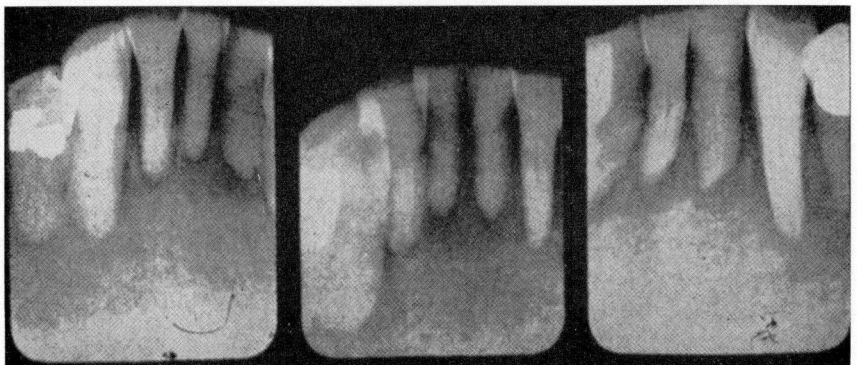

FIGURE 19. X-rays of case of Hand-Schüller-Christian disease showing diffuse involvement of alveolar bone in mandibular incisor area. (Sleeper, E. L., in Oral Surgery, Oral Medicine and Oral Pathology, Vol. 4, 1951.)

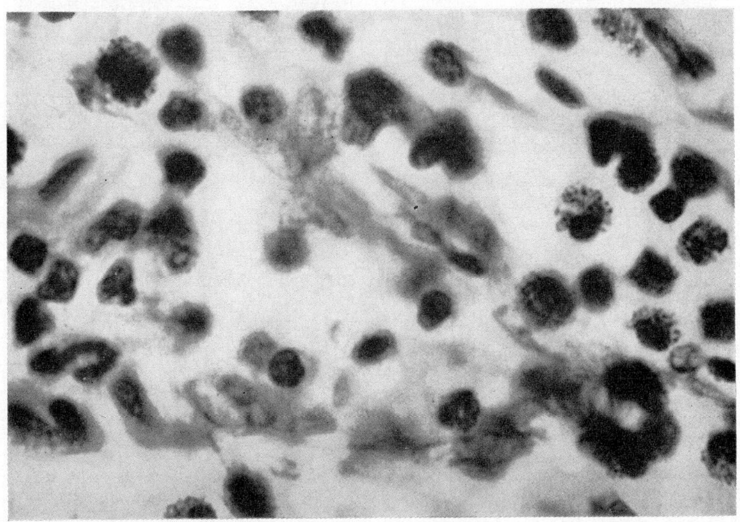

FIGURE 20. Eosinophilic granuloma. Although eosinophils may abound, they are not essential for the diagnosis of the disease. (Bernier, J. L.: The Management of Oral Disease, The C. V. Mosby Co., 1955.)

they are not considered absolutely diagnostic because other dental granulomas may also contain these cells (Fig. 20).

In Gaucher's disease there is rarefaction of the maxillary and mandibular bones and extensive chronic destructive periodontal disease (Fig. 21). The gingiva may become hemorrhagic due to an accompanying thrombocytopenia.[14]

Niemann-Pick disease is characterized by the presence of "foam cells" in the muscle tissue of the tongue and in the lingual nerve.[13]

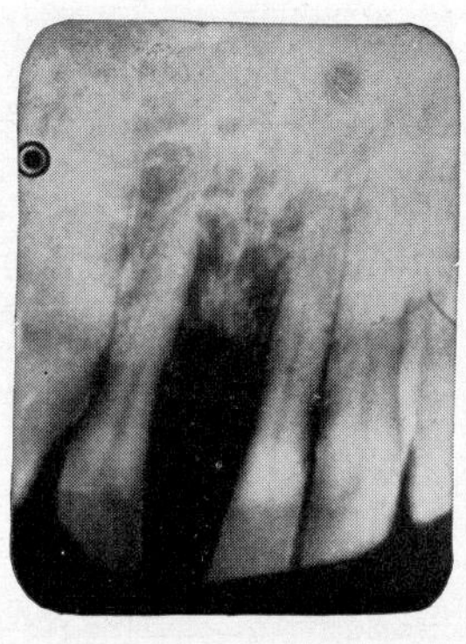

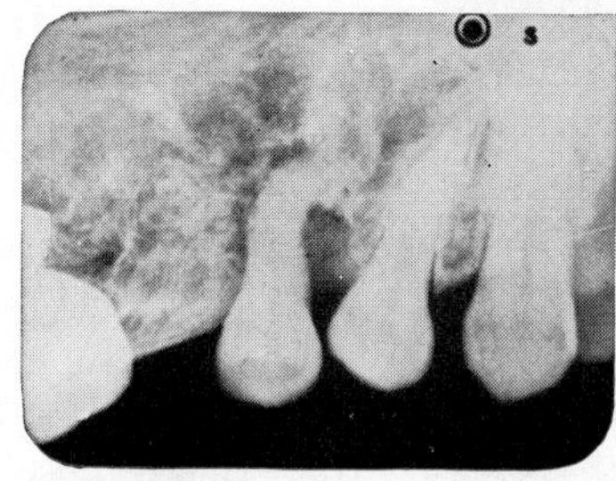

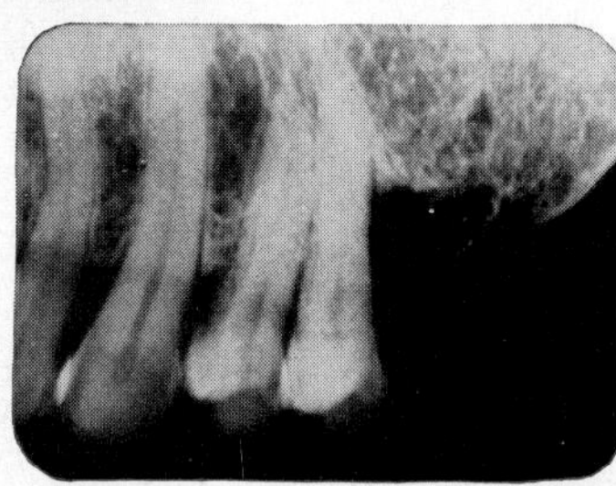

FIGURE 21. Osteoporosis in Gaucher's disease. (Courtesy Dr. David Weisberger, Harvard School of Dental Medicine.)

The oral mucous membranes develop a patchy, bluish-black pigmentation. The deciduous teeth may be slow to erupt and, because there may be a fatty infiltration of the supporting alveolar bone, the teeth become loose.

REFERENCES

1. Bernier, J. L.: The Management of Oral Disease. St. Louis, The C. V. Mosby Co., 1955.
2. Bloor, W. R.: Biochemistry of fats. Chem. Rev., *2:*243, 1925.
3. Boyd, J. D.: Dental caries as influenced by fat versus carbohydrate in the diet. Am. J. Dis. of Children, *67:*278, 1944.
4. Deuel, H. J.: The Lipids. Volume I. Chemistry. New York, Interscience Publishers, Inc., 1957.
5. Granados, H., and Dam, H.: Role of fat in incisor depigmentation of vitamin E deficient rats. Science, *101:*250, 1945.
6. Granados, H., Glavind, J., and Dam, H.: Observations on experimental

dental caries; effect of purified rations with and without dietary fat. Acta path. et microbiol. Scandinav., *25:*453, 1948.

7. Gustafson, G., Stelling, E., Abramson, E., and Brunius, E.: Experiments with various fats in a cariogenic diet. Experimental dental caries in golden hamsters. Acta Odont. Scand., *13:*75, 1955.
8. Gustafson, G., Stelling, E., and Brunius, E.: Experimental dental caries in golden hamsters. Experiments with dietary fats having different contents of unsaturated fatty acids. Brit. Dent. J., *95:*124, 1953.
9. Hess, W. C., Lee, C. Y., and Peckham, S. C.: The lipid content of enamel and dentin. J. D. Res., *35:*273, 1956.
10. Katz, L. N., and Stamler, J.: Experimental Atherosclerosis. Springfield, Ill., Charles C Thomas, 1953.
11. Kinsell, L. W., Friskey, R. W., Michaels, G. D., and Brown, F. R.: Effect of a synthetic triglyceride on lipid metabolism. Am. J. Clin. Nut., *4:*285, 1956.
12. Kummerow, F. A.: Fats and fatty acids in nutrition. Borden's Rev. of Nut. Res., *15:*1, 1954.
13. Pick, L.: Niemann-Pick disease and other forms of so-called xanthomatosis. (Dunham lecture.) Am. J. of Med. Sciences, *185:*601, 1933.
14. Rakower, W.: Oral manifestations of diseases of lipoid metabolism. N. Y. Dent. J., *24:*364, 1958.
15. Rosebury, T., and Karshan, M.: Susceptibility to dental caries in rat. Further studies of influence of vitamin D and of fats and fatty oils. J. D. Res., *18:*189, 1939.
16. Schweigert, B. S., Potts, E., Shaw, J. H., Zepplin, M., and Phillips, P. H.: Dental caries in the cotton rat. VIII. Further studies on the dietary effects of carbohydrate, protein, and fat on the incidence and extent of carious lesions. J. Nut., *32:*405, 1946.
17. Schweigert, B. S., Shaw, J. H., Zepplin, M., and Elvehjem, C. A.: Dental caries in the cotton rat. VI. The effect of amount of protein, fat, and carbohydrate in diet on the incidence and extent of carious lesions. J. Nut., *31:*439, 1946.
18. Shepro, M. J.: Oral manifestations of metabolic disturbances. J.A.D.A., *43:*543, 1951.
19. Sleeper, E. L.: Eosinophilic granuloma of bone. Its relationship to Hand-Schüller-Christian and Letterer-Siwe diseases, with emphasis on oral symptoms and findings. Oral Surg., Oral Med. and Oral Path., *4:*896, 1951.

Chapter IV

Proteins

“Plastic substances” was the name that Liebig, a German biochemist, gave to nitrogen-containing materials that served for building body tissues. Non-nitrogenous materials he called “respiratory substances.” Mulder, who was a contemporary of Liebig, gave the name “protein” (derived from the Greek word *protos*, meaning “first”) to a substance which turned out to be an artifact. Even though this substance was discarded, the generic name was retained for nitrogen-containing foodstuffs because they were considered of such prime importance.

Protein constitutes the major part of such fundamental cellular organic material as the cytoplasm and nucleus. The chromatin of the cell nucleus consists principally of desoxyribose nucleic acid, and the cell cytoplasm of ribose nucleic acid. Both of these compounds are nucleoproteins. In addition, protein serves as one of the essential components of such important substances as enzymes, hormones, hemoglobins, plasma proteins and antibiotics, and it contributes to ossein, collagen and dentin.

Carbohydrate and fat are composed entirely of carbon, hydrogen and oxygen which are oxidized to carbon dioxide and water. On the other hand, protein contains nitrogen and various combinations of other elements such as sulfur, phosphorus, iron, iodine, copper, manganese and zinc, besides carbon, hydrogen and oxygen. The essential chemical difference between protein and the other two major nutrients is that, in addition to carbon dioxide and water, protein end products always include ammonia.

CHEMISTRY

Chemical and Physical Properties

Proteins are large colloidal molecules, ranging in molecular weight from 5,000 to 25,000,000, that are formed from simpler units called amino acids. All proteins are characterized by the presence of alpha peptide bonds (—CONH—) which arise when the carboxyl group (—COOH) of one amino acid combines with the alpha amino group (—NH_2) of another amino acid with a resultant loss of one molecule of water.

Amino acids have the following typical formula

$$\begin{array}{c} H \\ | \\ R\text{—}C\text{—}COOH \\ | \\ NH_2 \end{array}$$

in which the R radical may be hydrogen, an aliphatic group (carbon atoms which form straight or branched chains), an aromatic group (carbon atoms which form closed rings), or a heterocyclic group (ring compounds which contain other atoms besides carbon atoms). The carbon atom adjacent to the terminal carboxyl group is called the alpha carbon atom. The number of amino acids linked together by peptide bonds will determine whether the compound is a dipeptide, tripeptide, proteose or peptone.

Physically, pure proteins are usually colorless, odorless and tasteless substances. When they are burned, however, they produce a distinctive odor, e.g., the burning of wool contrasted to the burning of cellulose. The salts of heavy metals, such as silver and mercury, will precipitate protein. This combining power of heavy metals with protein is the reason for use of egg whites or milk as an antidote in cases of metallic poisoning. In general, proteins are insoluble in the usual fat solvents (ether, acetone, chloroform, benzene, carbon tetrachloride) but vary in solubility in water, salt solution and alcohol. Under the influence of enzymes, or upon boiling with dilute acids or alkalis, they are hydrolyzed.

Classification

Proteins are classified as simple, conjugated and derived, based on solubility and other physical properties as well as on chemical

TABLE 9. PROTEIN CLASSIFICATION

	Food Protein	Body Protein
I. SIMPLE PROTEINS		
Albumin	egg albumin	
	legumelin (peas)	serum albumin
	leucosin (wheat)	
Globulins	edestin (wheat seed)	
	legumin (beans and peas)	serum globulin myosin
	tuberin (potato)	
Glutelins	glutenin (wheat)	
Prolamines	gliadin (wheat)	
	zein (maize)	
Histones	thymus histone	globin of hemoglobin
Protamines		protein or nucleo-protein
II. CONJUGATED PROTEINS		
Nucleoproteins	thymo-nucleic acid (thymus gland)	protein of cell nuclei gene of nucleus cytoplasm
	tritonucleic acid (wheat germ)	
Glycoproteins	mucins	mucus cartilage, bone tendon and intercellular spaces
Phosphoproteins	caseinogen (milk)	
	ovovitallin (egg yolk)	
Chromoproteins	flavoprotein	visual purple hemoglobin cytochrome
Lecithoprotein		cellular membranes
III. DERIVED PROTEINS		
a. Primary protein derivatives		
Proteans	casein (curdled milk)	fibrin (coagulated blood)
Metaproteans	(acid proteins, acid albumin, syntonic, alkali proteins, alkali albumins, and albuminates)	
Coagulated proteins	cooked egg albumin	
b. Secondary protein derivatives		
Proteoses		
Peptones		
Peptides		

composition. Simple proteins, such as albumins and globulins, yield primarily amino acids on hydrolysis. Conjugated proteins are compounds in which the protein molecule is attached to a nonprotein molecule or prosthetic group; for example, nucleoprotein, glycoprotein, hemoglobin, etc. Derived proteins are products resulting, usually, from the action of any kind of hydrolytic procedure on protein, e.g., proteose, peptide, coagulated protein. Table 9 shows examples of food and body proteins in each of these three main categories.

Properties of Amino Acids

Approximately twenty-one amino acids have been isolated from common plant and animal protein. Eight of these have been classified as indispensable for man; two more in addition to these are indispensable for the rat, while for the chick the number of essential amino acids is eleven. The remainder are termed nonessential. The term "nonessential" does not mean that they are not necessary to the body for its normal function but rather that they do not have to be provided *de novo* in the daily food; they can be produced by the body. A better term might be "synthesizable." Therefore, "essential" or indispensable amino acids are defined as those amino acids which must be supplied each day by the dietary because they are not synthesized by the body.

Amino acids are capable of existing in two different spatial forms which are mirror images of one another and which are designated by the letters D and L in front of the name of the amino acid. Most of the amino acids in living systems are in the L form. The D form is usually the result of a laboratory procedure such as extraction, processing or synthesis.

The necessity of ingesting certain amino acids daily was demonstrated by the classic experiments of Mendel in 1915.[17] He studied the growth of rats that were fed diets containing a single protein. When casein, which is very low in glycine, was used as the sole source of protein in the diet, satisfactory growth was obtained. However, when gliadin, which contains only a small amount of lysine, was the dietary protein, the animals barely maintained their weight. Furthermore, when zein, which is essentially devoid of lysine and tryptophan, was fed the animals did not grow and actually lost weight (Fig. 22). From these experiments it was deduced that glycine was not essential to the rat for growth and that lysine and tryptophan were the primary limiting amino acids of gliadin and zein. When zein was supplemented with lysine and trytophan and fed to the animals they grew very well.

It was by means of this type of animal experimentation that it was possible to demonstrate which amino acids were required in the daily ration of the rat for normal growth and the maintenance of good health. The ten amino acids that were found to be indispensable were isoleucine, leucine, lysine, methionine, phenylalanine, threonine, tryptophan, valine, histidine and arginine.

To determine those amino acids that were essential for man, various amino acid mixtures, each of which was limited with respect to one amino acid, were fed to a group of subjects and the ability of the subjects to maintain nitrogen balance was determined.[19]

Only eight amino acids—lysine, tryptophan, phenylalanine, leucine, isoleucine, threonine, methionine and valine—were found

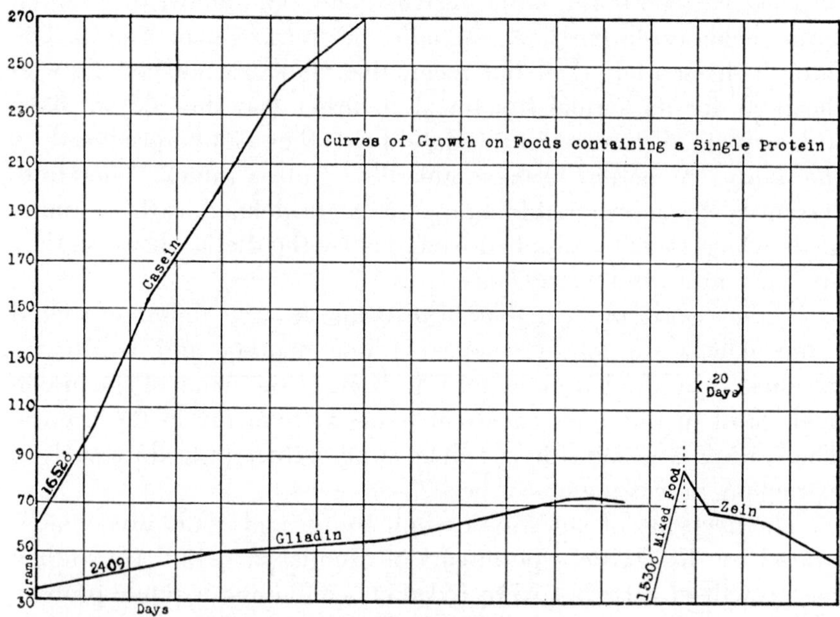

FIGURE 22. Showing typical curves of growth of rats on diets containing a single protein. On the casein food (devoid of glycine), satisfactory growth is obtained; on the gliadin food (deficient in lysine) little more than maintenance of body weight is possible; on the zein food (devoid of glycine, lysine, and tryptophan), even maintenance of body weight is impossible. (From Mendel, L. B.: J.A.M.A. *64*:1539, 1915.)

to be essential to maintain the nitrogen equilibrium. The minimum daily requirement for each of these eight indispensable amino acids for normal males was found to be:

L-isoleucine	0.70 Gm.	L-phenylalanine	1.10 Gm.
L-leucine	1.10 Gm.	L-threonine	0.50 Gm.
L-lysine	0.80 Gm.	L-tryptophan	0.25 Gm.
L-methionine	1.10 Gm.	L-valine	0.30 Gm.

However, to insure ample supply, Rose recommended that double these amounts be consumed daily.

The names of the remaining amino acids, which are nutritionally essential substances for man but are dispensable in the sense that, under normal conditions, they can be synthesized by the body, are:

glycine	glutamic acid	cystine
alanine	histidine	tyrosine
serine	norleucine	proline
aspartic acid	hydroxyglutamic acid	arginine
	hydroxyproline	

More recently, Block and his associates[8] have suggested that to the indispensable and dispensable classes of amino acids a third group, a semi-indispensable category, be added. This latter group would consist of arginine, tyrosine, cystine, glycine, serine and histidine. They are semi-indispensable because (1) they are not synthesized at an optimum rate, (2) they are essential only for a particular species, or (3) they can be spared if closely related amino acids are provided.

PHYSIOLOGY

Digestion

The first step in the digestion of protein takes place in the stomach, where the enzymatic action of pepsin is favored by the hydrochloric acid. The protein is split primarily into proteoses and peptones. Rennin found in infant's stomachs is an enzyme which acts on milk protein, casein, to form a more easily digested curd.

In the intestine, proteoses and peptones are broken down further by the enzyme trypsin, which is secreted by the pancreas. In addition to trypsin there are other hydrolytic enzymes secreted by the pancreas which aid in breaking down the complex protein molecule to simple peptides. Finally, from the villi of the wall of the small intestine there is liberated erepsin, containing the peptidase enzymes. This group of enzymes splits the peptides into amino acids (Fig. 23).

Absorption

After the amino acids are formed in the intestine, some are absorbed by simple diffusion, and others, after being phosphorylated, are actively absorbed. Simple diffusion is the passage of a nutrient from an area of high concentration to an area of low concentration. Active absorption allows material to be absorbed under any condition; no concentration gradient is required. The amino acids travel from the capillaries into the liver, through the portal system into the general circulation. Excess amino acids can be stored both in the liver and in muscle, but only in limited quantities.

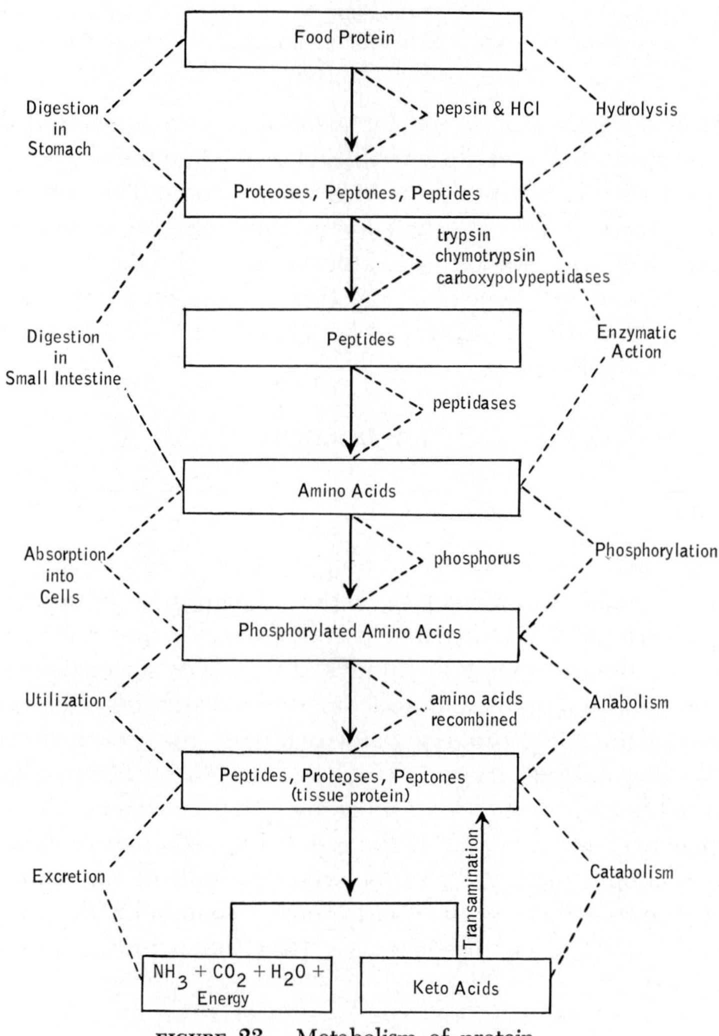

FIGURE 23. Metabolism of protein.

Sometimes proteins, instead of breaking down into amino acids, are absorbed as protein molecules. These molecular proteins cannot be utilized for the synthesis of body tissue but they can, and often do, lead to immunologic sensitization which may underlie many allergic phenomena.

Utilization

The body cells use the amino acids supplied them by the blood to form protein required for maintenance or growth. However, for optimum protein synthesis, all amino acids must be present simultaneously and in sufficient quantities. The energy necessary for this synthesis is provided by adenosine diphosphate (ADP) and adenosine triphosphate (ATP) through a complicated and not fully understood mechanism. According to one hypothesis, the specificity of proteins is maintained by their being formed as replicas of templates, or molds, each of which is specific for a particular protein. They, therefore, determine the kind of protein that is synthesized.

Those amino acids that are not utilized for protein synthesis for one reason or another may undergo an oxidative deamination, thus forming ammonia and alpha-keto acids; they may be decarboxylated into pharmacologically active amines; or they may eventually be converted to sugar and fat. There may also be some shifting of amino groups from an amino acid to keto acid; this is called transamination and makes possible the synthesis of additional tissue amino acids.

Excretion

The end products of protein metabolism, which are excreted in the urine, are urea, ammonia, creatinine, uric acid and amino acids.

Urea is formed in the liver from the ammonia which results from the deamination process. However, a very small amount of the metabolic ammonia is excreted as ammonium salts.

Uric acid is the chief metabolic end product of the metabolism of purines which may occur free in foods or may be derived from the nucleoproteins of food or body tissue.

Creatinine is the excretory form of creatine, which is formed in muscle from at least three different amino acids, arginine, glycine and methionine.

Amino acids may be present in the urine after excessive intake of protein or in certain pathologic conditions.

NUTRITIVE VALUE OF PROTEIN

To prevent or cure a protein deficiency, not only must adequate amounts of dietary protein be ingested, but it must be of high quality.

Qualitative Considerations

Protein can be derived from plant or animal foods. For example, egg, fish, fowl and meat are typical foods containing animal protein, while nuts, legumes and cereals contain plant protein. The origin and nutritive values of animal and plant protein differ greatly. Plant proteins are derived from inorganic substances, but animal proteins are formed from the digestion products of other proteins. On an equal weight basis, animal proteins are more nutritious than plant proteins.

Animal proteins usually contain all eight essential amino acids and, therefore, are considered "complete" proteins. On the other hand, the proteins of cereals or vegetables are termed "incomplete" because many of them lack one or more of the indispensable amino acids. If one vegetable or cereal lacks a number of essential amino acids which are present in another vegetable or cereal, the full complement of essential amino acids may be ingested by eating both foodstuffs at the same meal. However, it must be emphasized that amino acids are not stored for any appreciable length of time. Therefore, for the fabrication of tissue protein, all eight of the essential amino acids must be available at the site of synthesis simultaneously. In fact, the amount of tissue protein that is produced is limited by that essential amino acid which is present in the smallest amount. The benefits of the complementary feeding of plant proteins must have been instinctively appreciated by the Indians, because they served to the first white settlers a dish of maize and beans that had been cooked together in the same vessel. Corn, or maize, is deficient in tryptophan and lysine but contains the other six essential amino acids. Beans have plenty of tryptophan and lysine but lack arginine. Thus, when corn with its six essential amino acids was eaten with beans, which have the other two missing essential amino acids, there resulted a complete protein mixture containing all eight essential amino acids.

Quantitative Considerations

The nutritive value or quality of proteins is usually measured as protein efficiency ratio (P.E.R.), the ratio of gain in body weight to the protein consumed, or as biological value (B.V.) in terms of percentage of protein nitrogen utilized by the body. The product of B.V. and true digestibility gives a value for total utilization, or "net" utilization. Of all proteins, whole egg protein is usually considered the best (that is, the most complete) for man and is, therefore, used as a reference. Table 10 gives a summary of the nutritive

TABLE 10. NUTRITIVE VALUE OF SIX SELECTED PROTEINS

(Value expressed relative to egg white as 100.)

Animal	*Egg white*	*Whole egg*	*Beef*	*Casein*	*Peanut flour*	*Wheat gluten*
For Growth						
Rat	100	95	84	80	31	8
	100	90	78	71	56	41
For Maintenance						
Rat	100	87	73	54	49	69
Dog	100	76	68	64	49	39
Man	100	103	74	74	62	46

(Adapted from Block, R. J., and Mitchell, H. H.: The correlation of the amino acid composition of proteins with their nutritive values. Nut. Abst. and Rev., *16*:249, 1946–7.)

value of six proteins for rats, dogs and man. The value of egg white is expressed as 100, and the other protein foods are compared with it. Block and Mitchell[7] have devised a chemical method for measuring the nutritive value of a protein based upon a comparison of the amino acids present with those of whole egg. Agreement with the results of biological methods has been good.

PROTEIN REQUIREMENT AND NITROGEN EQUILIBRIUM

Protein Requirement

There are no large stores of protein in the body; therefore, an adequate daily intake is necessary. The recommended allowance for an active healthy adult is 1 Gm. of protein per kilogram of body weight per day. However, this allowance is much above the minimal amount that must be ingested before the nitrogen balance is disturbed. Diets which contain 0.5 to 0.8 Gm. of protein per kilogram of body weight have not produced a protein deficiency.

The protein requirement for the infant and child is comparatively greater than that for the adult because of their rapid growth. The one to three year old child is allowed 4 Gm. of protein per kilogram of body weight. For the next three years it is recommended that the protein allowance be reduced by 0.5 Gm. per kilogram of body weight. Starting at age six and for about every three years of increased age, the protein allowance can be reduced by about

0.5 Gm. until the adult allowance of 1 Gm. per kilogram of body weight is reached.

Nitrogen Equilibrium

Nitrogen equilibrium is a condition in which the nitrogen intake furnished by foods is equal to the nitrogen excreted in the urine and feces. If the nitrogen intake is greater than the output, the balance is positive, which indicates that anabolism (tissue synthesis) is taking place. This is the condition during growth and tissue repair. On the other hand, if the nitrogen intake is less than the output, a

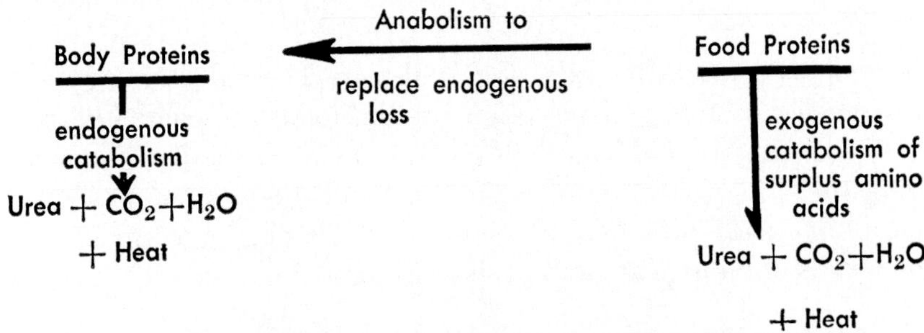

FIGURE 24. Protein metabolism, according to Folin.

condition of negative balance is produced, which means that catabolism (tissue breakdown) is occurring. Conditions which contribute to the negative nitrogen balance are (1) low calorie intake, (2) severe burns, and (3) hemorrhage.

Originally, it was believed that protein metabolism had an endogenous and an exogenous component. The metabolism of amino acids from foods was exogenous and that from body protein was endogenous. Actually, it was believed that the tissues slowly wasted away due to "wear and tear" and that constant replenishment was necessary to replace the lost protein (Fig. 24). Later Schoenheimer,[20] as a result of experiments with stable isotopes, showed that proteins are in a continuous dynamic state (Fig. 25). Amino acids are deposited and withdrawn from a metabolic pool contributed to by both food and tissue proteins; this allows for an interchange between "endogenous" and "exogenous" sources of protein.

If dietary protein is gradually reduced, the output of nitrogen

Diagrammatic scheme of Schoenheimer's hypothesis of the dynamic equilibrium in protein metabolism.

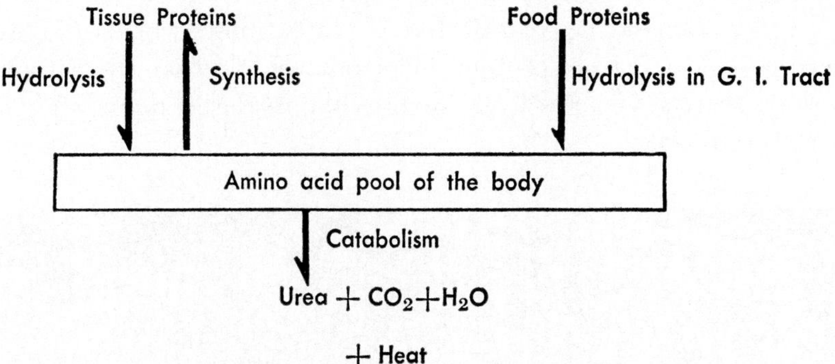

FIGURE 25. Protein metabolism, according to Schoenheimer.

will decrease correspondingly, maintaining an equilibrium. However, there is a point beyond which further reduction of dietary protein will lead to negative nitrogen balance and protein deficiency.

GENERAL SYSTEMIC PATHOLOGY OF PROTEIN DEFICIENCY

General Effects

Protein deficiency, if sufficiently severe and protracted, leads to poor growth and reproduction, poor wound healing, increased susceptibility to infection, liver injury, reduction in enzyme activity, atrophy of lymphoid tissue, interference with endocrine gland function, anemia and edema.[18]

There are skeletal changes which make for poor growth in a protein-deficient animal. Osteoblastic activity is interfered with and the result is osteoporosis. The arrangement and maturity of cartilage cells is an important criterion in determining the nutritional status of an animal. As seen in Figure 26, there is direct correlation between the length of time an animal is on a protein-deficient diet and the degree of cartilaginous change.[11]

Because protein deficiency is responsible for the slowing down of fibroblastic as well as osteoblastic activity, healing of soft tissue wounds and formation of bony callus in fractures are seriously retarded.

Cannon[9] has shown that there is a reduced capacity to produce antibodies and, therefore, an increased susceptibility to infection in protein-deficient animals. Inadequate dietary protein can adversely influence the response of the host to viral infection.

Liver damage, as manifested by fatty infiltration and fibrosis, can be expected from protein deficiency. In addition, the activity of certain enzymes in the liver, such as the oxidases, dehydrogenases, etc., is reduced.

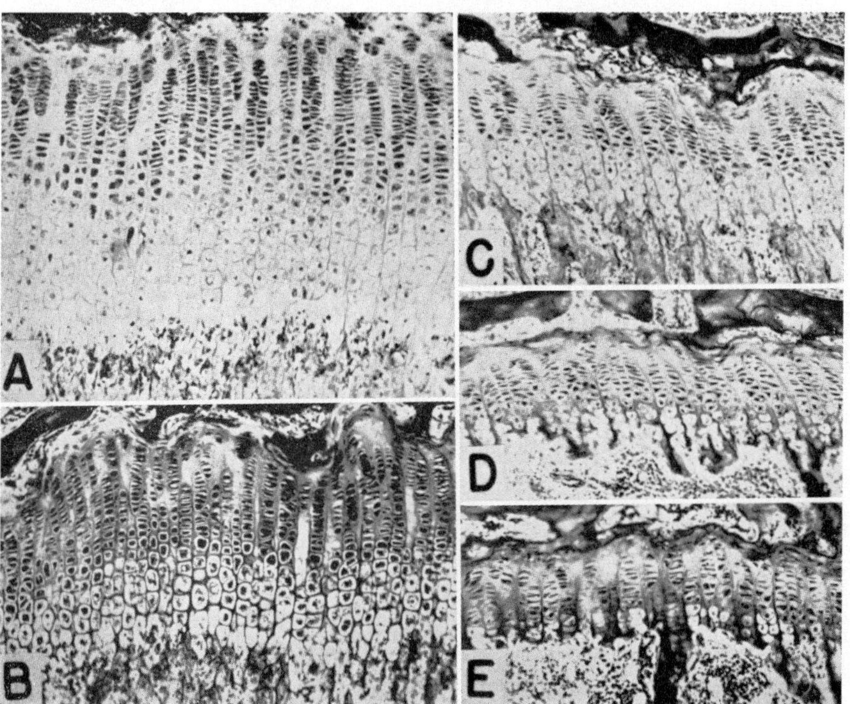

FIGURE 26. Protein deficiency. Epiphyseal cartilages, rat. Upper ends of the tibiae of rats placed on a diet adequate in all respects save that it contained no protein. A. Control, killed at start. B, C, D and E, animals killed at 7, 13, 18 and 21 days. (Follis, R. H.: Deficiency Disease. Springfield, Ill., Charles C Thomas, 1958.)

Hemoglobin will fail to regenerate during protein restriction, which will contribute to anemia. Sometimes hypoproteinemia will produce edema.

Kwashiorkor. Kwashiorkor is caused by an extreme deficiency of protein and is found in tropical regions such as South Africa and South and Central America where meat is scarce and cultivation of high quality protein cereals is impossible. This disease is fatal to infants. It is manifested by weakness, steatorrhea, skin pigmentation, ulcerative dermatitis, hepatomegaly and edema. There also may be fatty infiltration and cirrhosis of the liver, and atrophy of the intestinal mucosa.

EFFECTS OF PROTEIN DEFICIENCY ON TEETH, SALIVA AND PERIODONTIUM

Teeth

Normally, dental enamel contains about 1 per cent organic matter consisting of the eukeratin type of protein.[1] Human dentin consists of 21 to 22 per cent organic matter, of which only 1 or 2 per cent is not protein. The remaining 20 per cent is a collagen type of protein which, on analysis by two-dimensional paper chromatography, has been shown to contain twenty amino acids.[2]

Hypocalcification. Rats fed a tryptophan-deficient diet show an increased number of interglobular areas in the dentin. Proper calcification is prevented by depolymerization of the ground substance.[6]

Dental Caries. The incidence of smooth-surface caries in rat molars was significantly increased when a diet composed largely of processed cereal foods was used. McClure[15] noted that the cereal protein in the diet, particularly the lysine content, was inadequate for normal growth of the experimental animal. In a later experiment Bavetta and McClure[5] were able to change a protein-poor cariogenic diet to a cariostatic one by increasing the L-lysine component of the diet to the 1 per cent level. To determine the mode of action of lysine in inhibiting experimental caries, McClure[16] carried out further experiments in which 1.5 per cent L-lysine was added to food or to drinking water or administered by intubation or intraperitoneal injection. A reduction in caries was noted when L-lysine was provided by the first three routes; and, according to the investigator, this result was indicative of a systemic action. However, in apparent contradiction to this conclusion, injected L-lysine was not effective.

Saliva

Normally, there are at least sixteen different amino acids in human saliva.[14]

On the basis that ptyalin (the starch-splitting oral enzyme) is inhibited by tryptophan, Turner and Crowell[23] investigated the relationship between levels of tryptophan in the saliva and the incidence of caries. They found free tryptophan in the saliva from caries-immune subjects, but not in the saliva from patients with rampant caries. On the other hand, Stack[21] found no correlation between the DMF (defective, missing and filled teeth) rate and the presence of salivary tryptophan.

Green[13] suggested that the innate caries resistance shown by some people may be attributed to the presence of a bacteriolytic agent in the globulin fraction of their saliva which coincidentally contains tryptophan and some related compounds. This factor adversely affects the growth of the caries-promoting bacteria, lactobacilli and streptococci.

Periodontium

Protein deficiency primarily affects the matrix-forming cells such as fibroblasts and osteoblasts. Therefore, the many reports[10,12,22] of atrophic and degenerative changes in the periodontal membrane and alveolar bone of protein-deprived animals are not surprising. The microscopic bone picture which accompanies this deficiency

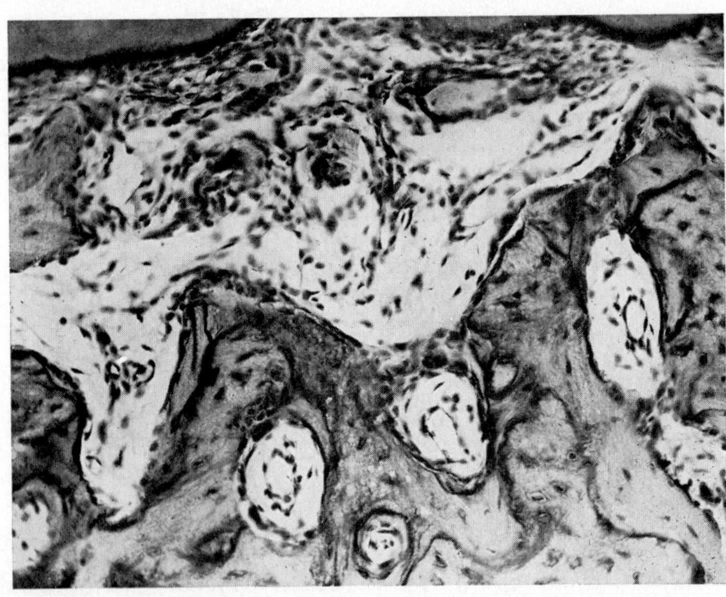

FIGURE 27. The effect of protein deprivation upon the periodontium of the albino rat. Bone shows marked diminution in osteoid and number of osteoblasts. (Glickman, I.: Clinical Periodontology. 1st ed.)

consists of increased size of cancellous bone spaces, less than normal amounts of osteoid tissue and fewer osteoblasts; this group of characteristics is referred to as osteoporosis (Fig. 27). Chawla and Glickman[10] also found retardation in deposition of cementum.

A tryptophan-deficient diet fed different groups of rats for varying periods of time resulted in osteoporosis of the alveolar bone. However, the prolongation of the deficiency did not produce an aggravation of the degenerative changes.[3] In an extension of this research in which effects of age were considered, it was found that the alveolar bone was affected most in the young and least in older animals. However, greater gingival changes were noted in the older animals.[4]

In protein-deprived rats, local irritation of the periodontal tissues produced by food impaction accentuated the resorption of the alveolar crest, downgrowth of the epithelial attachment and increase of the general inflammatory infiltrate.[22] These findings were in addition to the endosteal osteoporosis and increased cellularity of the periodontal membrane. However, this deficiency effect could be reversed if a normal diet complete in protein was fed.

REFERENCES

1. Battistone, G. C., and Burnett, G. W.: Studies of the composition of teeth. IV. The amino acid composition of human enamel protein. J. D. Res., *35:*260, 1956.
2. Battistone, G. C., and Burnett, G. W.: Studies of the composition of teeth. III. The amino acid composition of human dentinal protein. J. D. Res., *35:*255, 1956.
3. Bavetta, L. A., and Bernick, S.: Effect of tryptophan deficiency on bones and teeth of rats. II. Effect of prolongation. Oral Surg., Oral Med. and Oral Path., *9:*308, 1956.
4. Bavetta, L. A., and Bernick, S.: Effect of tryptophan deficiency on bones and teeth of rats. III. Effect of age. Oral Surg., Oral Med. and Oral Path., *9:*906, 1956.
5. Bavetta, L. A., and McClure, F. J.: Protein factors in experimental rat caries. J. of Nut., *63:*107, 1957.
6. Bernick, S., Bavetta, L. A., and Baker, R.: Histochemical and electron microscopy studies on tryptophan-deficient dentin. J. D. Res., *34:*671, 1955. Abstract.
7. Block, R. J., and Mitchell, H. H.: The correlation of the amino acid composition of proteins with their nutritive values. Nut. Abst. and Rev., *16:*249, 1946–7.
8. Block, R. J., Weiss, K. W., Almquist, H. J., Carroll, D. B., Gordon, W. G., and Saperstein, S.: Amino Acid Handbook. Springfield, Ill., Charles C Thomas, 1956.
9. Cannon, R. R.: The relationship of protein metabolism to anti-body production and resistance to infection. Adv. Protein Chem., *2:*135, 1945.

10. Chawla, T. N., and Glickman, I.: Protein deprivation and the periodontal structure of the albino rat. Oral Surg., Oral Med. and Oral Path., *4*:578, 1951.
11. Follis, R. H.: Deficiency Disease. Springfield, Ill., Charles C Thomas, 1958.
12. Frandsen, A. M., Becks, H., Nelson, M. M., and Evans, H. M.: The effects of various levels of dietary protein on the periodontal tissues of young rats. J. of Perio., *24:*135, 1953.
13. Green, G. E.: A bacteriolytic agent in salivary globulin of caries-immune human beings. J. D. Res., *38:*362, 1959.
14. Kirch, E. R., Kesel, R. G., O'Donnell, J. F., and Wach, E. C.: Amino acids in human saliva. J. D. Res., *26*:297, 1947.
15. McClure, F. J., and Folk, J. E.: Skim milk powders and experimental rat caries. Proc. Soc. Exper. Biol. & Med., *83:*21, 1953.
16. McClure, F. J.: Effect of lysine provided by different routes on cariogenicity of lysine-deficient diet. Proc. Soc. Exper. Biol. & Med., *96:*631, 1957.
17. Mendel, L. B.: Nutrition and growth. J.A.M.A., *64:*1539, 1915.
18. Pollack, H., and Halpern, S. L.: Therapeutic nutrition. Publication 234. Washington, D.C., National Academy of Sciences-National Research Council, 1952.
19. Rose, W. C.: Amino Acid Requirements of Man. Federation Proceedings, *8*:546, 1949.
20. Schoenheimer, R.: Dynamic State of Body Constituents. Cambridge, Harvard University Press, 1942.
21. Stack, M. V.: The independence of caries experience and salivary tryptophan content. J. D. Res., *33:*316, 1954.
22. Stahl, S. S., Miller, S. C., and Goldsmith, E. D.: Effects of protein deprivation on the periodontium of young adult male hamsters. J. D. Res., *37:*984, 1958. Abstract.
23. Turner, N. C., and Crowell, G. E.: Dental caries and tryptophan deficiency. J. D. Res.: *26:*99, 1947.

Chapter V

The Intermediary Metabolism and Interrelationships of Carbohydrates, Proteins and Fats

BY SANFORD MILLER, PH.D.

INTRODUCTION

"By its nature, life is unstable. An organism that is in a stable equilibrium with its environment is dead." In order to preserve life, energy must be expended to counteract the destructive forces which tend to destroy it. The sources of energy of the body have already been described as protein, fat and carbohydrate. This chapter will now consider briefly the manner in which these nutrients are utilized.

In living tissues, the bulk of energy derived from the metabolism of foodstuffs is liberated, not as a single burst of heat as occurs outside of the body, but rather as the result of a series of integrated reactions. Presented in this way, the potential energy of a foodstuff can eventually be utilized more efficiently by the body. Moreover, the organic products of these reactions are used to maintain the structure of the body. Protein, for example, is catabolized to amino acids which, in turn, are used for the replacement of worn existing tissue and for the growth of new structures. These series of reactions are known as the intermediary metabolism of a nutrient; similar pathways exist for every molecule utilized by the body.

Although we present the intermediary metabolism of proteins as example, none of these systems is isolated. All are related and, in fact, are intimately dependent upon one another. Deficiencies in one nutrient affect not only the systems of that material but alter the activities of nearly all of the pathways of metabolism and thus alter the economy of life.

In addition, life is dynamic. A cell once formed does not continue to exist for the life of the organism. A muscle protein does not remain forever. All constituents of the body are constantly in a state of flux, being broken down and resynthesized. It is the function of metabolism to maintain this activity by breaking down molecules, building them again, deriving energy, and preparing for excretion those portions the body cannot use.

Life, therefore, can be described as a series of dynamic, interrelated processes integrated through the common goal of maintaining the organism in the presence of an ever-changing environment. To understand life and the ills which beset it, some concept of the way in which metabolism works must be gained. To approach this concept, each major nutrient will be discussed in turn, with the understanding that all are intertwined and none can long operate without the others.

The discussion of carbohydrate oxidation which follows is presented in somewhat greater detail than would be expected in a book of this type. This has been done in order to emphasize the order and logic of metabolic activities. As discussed earlier, compounds are not "exploded" in the body to dissipate their energy as wasted heat but rather are taken apart relatively gently, each morsel extracted to its limit. While this has the advantage of extraordinary efficiency in converting chemical energy to other forms, it suffers from the serious disadvantage of offering many areas of potential difficulty. A partial deficiency in Mg^{++}, for example, will decrease the activity of all reactions in which Mg^{++} is a co-factor. Since energy produced in these reactions is needed for tissue synthesis, if affected, protein metabolism as well as fat utilization, absorption of nutrients, neurological activities and muscle movements will be altered. In fact, the entire normal operation of the body will be upset, all as a result of the partial lack of a nutrient required in minute quantities. The surprising point about metabolism, and thus life, is not that it occasionally suffers lapses, but rather that it can continue to operate at all under widely varying conditions and environments. The broad patterns of life appear, at first glance, to be composed of wild rugged strokes. On closer examination, each stroke is found to be composed of numbers of smaller lines, connected in an almost infinite number of combinations forming a fine filigree, which is the basic structure of life itself. To understand "normal" life, therefore, these interrelationships must be understood or, at least, their existence recognized. Finally, to understand the illnesses and abnormalities which influence it, life itself must be understood.

HIGH ENERGY BONDS[4]

Metabolism serves the dual function of either utilizing or producing energy. Energy, therefore, must be transferred to or from a reaction. The body uses an ingenious way of accomplishing this task. All molecules require energy to maintain their structure. This energy is generally contained in the bonds which hold the molecule together. The amount of energy which can be released when the bond is broken or, on the other hand, is necessary to synthesize the bond is a function of the structure and composition of the entire molecule. There are a number of compounds which have the fortunate ability of concentrating relatively large amounts of energy in a single bond or a few bonds. These are known as high energy compounds and the bonds as high energy bonds.

Of the many known high energy substances, two are important biologically. These are adenosine triphosphate (ATP) and creatine phosphate (CMP). ATP, in particular, is perhaps the body's most important means of transfering energy. The energy produced in an exergonic reaction (energy producing) is utilized by the body to synthesize ATP from either the monophosphate (AMP) or the diphosphate (ADP) form. The newly formed ATP can then carry this energy to a reaction that requires it (an endergonic reaction). While giving up its energy, the ATP is hydrolyzed to either ADP or AMP, depending on the reaction involved. As much as 22,000 calories can be transferred in this way by each mole of ATP. As far as is known, ATP is, in some way, formed in most exergonic reactions and utilized in most endergonic reactions. It is easy to see why this compound has been called "the common currency of energy."

ATP is relatively unstable and is not a good storage compound for energy; on the other hand, phosphocreatine (CMP) is. Surplus high energy phosphate is transferred from ATP to CMP and is stored as such. When energy is required, the phosphate group of CMP is utilized to reform ATP.

It can easily be seen from the foregoing discussion that a concept has been developed which may be stated as follows: reactions forming ATP are energy producers while those that utilize ATP require energy for their proper functioning. By this concept the reactions in which the energy of the body is produced can be determined.

CARBOHYDRATE METABOLISM

It is not within the scope of this book to discuss the complexities and details of intermediary metabolism. Since some knowledge of pathways is required, however, the major pathways of metabolism will be outlined in very broad form.

The major pathway for the utilization of carbohydrate in the body is its oxidation to CO_2 and H_2O, thus producing energy as a product. This sequence of catabolic reactions may be divided into anaerobic and aerobic phases, depending on whether or not oxygen is needed.

Anaerobic Metabolism[2,8]

In this series of reactions, hexoses (particularly glucose) are sequentially broken down to simpler triose forms as shown in Figure 28.

Glucose is phosphorylated to form glucose-6-phosphate. This is converted to fructose-6-phosphate which, in turn, is phosphorylated to form fructose-1,6-diphosphate. Fructose-1,6-diphosphate is then split to form two triose phosphates, D-glyceraldehyde-3-phosphate and dihydroxyacetone phosphate. The latter compound is eventually all converted to the glyceraldehyde form, which then first forms D-1,3 diphosphoglyceric acid and finally 3-phosphoglyceric acid. 3-phosphoglyceric acid is then transformed to pyruvic acid through 2-phosphoglyceric acid and enol phosphopyruvic acid. Under anerobic conditions, pyruvic acid is converted to lactic acid. This, in turn, is reconverted to pyruvate when sufficient oxygen is supplied. For each of these steps a specific enzyme is required as well as a

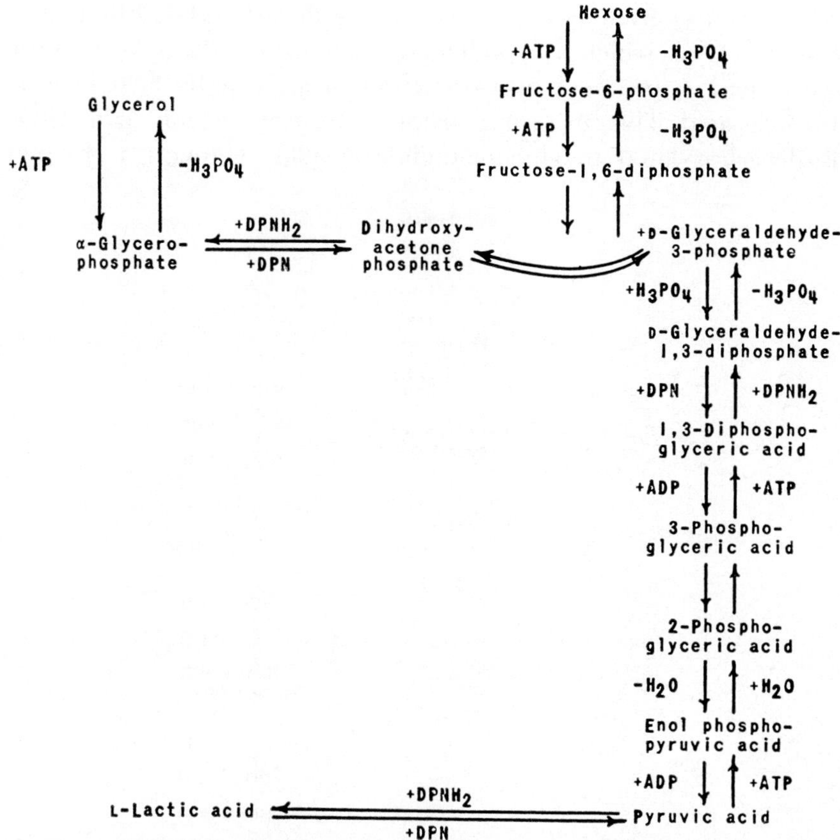

FIGURE 28. Meyerhof-Embden-Parns scheme of glycolysis. (Sourkes, T. L., in Bourne, G. H., and Kidder, G. W.: Biochemistry and Physiology of Nutrition. Vol. 1. New York, Academic Press, Inc., 1953.)

number of co-factors, such as Mg^{++} and K^+. In terms of energy, 2 moles of ATP are utilized in these reactions and 8 are produced, for a net gain of 6 moles of ATP.

Aerobic Metabolism[3]

The aerobic metabolism of carbohydrate is essentially the energy-producing phase of carbohydrate oxidation. Compared to the anaerobic phase, 30 moles or 5 times the amount of ATP are produced. During the course of these events, the pyruvate produced as a result of the anaerobic process is oxidized to CO_2 and H_2O through a cyclical sequence of reactions that is called the "Krebs" or "Tricarboxylic Acid" or "Citric Acid" cycle. (Fig. 29) Briefly, the reactions are: Pyruvic acid is oxidatively decarboxylated to an acetate fraction, which is condensed with oxalacetic acid to form citric acid. Citric acid proceeds through *cis*-aconitic acid to form isocitric acid. This, in turn, is oxidized to oxalosuccinic acid which is decarboxylated to alpha-ketoglutaric acid. Through a complex

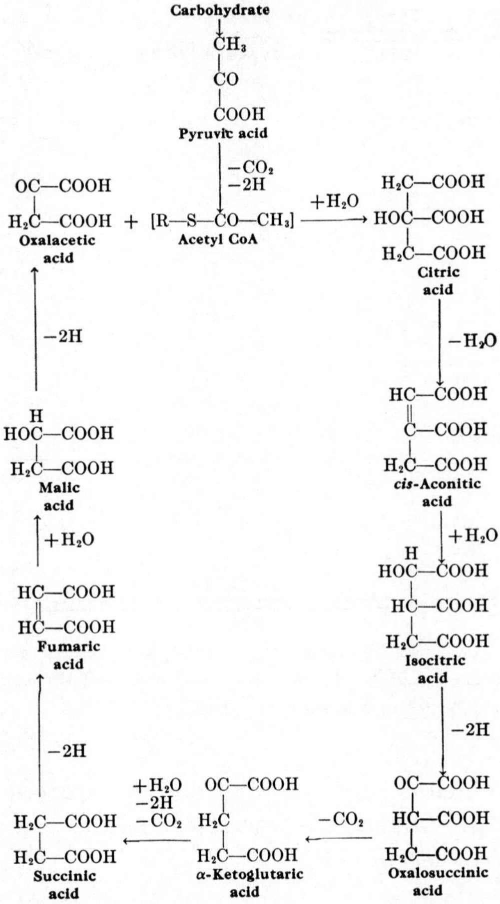

Carbohydrate

CH_3–CO–COOH
Pyruvic acid

$-CO_2$, $-2H$

OC—COOH / H_2C—COOH (Oxalacetic acid) + [R—S—CO—CH_3] (Acetyl CoA) $\xrightarrow{+H_2O}$ H_2C—COOH / HOC—COOH / H_2C—COOH (Citric acid)

$-H_2O$

HC—COOH / C—COOH / H_2C—COOH (*cis*-Aconitic acid)

$+H_2O$

H / HOC—COOH / HC—COOH / H_2C—COOH (Isocitric acid)

$-2H$

OC—COOH / HC—COOH / H_2C—COOH (Oxalosuccinic acid)

$-CO_2$

OC—COOH / H_2C / H_2C—COOH (α-Ketoglutaric acid)

$+H_2O$, $-2H$, $-CO_2$

H_2C—COOH / H_2C—COOH (Succinic acid)

$-2H$

HC—COOH / HC—COOH (Fumaric acid)

$+H_2O$

H / HOC—COOH / H_2C—COOH (Malic acid)

$-2H$

(to Oxalacetic acid)

FIGURE 29. Aerobic carbohydrate metabolism. (Krebs or tricarboxylic acid or citric acid cycle.) (Hawk, P. B., Oser, B. L., and Summerson, W. H.: Practical Physiological Chemistry, 13th ed. The Blakiston Co., Inc., N. Y.)

subpathway, alpha-ketoglutaric acid is decarboxylated to form succinic acid which is then oxidized to fumaric acid. With the addition of H_2O, fumaric acid forms malic acid which is then dehydrogenated to again form oxalacetic acid. This is again available for condensation with an acetate fraction to start the cycle again. A number of co-factors are necessary for these reactions. In addition to the specific enzymes, thiamine, phosphate, Mg^{++} and diphosphopyridine nucleotide are among the necessary factors. The over-all reaction of 1 mole of glucose produces 6 moles of H_2O, 6 moles of CO_2 and 38 high energy bonds or about 456,000 calories. Since glucose can potentially produce 686,000 cal./mole, the body has an efficiency of about 67 per cent in this conversion of nutrients to energy, a considerably greater efficiency than is found in any other energy conversion system.

Alternate Pathways

While the sequence of events discussed thus far depicts the major pathways of carbohydrate metabolism, a number of alternate reactions have been found. For example, glucose can be converted to glycogen for storage, to fatty acids or to amino acids. Glucose and similar sugars are integral parts of a number of structural and biologically active molecules, such as mucopolysaccharides, riboflavin and nucleic acids. It is obvious that the importance of carbohydrate cannot be overestimated, nor can its key place in nutrition be ignored.

LIPID METABOLISM

The major function of the lipids in metabolism is as a source of fuel. Not only do they supply more than twice the amount of energy per unit weight than do the carbohydrates, but they also can be stored easily and are labile enough to be available quickly when needed. Nevertheless, carbohydrate, not fat, is the preferred energy source. For this reason, lipid must be metabolically converted to a form which can enter some steps in the carbohydrate metabolic cycle before it can fulfill its function. A serious complication in a discussion of the lipids is the multiplicity of chemical forms which comprise the lipid class. Compounds as diverse as the steroids, waxes and fats are all members of this group. The lipids are by far the most heterogeneous and least understood of all the nutrients.

Among the lipid family, only the fatty acids have a completely "lipid" metabolism. Most of the other members enter into these pathways only as they are incorporated into the fatty molecule. Moreover, the fatty acids are the prime lipid source of energy, and their metabolism offers the clearest example of the interrelationships among the various metabolic pathways. For this reason, the following discussion of lipid metabolism will be concerned with the oxidation of fatty acids to carbon dioxide, water and energy, as well as with the manner in which this pathway is related to carbohydrate metabolism.

Oxidation of Fatty Acid[5,6]

Briefly, the metabolism of fatty acids begins with the splitting of triglyceride molecules, consisting of glycerol and three fatty acid molecules, to their constituent parts. The fatty acids are then oxidized sequentially into a series of 2-carbon acetate fragments. These, under the proper conditions, can condense with oxalacetic acid and enter the "Krebs cycle" in the same manner as did the 2-carbon fragments from pyruvate. In this way, the body can utilize its lipids for energy.

The rate at which the "Krebs cycle" can accept and oxidize the 2-carbon fragments from fatty acids is dependent primarily on the amount of carbohydrate fragments entering the cycle. In abnormal conditions such as diabetes, carbohydrate is not well utilized. The 2-carbon fragments derived from fatty acids begin to accumulate and, in fact, condense to form 4-carbon acetoacetate fragments. Some of these are converted to β-hydroxy butyric acid and acetone. These three compounds are known as ketone bodies and are responsible, in part, for the acidosis found in diabetes.

It is in this way, therefore, that the fats are related to the carbohydrates. It is easily seen that a defect in one pathway may affect the other.

PROTEIN METABOLISM

Of all the nutrients, the metabolism of the proteins is by far the most difficult to discuss in the brief space available in this book. Not only are the amino acids, which are the building blocks of protein, metabolically interrelated with fat, carbohydrate and other metabolites, but the whole protein itself forms the structural framework and active machinery of the body. Protein forms the walls and membranes of the cells, as well as many of the regulators of metabolism, the hormones, and the body's catalysts, the enzymes. For each facet of protein function, a different pathway must be considered. For these reasons, no attempt will be made to outline the systems involved. Only the broadest areas will be discussed.

The Dynamic State of Proteins and the Metabolic Pool[9]

As with the other nutrients, body protein is constantly being broken down to its constituent amino acids. These amino acids then enter into a "metabolic pool" where they are joined by amino acids derived from the proteins of the diet. Some amino acids of this mixed pool of amino acids are catabolized to urea and excreted. Others are converted to carbohydrate intermediates and oxidized via the Krebs cycle to CO_2 and H_2O (the glucogenic amino acids). Still others are metabolized to lipid intermediates and are metabolized through fat pathways (ketogenic amino acids). Protein synthesis also draws upon this pool for its necessary amino acids. It is obvious that the constant turnover of protein and its multiplicity of uses makes protein metabolism an area that is sensitive to deficiency. The current status of world protein malnutrition substantiates this.

Amino Acids[7]

The variety of amino acids which make up the protein molecule have many different structures. They are all related by the fact that they are alpha amino acids, i.e., they have the group, —$CH(NH_2)COOH$, as part of their structure. The variation in structure allows for many different pathways. Alanine, aspartic acid and glutamic acid are glucogenic, while leucine and tyrosine are ketogenic. Methionine is a high energy compound that transfers its energy through the methyl group. Tyrosine forms adrenaline, melanin (the pigment of the body) and thyroxine. Many more examples could be given to emphasize the importance of these substances.

There are, however, certain reactions that are common to most amino acid pathways. These are: deamination, the removal of the alpha amino group; transamination, the transfer of the alpha amino group from an amino acid to another compound, usually a keto acid; and decarboxylation, the removal of CO_2 from the compound. Most of the amino acids undergo one or more of these reactions at some point in their metabolism.

Protein Synthesis[1]

The synthesis of proteins is a little understood phenomenon. There are almost as many hypotheses available as there are workers in the field. One theory is that small amino acid chains (peptides) are synthesized simultaneously. These are joined into larger polypeptide chains which, in turn, are twisted and coupled to form the final macromolecule. In any case, it is known that all of the necessary amino acids must be supplied at the same time to the proper catalytic surfaces. The essential amino acids must all be present together in the diet for synthesis to function effectively. When this is not done, a protein deficiency can be developed. It is apparent that not only is the total quantity of protein supplied important, but the amino acid pattern of that protein must be considered. It is the function of nutrition, therefore, to determine these facts based upon a consideration of the total metabolism of the organism. Both quantitative and qualitative details must be evaluated before a full understanding of this basic area of life can be reached.

METABOLIC INTERRELATIONSHIPS OF CARBOHYDRATES, PROTEINS AND FATS

In our preceding discussions of the intermediary metabolism of the three basic nutrients, many points of similarity between the three

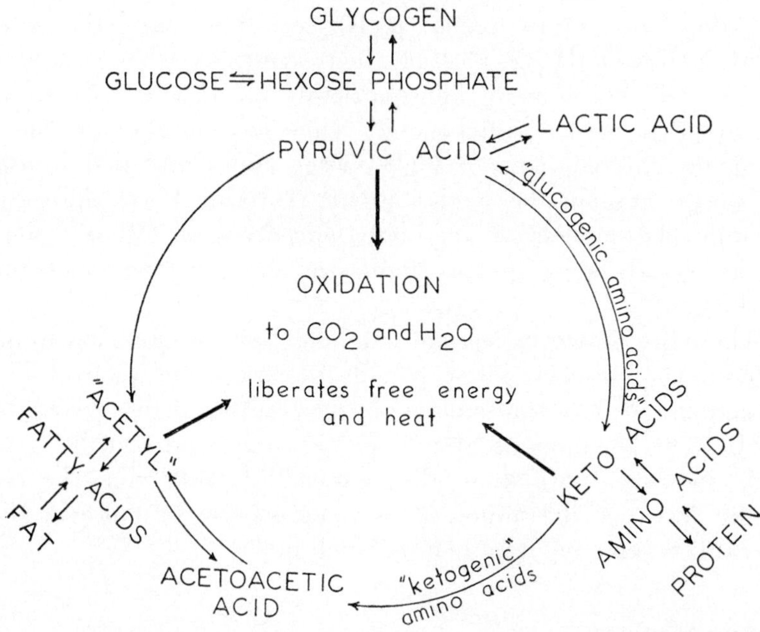

FIGURE 30. Diagram to illustrate possible interconversions among the three classes of foodstuffs. Most of the interconversions take place in the liver, while the oxidations are presumed to occur in all tissues. (Adapted from Long, in Duncan, G. G., "Diseases of Metabolism." 2nd ed. W. B. Saunders Co., 1947.)

systems should have become evident. It seems proper that this should be true. In order for the organism to survive the vagaries of an ever-changing environment, some mechanism should be available which would allow the organism to adapt to and survive the stresses of life. The presence of interrelationships among the various nutrients is such a mechanism. With these systems the organism can at least partially correct for deficiencies in one or more metabolites and, in this way, weather the almost continual attacks upon its biological integrity. The following remarks will attempt to consider these interactions and to indicate their role in the maintenance of life.

The Interplay of Carbohydrates with Proteins and Fats

Since the ultimate metabolic fate of many nutrients is metabolism through the Krebs cycle, the carbohydrates, which play a key role in maintaining this cycle, occupy a central place in the over-all plan of metabolic events. Pyruvate, a product of anaerobic carbohydrate metabolism, is the important point in these relationships. This compound can be carboxylated to oxalacetic acid which, it may be recalled, is an important component of the Krebs cycle. On the other hand, it can be decarboxylated to 2-carbon acetate fragments which, in addition to entering the Krebs cycle, can also be used to synthesize fatty acids and thus contribute to fat synthesis. Furthermore, it is possible for pyruvate to be metabolized to amino acids such as alanine and enter into protein metabolism.

While the 2-carbon fragments derived from fatty acids cannot be used directly for the synthesis of carbohydrate, the glycerol moiety of fats can enter directly into carbohydrate pathways. While this is generally not an important source of carbohydrate, it does represent an available pathway in time of need.

Certain of the amino acids can directly enter carbohydrate systems. Alanine, as has been indicated, is convertible with pyruvate. Through the Krebs cycle, glutamic and aspartic acids can eventually be converted to carbohydrate. These events are not of major importance under ordinary conditions but may play an important part when carbohydrate is deficient.

The Interplay of Fats with Carbohydrates and Proteins

The fats do not contribute any significant amounts of material for carbohydrate or protein synthesis. There are, of course, some indirect relationships through glycerol to trioses and through the Krebs cycle to alpha keto acids and then to glutamate or aspartate. On the other hand, both protein and carbohydrate can enter easily into fat pathways.

Carbohydrates can be used for fat synthesis in three ways. Cerebrosides and similar compounds have carbohydrate molecules as integral parts of their structure. Glycerol is easily formed from the triose fragments of carbohydrate metabolism. The major influence of carbohydrates on fats is, however, through 2-carbon fragments. Through the decarboxylation of pyruvate to acetate, fatty acid structures can be formed. This is the general case under conditions of caloric oversupply and represents the pathway of fat accumulation in these circumstances. It is in this way that excess carbohydrate is converted to fat and deposited, leading to obesity.

The amino acids can contribute to fat synthesis in two ways. First, components of phospholipids such as choline and ethanolamine are derived from amino acids. Secondly, amino acids such as tyrosine and phenylalanine can form 2-carbon fragments and thus enter lipid pathways. For many of these pathways, mechanisms are obscure. It is obvious, however, that the presence or oversupply of fats can markedly alter the activities of both proteins and carbohydrates.

The Interplay of Proteins with Carbohydrates and Fats

The important position of the proteins in metabolic events has been emphasized many times thus far. As enzymes and hormones the proteins are catalysts and regulators of all metabolism. There are, however, a number of specific actions of the proteins and their components which should be mentioned.

The relationship of certain of the amino acids to carbohydrate through pyruvate and the alpha keto acids has been discussed earlier. It is also interesting to note that the alpha keto acids are, in addition to their role as carbohydrate precursors, important stimulators of Kreb cycle activity. For example, it is known that the feeding of these materials with fats can reduce ketogenesis to approximately the same degree as does carbohydrate. It is obvious, therefore, that these intermediates are important in the conversion of food materials to energy.

Carbohydrate has a number of specific actions on protein metabolism. Sugars are apparently more efficient in sparing protein than are fats. The decrease in nitrogen excretion seen upon feeding fats or carbohydrates to caloric-deficient animals is an example of this specific effect of sugars. Certain carbohydrates are known to facilitate protein absorption and utilization. The mechanism of the events is unknown.

The implication of these metabolic interactions among the various nutrients is not only of academic interest, since dietary formulations must be based on a careful consideration of this point. In addition, many of the symptoms of certain pathologies can be interpreted with this knowledge. As with all else in metabolism, each is dependent on the other. Consideration of all aspects of metabolic activity is a necessary prerequisite for a clear understanding of life.

REFERENCES

1. Borsook, H., and Deasy, C. L.: The Biosynthesis of Protein; in Bourne, G. H., and Kidder, G. W., ed.: Biochemistry and Physiology of Nutrition, Vol. 1. New York, Academic Press, Inc., 1953.
2. Dickens, F.: Anaerobic glycolysis, respiration and the Pasteur effect. Enzymes, *2* (Part 1):624, 1951.
3. Krebs, H.: The intermediary stages in the biological oxidation of carbohydrates. Ad. in Enzymology, *3:*191, 1943.
4. Lipmann, F.: Metabolic generation and utilization of phosphate bond energy. Ad. in Enzymology, *1:*99, 1941.
5. Mackay, E. M., Barnes, R. H., Carne, H. O., and Wick, A. N.: Ketogenic activity of acetic acid. J. Biol. Chem., *135:*157, 1940.
6. Mackay, E. M.: Significance of ketosis. J. Clin. Endocrin., *3:*101, 1943.
7. Meister, A.: Amino Acids; in Bourne, G. H., and Kidder, G. W., ed.: Biochemistry and Physiology of Nutrition. Vol 1. New York, Academic Press, Inc., 1953.
8. Nord, F. F., and Weiss, S.: Yeast and mold fermentation. Enzymes, *2* (Part 1):684, 1951.
9. Rittenberg, D., and Shemin, D.: The metabolism of proteins and amino acids. Ann. Rev. Biochem., *15:*247, 1946.

Chapter VI

Principal Minerals, Water and Electrolytes (Na, Cl and K)

Mineral Composition of the Body

Hydrogen and oxygen, combined in the form of water, constitute two-thirds of the body weight. Nitrogen and carbon are two other elements that form a large percentage of body tissues.

Although the remaining mineral elements in the body contribute only about 2 or 3 per cent to the total body weight, they are indispensable for maintaining the health and well-being of the individual. There are 7 principal minerals, namely, calcium, phosphorus, magnesium, sodium, potassium, chlorine and sulfur. In addition, there are 6 essential elements which, at very low concentrations, affect normal growth, development and reproduction of living organisms. These are the so-called "trace" elements; they will be discussed in greater detail in the chapter that follows.

The approximate percentage of each of the seventeen essential elements as found in the human body is listed in Table 11.

Functions of the Mineral Elements

The principal minerals have several functions, a primary one being to impart rigidity and strength to bones and teeth.

Other important functions, such as those associated with the permeability of cell membranes, the elasticity of muscle and the

TABLE 11. APPROXIMATE ELEMENTARY COMPOSITION OF THE BODY

Element	*Percentage*
Oxygen	65.
Carbon	18.
Hydrogen	10.
Nitrogen	3.
Calcium	2.[a]
Phosphorus	1.1[b]
Potassium	0.35
Sulfur	0.25
Sodium	0.15
Chlorine	0.15
Magnesium	0.05
Iron	0.004
Manganese	0.00013
Copper	0.00015
Iodine	0.00004
Cobalt	[c]
Zinc	[c]
Others of more doubtful status	

[a] Estimates vary widely.
[b] Percentage varies with that of calcium.
[c] Believed to be essential, but quantitative data are not yet at hand.
(From Sherman and Lanford: Essentials of Nutrition. By permission of The Macmillan Co., Publishers.)

irritability of nerves, are dependent upon a delicate electrolytic balance of such ions as calcium, sodium, potassium, etc.

Effect of Mineral Deficiency on Growth and Development

When mineral intake is below the required level, growth and development cease.[2] Rats that are fed a diet completely adequate in all nutrients except minerals will be stunted in growth. When this mineral-deficient diet is enriched with a complete salt mixture, the growth process is resumed.

Effect of General Mineral Deficiency on Teeth

Tooth Formation. Arnim et al.[1] have demonstrated in rats that during periods of stress brought on by a general mineral deficiency, labile alveolar bone, in preference to the growing tooth, suffers the loss of minerals. If the deficiency is a low grade chronic type, the amount of dentin of the growing tooth is decreased and the predentin becomes wider than normal. However, neither the enamel nor the completely matured tooth is affected by any systemic mineral deficiency.

Dental Caries Incidence. Much research on the effects of minerals on dental caries incidence has dealt with single elements or compounds. Ordinarily, these elements occur as mixtures of organic and inorganic compounds in water, food and condiments of the diet. Therefore, it appeared to Nizel and Harris[8] that it would be more pertinent and practical to determine whether alterations in

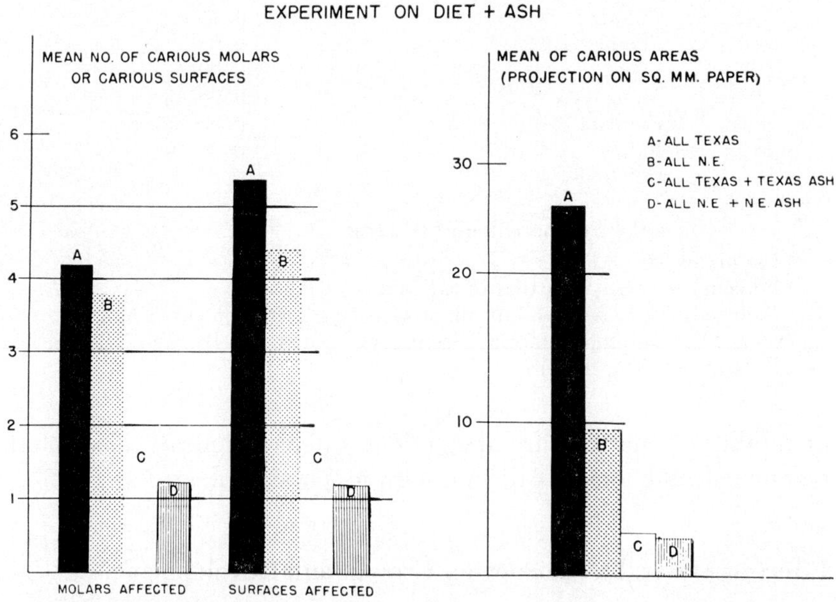

EXPERIMENT ON DIET + ASH

MEAN NO. OF CARIOUS MOLARS OR CARIOUS SURFACES

MEAN OF CARIOUS AREAS (PROJECTION ON SQ. MM. PAPER)

A- ALL TEXAS
B- ALL N.E.
C- ALL TEXAS + TEXAS ASH
D- ALL N.E. + N.E. ASH

MOLARS AFFECTED SURFACES AFFECTED

FIGURE 31. A bar graph depicting the comparative caries experience of hamsters fed a cariogenic diet and a cariogenic diet with ash supplement during pre- and postweaning periods.

the natural presence and ratios of all the mineral elements in foods had an effect on dental caries incidence. This approach was made by studying the effects of the ash of foodstuffs in an otherwise cariogenic diet fed to Syrian hamsters.

In 1952 Nizel[6] reported that the ash of foodstuffs used as a supplement in a cariogenic diet decreased its cariogenicity (Fig. 31). However, when identical natural ash supplements were introduced into the diet of hamsters, in one group at eight days of age, and in another group at twenty-one days of age, the caries score was found to be significantly lower in the group fed at an earlier age. Confirmation of the marked caries inhibitory effect of ash supplements when fed to hamsters during the development and calcification of their molars was obtained in a subsequent experiment.[7]

Other investigators,[10] using the Norway rat as an experimental animal, substituted the ash from a protective natural diet for the reagents in a purified diet and fed a dam and her four succeeding litters this mineral-rich experimental diet during various periods of tooth development. The group fed the natural ash supplement had a significantly lower caries incidence.

Shaw[9] demonstrated that a purified diet supplemented with a 3 to 5 per cent more soluble reagent salt mixture than the usual 2 per cent reagent salt mixture had no effect on the incidence of caries in fully erupted rat molars. However, both McClure et al.[5] and Constant et al.[3] were successful in reducing caries with synthetic salt mixtures. McClure found that the caries score in animals fed a supplement of 4 per cent Osborne-Mendel salts was 67.9 per cent lower than that of an unsupplemented control group. Constant et al.[4] found that basic inorganic salt (oxides) could reduce dental caries in cotton rats, but that acidic inorganic, basic organic, and acidic organic salt mixtures were ineffective.

REFERENCES

1. Arnim, S. S., Clarke, M. F., Anderson, B. G., and Smith, A. H.: Dental changes in rats consuming diet poor in inorganic salts. Yale J. Biol. & Med., *9*:117, 1936.
2. Clarke, M. F., Bassin, A. L., and Smith, A. H.: Skeletal changes in the rat induced by a ration extremely poor in inorganic salts. Am. J. Physiol., *11*:556, 1936.
3. Constant, M. A., Sievert, H. W., Phillips, P. H., and Elvehjem, C. A.: Dental caries in the cotton rat. XIV. Further studies of caries production with special reference to the role of minerals, fat and the stage of refinement of cereals. J. Nut., *53*:17, 1954.
4. Constant, M. A., Sievert, H. W., Phillips, P. H., and Elvehjem, C. A.: Dental caries in the cotton rat. XV. The effect of tooth maturity and minerals on caries production by semi-synthetic diets. J. Nut., *53*:29, 1954.
5. McClure, F. J., Folk, J. E., and Rust, J. D.: Smooth surface caries in white rats; effects of fluoride, iodoacetate, penicillin, Crisco, butterfat, and a salt mixture. J.A.D.A., *53*:1, 1956.
6. Nizel, A. E.: The cariogenic properties of similar foodstuffs grown in high and low caries areas: the influence of trace elements. Thesis, Tufts Univ. School of Dent. Med., May, 1952.
7. Nizel, A. E., and Harris, R. S.: Cariostatic effects of ashed foodstuffs fed in the diet of hamsters. J. D. Res., *32*:672, 1953. Abstract.

8. Nizel, A. E., and Harris, R. S.: Effects of ashed foodstuffs on dental decay in hamsters. J. D. Res., *34*:513, 1955.
9. Shaw, J. H.: Ineffectiveness of certain essential nutrients in prevention of tooth decay in cotton rat molars. Proc. Soc. Exper. Biol. & Med., *70*:479, 1949.
10. Sognnaes, R. F., and Shaw, J. H.: Experimental rat caries. IV. Effect of a natural salt mixture on the caries conduciveness of an otherwise purified diet. J. Nut., *53*:195, 1954.

CALCIUM

Chemistry

The principal mineral element in the body is calcium. Over 99 per cent is found in bones and teeth, while the remainder is distributed in the soft tissues and body fluids.

The skeleton of a 70 kg. man contains about 1200 grams of calcium. In the serum, calcium is found in ionized and un-ionized forms. Sixty to 70 per cent of this calcium is ionized and diffusible, while the remaining 30 to 40 per cent is nondiffusible and unionized, occurring principally as calcium proteinate. Both these types of calcium together usually amount to 9 to 11.5 mg. per 100 ml. of blood serum. The primary bone salt is probably a tricalcium phosphate derivative, $3Ca_3(PO_4)_2.Ca(OH)_2$, or hydroxyapatite containing an excess of phosphate on its surface. Because the surface area of bone is large and because the opportunity for physical adsorption on the surface is great, many salts and ions have been found associated with this molecule, e.g., magnesium carbonate and citrate, and chloride and fluoride ions.

Teeth resemble bone chemically, for the mineral portion of each has an apatite structure. Actually, the enamel consists of a matrix of keratin and mucopolysaccharide impregnated with a hydroxyapatite, $Ca_{10}(PO_4)_6.(OH)_2$. The chemical structure of dentin resembles that of bone more closely than does enamel, consisting, for the most part, of collagen and chondroitin sulfuric acid but with a smaller amount of inorganic hydroxyapatite.

Physiology

Function. The main function of calcium is to contribute to the rigidity and strength of bones and teeth.

Cell permeability, particularly of the capillary vessels, is dependent on calcium. The intercellular cement substance is a calcium proteinate and its integrity, which affects tissue permeability, depends on the presence of the calcium ion.

Normal muscular contraction, as well as voluntary and autonomic nerve transmission, also depends on the level of the serum calcium. If it falls considerably below a critical level, there is an increase in nerve and muscle irritability; very low serum values may be accompanied by tetanic convulsions. However, this is not a simple relationship; other ions are involved.

Calcium has been shown to activate many enzymes. It also plays a role in the blood-clotting mechanism. Calcium is required along with prothrombin and thromboplastin to form thrombin, which then can transform fibrinogen to fibrin. Therefore, prolonged clotting time could conceivably be attributed to an insufficiency of available calcium.

Metabolism. The amount of serum calcium depends not only on the availability and proper utilization of dietary calcium but also on the extent of the calcification and decalcification process of bone. The total serum calcium is about 10 mg. per 100 ml. Seventy per cent is derived by simple solution from the intercrystalline soluble material of bone. As the level of calcium diminishes through chemical and physical factors, more is dissolved out of the bone into the surrounding fluid and blood. The remaining 30 per cent is derived from the less soluble crystalline hydroxyapatite. According to McLean, the calcium from the hydroxyapatite crystals is released by the action of the parathyroid hormone through a "feedback mechanism" (Fig. 32).

Absorption. Only 20 to 30 per cent of the ingested calcium is usually absorbed by man. However, many factors influence this amount. For example, children suffering from a calcium deficiency show a greater percentage of absorption.

Calcium is present in both organic and inorganic form in food. The organic form is first converted to the inorganic form in the gastrointestinal tract before it is absorbed. The calcium in milk, milk products and eggs is better absorbed than that in vegetables and meats.

There are several factors which influence the rate of absorption of calcium into the blood stream from the duodenum. Some of these are (a) the calcium, phosphorus and vitamin D levels of the diet and the ratio of these factors to each other, (b) gastric and intestinal acidity, and (c) other food factors such as the presence of fats, minerals, oxalates, phytates, lactose and protein. It should also be noted that parathyroid secretion affects the mobilization of calcium from bone.

The calcium:phosphorus ratio considered optimum for absorption and utilization during periods of growth is between 1:1 and 2:1; this is the approximate Ca:P ratio of cow and human milk,

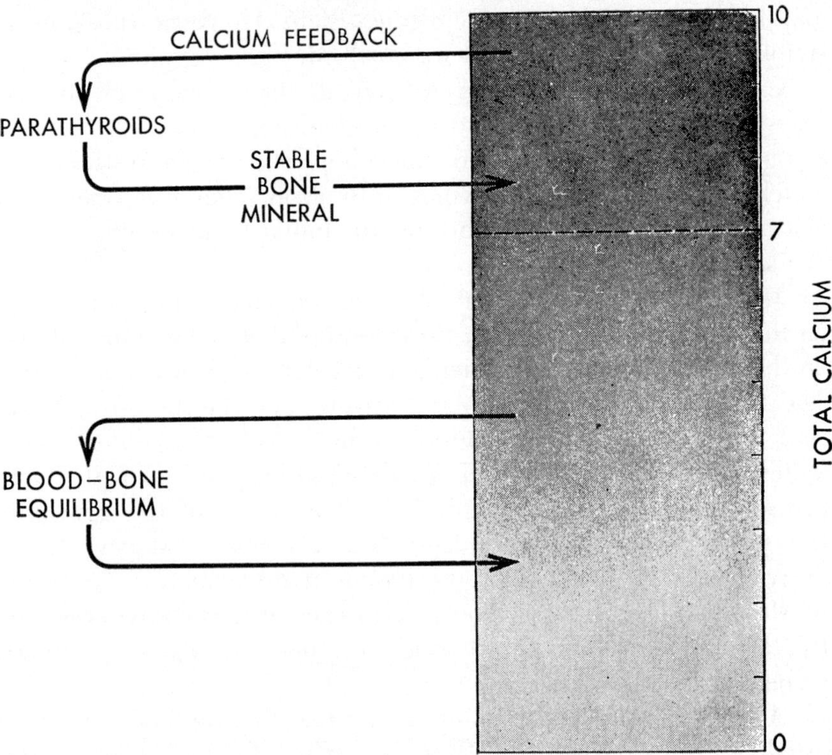

FIGURE 32. Diagram of feedback mechanism regulating the level of calcium in the blood. The normal concentration of calcium in the blood plasma is about 10 mg. per 100 ml. Seven milligrams of this is supplied by the more soluble fraction of bone mineral between the hydroxyapatite crystals. The parathormone promotes the release of calcium from the hydroxyapatite crystals, the stable crystalline reserve, and also from the intercrystalline substance when the calcium level falls below 7 mg. (From McLean, F. C.: Scient. Am. *192*:84, 1955.)

respectively. The interdependence of these mineral nutrients is such that a deficiency or an excess of one will create a similar condition with respect to the other. Milk and milk products, as well as green leafy vegetables, contain these optimal Ca:P ratios and, therefore, should be recommended in preference to calcium pills.

Proper gastric acidity is necessary for the conversion of insoluble basic calcium salts to the chloride and acid phosphates, in which forms calcium is better absorbed. The hydrochloric acid of the stomach dissociates calcium from insoluble compounds such as calcium carbonate. Therefore, sufficient quantities of this acid are needed to ensure this dissociation process. Improved calcium absorption may also result from feeding lactose, probably owing to its stimulation of lactic acid fermentation with increased acidity in the intestinal tract.

Insoluble calcium compounds are formed when excess oxalic acid, phytic acid and fats are ingested. Calcium combines readily with free oxalic acid that is present in spinach, rhubarb and pineapple to form the insoluble and unavailable calcium oxalate. The bran of wheat, which is the outer layer of the wheat seed and is included in the ordinary bran cereals and bread products, contains phytic acid, the hexaphosphoric acid ester of inositol. Calcium combines with phytic acid to form the insoluble calcium phytate compound. If the intake of fat is excessive, an insoluble fatty acid calcium complex is formed. In steatorrhea, celiac disease and sprue, where fat metabolism is abnormal, excretion of insoluble calcium soaps commonly occurs. The role of these various factors in the absorption, utilization and excretion of calcium is diagrammatically illustrated in Figure 33.

Requirement. The recommended allowance for the average adult in the United States has been set by the Food and Nutrition Board[12] at 0.8 gram per day. This allowance is based on balance studies in adults in the United States. However, Hegsted et al.[19] have shown that most of the world population living on intakes of less than 0.5 gram per day do not show signs of calcium deficiency. According to these authors, the true minimum requirement is 0.2 to 0.3 gram per day, and the body can adjust to this level without showing any pathology. However, gradual reduction over long periods of time is required to insure proper adaptation of the organism. If there is an abrupt change from a high to a low calcium diet, a negative calcium balance will result. Ohlson[34] concluded that we do not have a definitive test for good calcium nutrition because people are different. The calcium allowance is just a guide and should be construed only as the "level of nutrient intake appearing desirable for use in planning diets and food supplies"[12] of population groups, not individuals.

The recommended allowance of 0.8 gram should be increased during periods of increased stress, such as spurt growth, pregnancy and lactation. For children, 1.0 to 1.4 grams is recommended; during the latter half of pregnancy and lactation 1.5 to 2 grams is recommended. Since a quart of milk contains 1.2 grams of calcium, at least two cups of milk a day for adults, 4 cups for children and pregnant women and 6 cups for the lactating mother are most desirable. Unfortunately, many Americans do not consume the amount of milk and green leafy vegetables that contain the recommended

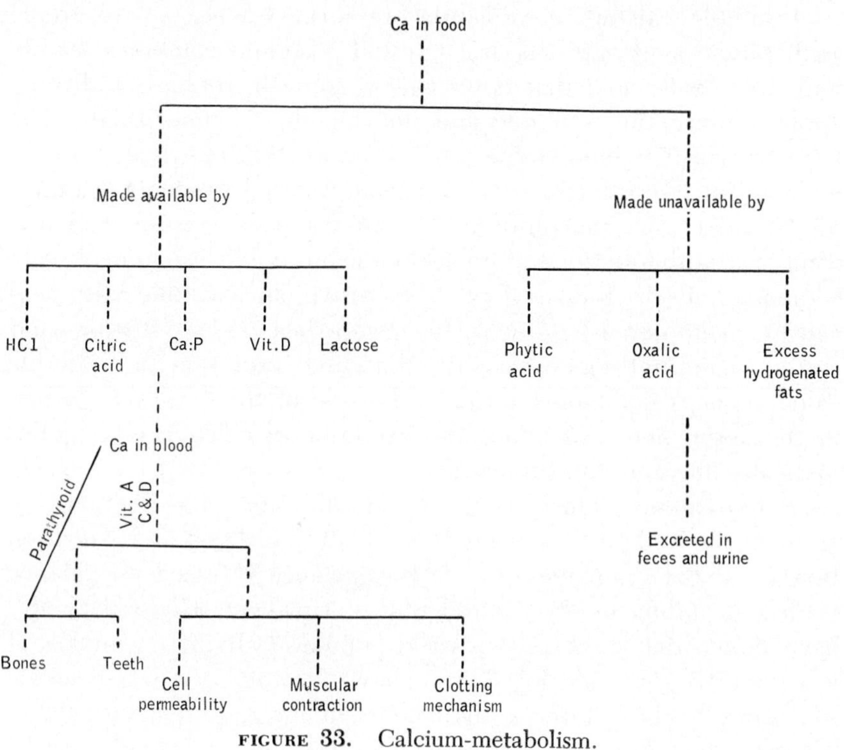

FIGURE 33. Calcium-metabolism.

daily calcium intake. As a result, calcium is one mineral element that is often deficient in the diet, according to the standards of the Food and Nutrition Board of the National Research Council.

General Systemic Pathology of Abnormal Calcium Metabolism

Hypercalcemia. Hypercalcemia and hypercalcuria may be caused directly by excessive activity of the parathyroid glands, or indirectly by a chronic renal disease. Increased parathyroid function may result from a tumor which is usually benign in nature. A secondary hyperparathyroidism may follow chronic renal insufficiency and is actually a compensatory mechanism to counteract the low serum calcium which develops as a result of kidney failure.

Increases in serum calcium are also seen in conditions of osteoporosis, which may result from the aging process, immobilization of bone after injury or paralysis, increased intake of vitamin D through vitamin concentrates, or diffuse neoplastic destruction of bone.

In hypercalcemia, deposits of calcium may be found in such soft tissues as the lungs, kidneys and stomach. There are also several types of abnormal calcifications which occur as amorphous basophilic aggregations of granular precipitate in the interstitial tissues. These may be found in injured or dead tissue, such as blood vessel walls, skin, subcutaneous tissues, tendons and muscles.

Hypocalcemia. Rickets will develop in children, and osteomalacia in adults, when the serum calcium is decreased so that the product of calcium $\times$ phosphorus is less than 30. (The normal level of serum calcium is approximately 10 mg. per milliliter and that of serum phosphorus is 3 mg. per milliliter of blood.) Further description of both of these classic nutritional deficiencies will be found in the chapter on vitamin D.

Tetany, which is physiologic rather than pathologic in nature, is caused by a hypocalcemia. The lowered serum calcium causes an increase in the permeability of the cell membranes and increased myoneural irritability. This results in muscular spasms, particularly in the extremities, trunk and larynx.

Some Bone Tumors and Calcifications Found in the Mouth

Osteitis Fibrosa Cystica (von Recklinghausen's Disease). Very often the first sign of hyperparathyroidism is a tumor of the jaw, malocclusion due to prognathism, alveolar atrophy, and looseness and spreading of the teeth. This may be accompanied by complaints of deep boring pain in the long bones or pelvis. X-rays show diffuse osteoporosis involving the entire skeleton. In the jaws, the alveolar bone has a mottled appearance, the periodontal membrane space is widened, and the lamina dura is missing because of the thinning of the bone trabeculae (Fig. 34). In general, there is excessive osteoblastic and osteoclastic activity accompanied by foci of fibrous proliferation (brown tumors). The teeth may show severe enamel hypoplasia. The blood picture shows an elevated serum calcium, lowered serum phosphorus, and an elevated serum alkaline phosphatase. Urinary excretion of calcium and phosphorus is increased; this may produce renal calculi.

Osteitis Deformans (Paget's Disease). This disease is an acquired disorder of unknown etiology in which there is a replacement of normal bone by osteoid tissue. Actually, this disease produces no alterations in calcium or phosphorus metabolism but, owing to increased osteoblastic activity, laboratory examination of the serum will show a high serum alkaline phosphatase. Clinically, when many bones (polyostotic) are involved, the skull is enlarged

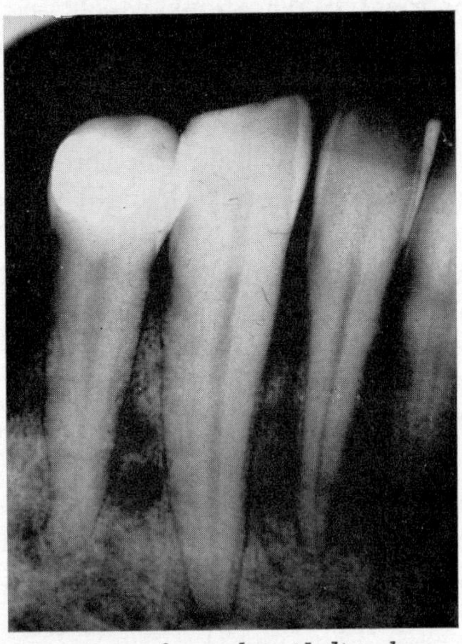

FIGURE 34. X-ray appearance of parathyroid disturbance in teeth. (Courtesy Dr. G. Sklar.)

and the tibia and femur are bowed. As a monostotic disease, in which there is an enlargement and "cotton wool" appearance of the mandible (Fig. 35), a diagnosis differentiating between osteitis deformans and fibrous dysplasia is sometimes difficult.

Myositis Ossificans of the Masseter Muscle. This condition may result from a traumatic injury to the muscle, such as a gunshot wound. The hemorrhage following the injury is organized to form granulation tissue, which becomes fibrous and then calcified. Because it involves a major muscle of mastication, there may be limited opening and, sometimes, complete immobilization of the jaw (Fig. 36).

Sialolithiasis. Salivary calculi result from the calcification of a nidus of food debris, epithelial remnants and bacteria. These calculi

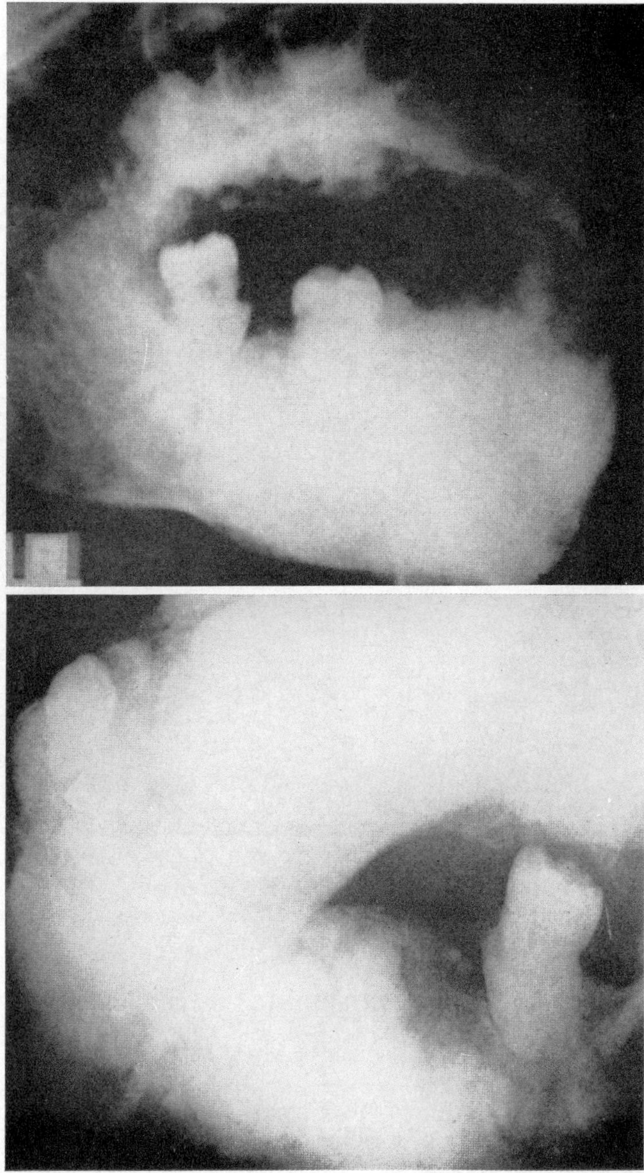

FIGURE 35. Osteitis deformans (Paget's disease) of the mandible. (Bernier: The Management of Oral Disease, C. V. Mosby Co., 1955.)

will produce sialadenitis, which is characterized by swelling, pain and redness of the orifice of the salivary gland. As the disease progresses, the gland enlarges. These salivary stones may sometimes be expressed manually, but more often they must be removed surgically.

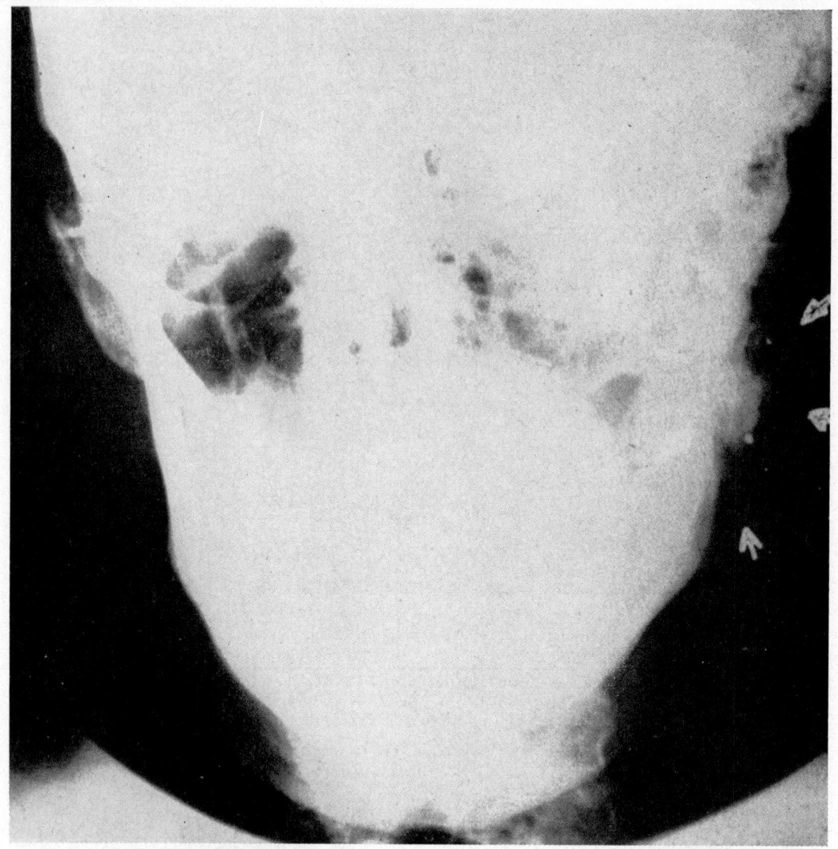

FIGURE 36. Radiograph, showing ossified mass along ramus of right mandible. (X-ray was underexposed to bring out the mass in better detail.) (Nizel, A. E., and Prigge, E. K., in J. of Oral Surgery, Vol. 4, No. 1, Jan. 1946.)

PHOSPHORUS

Chemistry

Occurrence. The foods richest in calcium and protein are the best sources of phosphorus.

About 80 per cent of the total 600 grams of phosphorus found in the body is in the bones and teeth in combination with hydroxyapatite. In muscle and brain tissue, there are about 57 and 5 grams of phosphorus, respectively. In these latter tissues it occurs in organic combination with carbohydrates, fats and proteins, forming such compounds as nucleoprotein, lecithin and cephalin.

Many enzyme systems which are involved in the phosphorylation of glucose, amino acids and fatty acids are activated by phosphates. In addition, the enzymes adenosine diphosphate (ADP) and adenosine triphosphate (ATP) play a vital role in muscle contraction and energy transfer.

Inorganic phosphate is made available for the calcification process by the action of serum alkaline phosphatase. The former is found in blood, bones, ossifying cartilage, kidney and lungs; the latter is found in blood, prostate, liver and kidney.

Physiology

Absorption and Excretion. The absorption and excretion of phosphorus is related to the calcium and vitamin D levels of the diet. If the desired 1:1 ratio between calcium and phosphorus is maintained, 70 per cent of the ingested phosphorus is absorbed. Phosphorus is not absorbed in the form of phytin or as an insoluble salt with Al, Mg, Ca, and Fe.

Requirements. The daily requirement of phosphorus for children and for women during the latter part of pregnancy and lactation, as recommended by the Food and Nutrition Board, is about the same as that for calcium. In adults the recommended phosphorus intake is approximately 1.5 times that for calcium.

General Systemic Pathology of Abnormal Phosphorus Metabolism

Parathyroid disturbances resulting from chronic renal disease may indirectly raise the serum phosphorus level. The anterior pituitary also affects the serum phosphorus level, which is elevated during acromegaly.

As in the case of calcium pathology, rickets and osteomalacia will result if there is disturbance in the Ca:P ratio due to either an excess or a deficiency of phosphorus.

RELATION OF CALCIUM AND PHOSPHORUS LEVELS TO TOOTH FORMATION AND TO DENTAL CARIES

Tooth Formation

It has been demonstrated that fully matured adult enamel and dentin are influenced not at all,[23] and newly erupted maturing tooth components only slightly, by the withdrawal or addition of minerals to the diet. For example, the stress of increased calcium needs during pregnancy[48] does not influence the caries susceptibility of the mother's own teeth, and the aphorism "a tooth for every child" is not valid.

On the other hand, the unerupted developing tooth can be greatly influenced by varying dietary levels of calcium and phosphorus.[15]

According to the calcio-protective law of Erdheim,[11] dentin has a distinct priority over bone for the available calcium. For example,

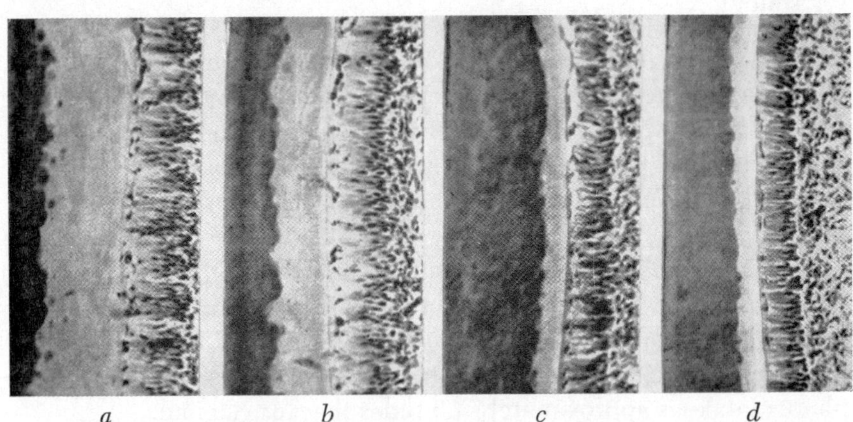

FIGURE 37. Longitudinal sections of the dentine and odontoblasts from the basal end of the upper incisor teeth of four rats. *a*, from the rat getting diet containing 0.08 per cent Ca, 0.16 per cent P; *b*, from the rat getting diet containing 0.12 per cent Ca, 0.24 per cent P; *c*, from the rat getting diet containing 0.20 per cent Ca, 0.4 per cent P; *d*, from the rat getting diet containing 0.30 per cent Ca, 0.6 per cent P. Note the very wide predentine in *a* and the improvement in calcification as the Ca and P contents of the diet were raised; *d* is normal in appearance. (Gaunt, W. E., and Irving, J. T., in Journal of Physiology, Vol. 99, No. 1, 1940.)

when high levels of calcium and phosphorus were fed to one group of rats and lower levels, but at the same ratio to each other, were fed to another group (0.32:0.08 vs. 1.20:0.30), there was no difference in the ash of the incisor teeth but a very significant difference in the bone ash.[15]

With drastic deficiencies of either total mineral intake or of individual elements, such as calcium or phosphorus, the dentin formation is irregular and the predentin width is considerably increased.[14] Normally, the predentin, which is the unmineralized matrix, is 10 to 20 microns in width; in calcium and phosphorus deficiency, it is 90 to 100 microns in width. In Figure 37 are histologic sections showing the comparative effects of varying amounts of minerals on the developing dentin.

Calcium and Dental Caries

A comparative analysis of the calcium contents of carious and noncarious teeth, performed as far back as 1895 by Black[6] and later confirmed by others,[3] indicated no difference between them.

Enamel hypoplasia is a reflection of faulty calcium metabolism. Mellanby[30] proposed the thesis that hypoplastic enamel was caries susceptible, thus implying that faulty calcium metabolism influences caries production. Two other investigations[9,18] have correlated caries incidence and hypoplastic enamel in children with high serum calcium to low serum phosphorus ratios. In calcium balance studies done by Boyd et al.[7] it was demonstrated that the incidence of dental caries was decreased if the absorption, utilization and retention of calcium were optimal.

However, Schour[40] is convinced that the quality of the calcified structure of the tooth is not significantly related to the incidence of caries. He has demonstrated that hypoplasia corresponds to the incremental growth patterns of the tooth and is not associated with pits and fissures, as is caries. According to McKay,[29] mottled enamel was not more susceptible to decay than ordinary enamel even though there were imperfections present which reflected disturbed calcium metabolism. Likewise, Albright et al.[2] have shown that patients with parathyroid tumors who had generalized decalcification showed no evidence of any dental decalcification. In short, in these studies an altered calcium metabolism did not contribute to caries etiology.

Actually, the matter of caries susceptibility in hypoplastic teeth has been best explained by McCall and Krasnow,[25] who suggested that the hypoplasia in the deciduous teeth was different from that in the permanent ones. When the hypoplastic deciduous tooth erupts, it is smooth, lacks density, and is soft and chalky. Because of these physical properties, it is highly susceptible to caries. On the other hand the hypoplastic permanent teeth are pitted and grooved, but the defective enamel has the normal density. Therefore, its physical properties are not sufficiently changed to make it more prone to caries. The factor that makes it susceptible to decay is that there is retention and stagnation of food in the deep pits and grooves of the defective enamel surface.

Calcium and phosphorus medication was in vogue for the treatment of dental caries in the early thirties. However, this practice was short-lived. Malan and Ockerse[24] conducted a 3 year experiment with daily supplements of 0.5 gram of calcium and 0.5 gram of phosphorus in the diet of schoolchildren. There was no significant difference in caries susceptibility in either the deciduous or permanent dentition between those children whose diets were supplemented with calcium and phosphorus and those whose diets were not supplemented. In 1936 the Council on Dental Therapeutics[8] expressed the opinion that calcium and phosphorus medication was unnecessary and there was no evidence that such supplements prevented decay in children or adults or that they promoted the development of noncarious teeth.

Some indirect evidence that calcium intake might have been related to lower than average incidence of caries in schoolchildren was presented by East.[10] He did a survey in 109 cities in the United States and found a positive correlation between increased water hardness, due to calcium carbonate in the city water supplies, and lowered caries incidence.

Phosphorus and Dental Caries

Lennox,[22] in 1930, without benefit of comparative detailed dental examination records of caries experience between control and experimental groups and without consideration of other nutrients in the diet, suggested that phosphorus deficiency in foods and soils was the cause for dental caries in South African natives. At about this time Klein and McCollum[21] and others,[1,26] by means of animal feeding experiments, demonstrated that increased phosphorus intake might be caries inhibitory. Only Shelling and Asher[41] took exception to the phosphorus deficiency–increased caries theory.

In the late thirties and early forties an English investigator, T. W. B. Osborn, conducted a series of very interesting in vitro experiments with inorganic and organic phosphate compounds.[36,37,38] These experiments were motivated by a clinical observation made by himself and Noriskin.[35] They found that Bantus who adhered to their native food habits had a lower caries incidence than those of the same tribe who ate refined European bread. What "protective agent" was absent in this refined bread? To answer this question, Osborn used W. D. Miller's technique of measuring decalcification when a tooth was incubated in saliva and bread. The rate of decalcification of the group of teeth that were immersed and incubated in a refined carbohydrate-saliva mixture was greater than that of another group of teeth that were immersed and incubated in a crude carbohydrate-saliva mixture. This result was explained by the hypothesis that calcium and phosphate ions, released on incubation, somehow interfered with the decalcification. Originally, inorganic phosphates were found to be less effective than organic phosphates in reducing in vitro decalcification, but later the experimenters were able to show that inorganic phosphates were effective in the presence of organic calcium compounds. The final conclusion was that the protective mechanism was not the liberation of the phosphorus, as was originally suggested, but rather the release of calcium ions from organic compounds.

More recently, Jenkins et al.,[20] using better chemically controlled procedures, confirmed Osborn's findings. By using powdered calcium phosphate rather than teeth, they eliminated the extreme variations in solubility that occur among different teeth and even in different portions of the same tooth. The amount of calcium dissolved out of the saliva-incubated mixture in the presence of brown flour was only about two-thirds of that dissolved in the presence of white flour. This difference was explained by the fact that organic phosphates, including phytate, were the active substance in the brown, unrefined flour that reduced the solubility of calcium phosphate. The investigators suggested, furthermore, that the phytate attached itself to the tooth and acted either as a protective coating or formed a less soluble complex.

During the last ten years several laboratories have investigated the relation of inorganic phosphate compounds to dental caries incidence. In 1948 Sobel and Hanok[43] proposed the hypothesis that there is "a relationship between the inorganic composition of teeth and the fluid from which the tooth salts precipitate and that the composition of this fluid, in turn, is related to the blood serum." Sobel[42] later reported that a high ratio of calcium to phosphorus in the diet produced a correspondingly high carbonate to phosphate ratio in the teeth which made them more caries susceptible. Conversely, if the calcium and phosphorus components of the diet were so manipulated that a low carbonate to phosphate ratio was obtained, the experimental animals on this diet had comparatively little decay. More recently, Sobel and Hanok[44] have postulated that hereditary, as well as environmental, differences in the "local factor(s)" of calcification influence caries susceptibility.

By varying the dietary phosphate so that the Ca:P ratio decreased from 1:0.5 to 1:1 to 1:2, Wynn et al.[47] showed that there was a corresponding decrease in the cariogenicity of high sucrose diets. However, unlike Sobel, they found that the calcium and phosphorus contents of the carious and noncarious enamel and dentin of the teeth were the same and were independent of a high or low Ca:P ratio in the diet. More recently they[16] have concluded from further experiments that the reduction in cariogenicity in their sucrose diets was due to the actual calcium and phosphorus content of the diet, not to the Ca:P ratio.

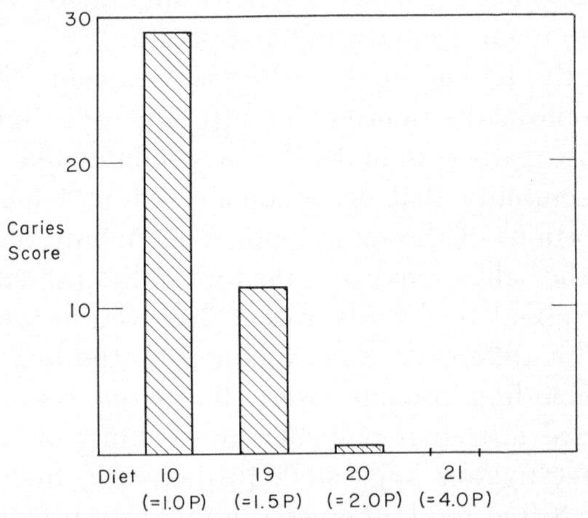

FIGURE 38. Bar graph showing differences in caries scores in groups of hamsters fed varying levels of a metaphosphoric acid supplement. 1.0 P is the control group; 1.5 P, 2.0 P, and 4.0 P groups were fed one and a half, twice and four times, respectively, more phosphates than the control group.

Stralfors[46] postulated that the addition of calcium or phosphate to the dental plaque decreased the local carious process after he demonstrated that 5 per cent $Ca_3(PO_4)_2$ or 1 per cent $CaHPO_4$ or 5 per cent Na_3PO_4 could reduce caries significantly in hamsters. Others like McClure et al.[27,28] have shown that 2 per cent disodium orthophosphate is invariably an effective cariostatic supplement in otherwise cariogenic diets. On the other hand, $CaHPO_4$ as a supplement is able to inhibit caries in only very particular situations.[4,28]

Harris et al.[17] used KH_2PO_4 (mono-potassium orthophosphate) and Nizel et al.[31,32] used HPO_3 (metaphosphoric acid) as phosphate supplements in diets fed hamsters. Both of these phosphate compounds were significantly effective in reducing caries incidence.

When a 2 per cent analytical grade HPO_3 (which was impure and probably was Na_2O-H_2O-P_2O_5) was fed as a supplement to Syrian hamsters postweaning, there was a 70 per cent reduction in dental caries. If this same supplement was fed preweaning, the reduction was over 90 per cent. When metaphosphoric acid was added to a cariogenic diet at a 4 per cent level and fed to 8 day old Syrian hamsters for 100 days, not a single carious lesion was found in any of the molars (Fig. 38). Furthermore, these teeth had a more

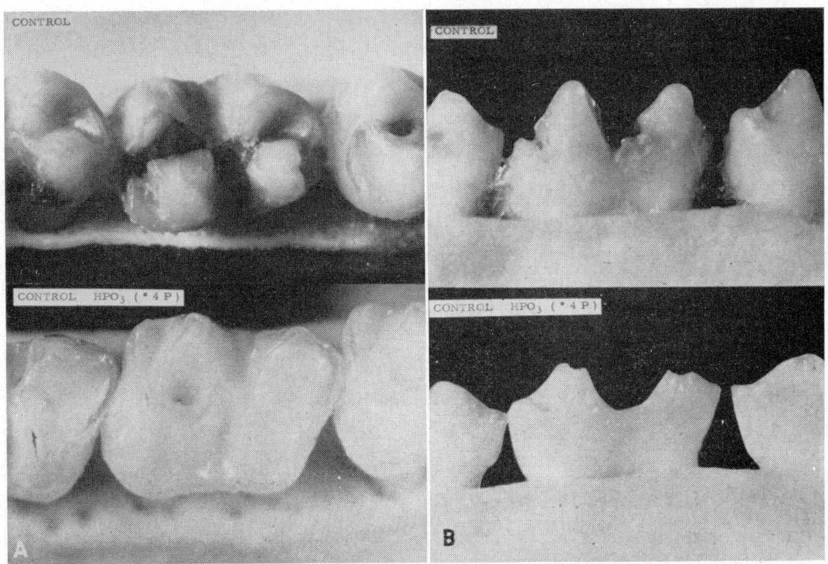

FIGURE 39. *A*, Occlusal view of hamster molars—note morphologic as well as caries difference between group on control diet and experimental (control + HPO_3) diet. *B*, Lateral view of same teeth.

lustrous, pearly white appearance and the grooves and fossae of the occlusal surfaces were shallower than those of the control group. Usually, the cusps of hamster molars are sharply pointed and cone shaped, but in the phosphate-supplemented group the cusps were more rounded and in some instances the occlusal surface was practically a flat plane (Fig. 39). However, there was no exposure of yellow dentin as seen in attrition. Whether this is a systemic, a local or a combination effect is currently being investigated.

If human clinical control studies which are currently under way confirm these animal and in vitro studies, optimal levels of phosphorus may prove to be as important as fluorine in the prevention of dental caries.

CALCIUM AND PHOSPHORUS AND THE PERIODONTIUM

Alveolar bone is composed of cancellous bone and is continuously being built up and resorbed. For this reason a calcium or phosphorus deficiency will affect the alveolar bone readily. The deficiency can be brought on as a result of (1) inadequate intake in the diet, or (2) systemic conditioning factors such as digestive disturbances and hormonal imbalance, or (3) such conditioning factors as inflammation.

Becks and Weber[5] demonstrated that the marrow spaces became hemorrhagic and filled with uncalcified fibro-osteoid tissue when calcium-deficient experimental diets were fed to rats. The alveolar bone underwent excessive resorption and the teeth became loose. Calcium deficiency, however, was shown not to be the critical factor for the development of gingivitis in monkeys.[13] Only 1 out of 4 *Macaca rhesus* monkeys developed a gingivitis on a calcium deficiency, but when both vitamin C and calcium were deficient, all of them developed extensive gingival lesions. Vitamin C, not calcium, evidently was the critical nutrient for gingival health.

Systemic conditioning factors like achlorhydria which will interfere with calcium absorption have been shown by Radusch[39] to influence alveolar resorption. Endocrine disturbances involving parathyroid hormone, estrogen, thyroid and adrenal hormones can all affect calcium metabolism of the alveolar bone. Most of these systemic disturbances manifest themselves by disintegration or disappearance of the lamina dura.

Inflammation of the periodontium is produced for the most part by such local irritants as calculus, which is composed chemically of:

$CaPO_4$	67.18%
$CaCO_3$	8.13%
CaFl	1.55%
$MgPO_4$	1.07%
Organic matter	22.07%

Inflammation produces a lowered *p*H which not only demineralizes the matrix but also activates proteolytic enzymes. Calcium salts are only stable within the matrix at a *p*H of 7.4.[45] It is possible for calcium to be withdrawn from bone in three ways: (1) by a simple chemical withdrawal which leaves the matrix intact; (2) by osteoclasts together with the matrix, a process otherwise known as osteoclastic absorption; and (3) without osteoclasts but conjointly with the matrix, a process otherwise known as halisteresis.

REFERENCES

1. Agnew, M. C., Agnew, R. S., and Tisdall, F. F.: The production and prevention of dental caries. J.A.D.A., *20:*193, 1933.
2. Albright, F., Aub, J. C., and Bauer, W.: Hyperparathyroidism: common and polymorphic conditions as illustrated by seventeen proven cases from one clinic. J.A.M.A., *102:*1276, 1934.
3. Armstrong, W. D., and Brekhus, P. J.: Chemical constitution of enamel and dentin; principal components. J. Biol. Chem., *120:*677, 1937.
4. Barnard, P., and Johansen, E.: The effect of 2% $CaHPO_4$ dietary supplement on experimental dental caries in the rat. J. D. Res., *37:*34, 1958.
5. Becks, H., and Weber, M.: Influence of diet on bone system with special reference to alveolar process and labyrinthine capsule. J.A.D.A., *18:* 197, 1931.
6. Black, G. V.: An investigation of the physical characters of the human teeth in relation to their diseases and to practical dental operations together with the physical characters of filling-materials. D. Cosmos, *37:*353, 1895.
7. Boyd, J. D., Drain, C. L., and Stearns, G.: Metabolic studies of children with dental caries. J. Biol. Chem., *103:*327, 1933.
8. Council on Dental Therapeutics: Calcium and phosphorus compounds in dentistry. J.A.D.A., *23:*139, 1936.
9. Dobbs, E. C.: Studies of blood calcium and phosphorus from a dental aspect. D. Cosmos, *74:*867, 1932.
10. East, B. R.: Association of dental caries in school children with hardness of communal water supplies. J. D. Res., *20:*323, 1941.
11. Erdheim, J.: Rachitis und Epithelkörperchen. Denkschr d.k. Akad. d. Wissensch. math. Naturw. Klasse, *90:*363, 1914.
12. Food and Nutrition Board: Recommended Dietary Allowances, Revised. Nat'l Acad. Sc.-Nat'l. Res. Council, Pub. No. 589, 1958.
13. Fraser, H. T., and Topping, N. H.: Mouth lesions in monkeys associated with chronic deficiency of calcium, vitamin C and both calcium and vitamin C. Pub. Health Rep., *57:*968, 1942.
14. Gaunt, W. E., and Irving, J. T.: Influence of calcium and phosphorus on tooth formation. J. Physiol., *95:*51P, 1939.
15. Gaunt, W. E., and Irving, J. T.: Influence of dietary calcium and phosphorus upon tooth formation. J. Physiol., *99:*18, 1940.
16. Haldi, J., Wynn, W., Bentley, K. D., and Law, M. L.: Dental caries in the albino rat in relation to the chemical composition of the teeth and of the diet. J. Nut., *67:*645, 1959.
17. Harris, R. S., Nizel, A. E., and Gardner, D. S.: Effects of food ash and trace minerals upon dental caries in hamsters. 4th Internat. Cong. Nut., Paris, France, p. 195, 1957.
18. Hawkins, H. F.: What is the cause of caries and systemic pyorrhea? J.A.D.A., *18:*943, 1931.
19. Hegsted, D. M., Moscoso, I., and Collazos, C.: A study of the minimum calcium requirements of adult men. J. Nut., *46:*181, 1952.
20. Jenkins, G. N., Forster, M. G., Spiers, R., and Kleinberg, I.: The influence of refinement of carbohydrates on their cariogenicity, in vitro experiments on white and brown flour. Brit. D. J., *106:*195, 1959.
21. Klein, H., and McCollum, E. V.: A preliminary note on the significance of the phosphorus intake in the diet and blood phosphorus concentra-

tion, in the experimental production of caries immunity, and caries susceptibility in the rat. Science, *74:*662, 1931.

22. Lennox, J.: Observations on diet in its relation to dental disease. S. African D. J., July, Aug., Sept., 1930.
23. Lund, A. P., and Armstrong, W. D.: The effect of a low calcium and vitamin D free diet on the skeleton and teeth of adult rats. J. D. Res., *21:*513, 1942.
24. Malan, A. L., and Ockerse, T.: Effect of calcium and phosphorus intake of school children upon dental caries, body weights, and heights. S. African D. J., *15:*153, 1941.
25. McCall, J. O., and Krasnow, F.: The influence of metabolism on teeth. J. Ped.,*13:*498, 1938.
26. McClendon, J. F., and Foster, W. C.: Effect of dietary fluorine in delaying dental caries. J. D. Res., *21:*139, 1942.
27. McClure, F. J.: Wheat cereal diets, rat caries, lysine and minerals. J. Nut., *65:*619, 1958.
28. McClure, F. J., and Muller, A.: The caries inhibiting effect of dibasic sodium phosphate and dibasic calcium phosphate added to wheat flour and bread diets. J.A.D.A., *58:*36, 1959.
29. McKay, F. S.: The establishment of a definite relation between enamel that is defective in its structure, as mottled enamel, and the liability to decay. D. Cosmos, *71:*747, 1929.
30. Mellanby, M.: Influence of diet on caries in children's teeth. London, Medical Res. Council, Special Report, Series No. 221, 1936.
31. Nizel, A. E., and Harris, R. S.: Effect of different dietary levels of metaphosphoric acid on hamster caries. J. D. Res., 1959 (in press).
32. Nizel, A. E., Keating, N., Sundstrom, C., and Harris, R. S.: Effect of phosphate supplement to diet on development of hamster caries. J. D. Res., *37:*35, 1958.
33. Nizel, A. E., and Prigge, E. K.: Trismus due to myositis ossificans traumatica: report of a case. J. Oral Surg., *4:*93, 1946.
34. Ohlson, M. A.: The calcium controversy. J. A. Diet. A., *31:*333, 1955.
35. Osborn, T. W. B., and Noriskin, J. N.: The relation between diet and caries in South African Bantu. J. D. Res., *16:*431, 1937.
36. Osborn, T. W. B.: Further studies on the in vitro decalcification of teeth. J. D. Res., *20:*59, 1941.
37. Osborn, T. W. B., Noriskin, J. N., and Staz, J.: A comparison of crude and refined sugar and cereals in their ability to produce in vitro decalcifications of teeth. J. D. Res., *16:*165, 1937.
38. Osborn, T. W. B., Noriskin, J. N., and Staz, J.: Inhibition in vitro of decalcification in teeth. J. D. Res., *16:*545, 1937.
39. Radusch, D. F.: Relationship of gastro-acidity to periodontoclasia. J. Periodont., *18:*110, 1947.
40. Schour, I.: Calcium metabolism and teeth. J.A.M.A., *110:*870, 1938.
41. Shelling, D. H., and Asher, D. E.: Calcium and phosphorus studies. VIII. Some observations on the incidence of caries-like lesions in the rat. J. D. Res., *13:*363, 1933.
42. Sobel, A. E.: Composition of teeth in relation to caries susceptibility. Trans. 4th Macy Conf. on Metabolic Interrelations, *4:*261, 1952.
43. Sobel, A. E., and Hanok, A.: Calcification of teeth. I. Composition in relation to blood and diet. J. Biol. Chem., *176:*1103, 1948.
44. Sobel, A. E., and Hanok, A.: Calcification. XVI. Composition of bones and teeth in relation to blood and diet in the cotton rat. J. D. Res., *37:* 631, 1958.

45. Stahl, S.: Roentgenographic and bacteriologic aspects of periodontal changes in diabetes. J. Periodont., *19:*130, 1948.
46. Stralfors, A.: Karieshamming genom fosfater. Svensk Tandak Tidskrift, *49:*108, 1956.
47. Wynn, W., Haldi, J., Bentley, K. D., and Law, M. L.: Dental caries in the albino rat in relation to the chemical composition of the teeth and of the diet. II. Variations in the Ca:P ratio of the diet induced by changing the phosphorus content. J. Nut., *58:*325, 1956.
48. Ziskin, D. E., and Hotelling, H.: Effects of pregnancy, mouth acidity, and age on dental caries. J. D. Res., *16:*507, 1937.

MAGNESIUM

Chemistry

Occurrence. Magnesium is found in all green plants because it is an essential component of chlorophyll. Cereals and nuts are a good source of this mineral and it also occurs in small amounts in meats and milk. Magnesium is widely distributed in tissues. Its concentration in the intracellular fluids is exceeded only by that of potassium. Three-fourths of the magnesium in the body is in the organic tissues of bone, but it also occurs in muscle and nerve tissue. The amount of magnesium present in tissues is intimately related to the amount of available calcium and phosphorus. If the calcium concentration is low, magnesium can replace it; it also can be mobilized from bone. Yet, excess magnesium inhibits the calcification process.

Physiology

Functions. Magnesium ions act as catalysts for many cellular reactions. As part of the enzyme systems involving inorganic pyrophosphatase and carboxylase, they aid in the intermediate metabolism of sugar.

Magnesium affects muscle and nerve tissue. In large amounts it has an anesthetic and anticonvulsant effect, whereas low concentrations cause hyperirritability or convulsions.

General Systemic Pathology of Magnesium Deficiency

Magnesium deficiency is very rare in man. When caused experimentally it is said to produce weakness.[6]

McCollum and Orent[13] found that the vessels in the skin of animals became dilated as a result of magnesium deficiency. Convulsive seizures consisting of spasticity and hyperextension usually followed this vasodilation and hyperemia. After a period of relaxation, the animals became rigid. Some animals died and others recovered. Those that recovered developed edema of the paws and ears, and kidney disorders.

Oral Pathology of Magnesium Imbalance

Gingiva. In a study on the effects of magnesium deficiency on the teeth and their supporting structures in rats, Klein et al.[11] found that the gingivae hypertrophied, that the teeth became loose, and that there was generally evidence of chronic destructive periodontal disease.

Teeth. Becks and Furuta,[2,3,4] in a series of studies on the effects of magnesium deficiency on the incisor teeth of the growing rat, noted (1) degenerative changes in the enamel epithelium, (2) degeneration of ameloblasts on the labial side of anterior teeth, with subsequent enamel hypoplasia, (3) striation of the dentin due to odontoblastic degeneration and irregular dentin formation, and (4) pathologic calcification of the pulp. Others[5,7,9] have noted similar histologic changes.

In magnesium deficiency the magnesium content of labile bone is reduced, but that of a rat's incisor tooth remains constant.

Dental Caries. Increased amounts of magnesium have been found in carious teeth.[10,16] However, Howe[8] pointed out that the method for determining the magnesium content of teeth is the most unreliable of all the methods for measuring inorganic elements. Murray et al.[14] and Armstrong et al.[1] have found marked differences between the magnesium content of sound and carious teeth.

Epidemiologically, Ockerse[15] reported no correlation between the magnesium content of soils and water and the magnesium content of enamel and dentin.

In testing the relation of the various minerals in food and drinking water to the incidence of rat caries, McClure[12] found that magnesium chloride was among the substances that were without effect.

REFERENCES

1. Armstrong, W. D., and Brekhus, P. J.: Chemical constitution of enamel and dentin; principal components. J. Biol. Chem., *120*:677, 1937.
2. Becks, H., and Furuta, W. J.: Effect of magnesium deficient diets on oral and dental structures. I. Changes in the enamel epithelium. J.A.D.A., *26*:883, 1939.

3. Becks, H., and Furuta, W. J.: Effects of magnesium deficient diets on oral and dental structures. II. Changes in the enamel structure. J.A.D.A., *28:*1083, 1941.
4. Becks, H., and Furuta, W. J.: Effects of magnesium deficient diets on oral and dental structures. III. Changes in the dentine and pulp tissue. Am. J. Ortho., *28:*1, 1942.
5. Duckworth, J., and Godden, W.: The influence of diets low in magnesium upon the chemical composition of the incisor teeth of the rat. J. Physiol., *99:*1, 1940.
6. Fitzgerald, M. G., and Fourman, P.: An experimental study of magnesium deficiency in man. Clin. Sc., *15:*635, 1956.
7. Gagnon, J. A., Schour, I., and Patros, M. C.: Effect of magnesium deficiency on dentine apposition and eruption in incisor of rat. Proc. Soc. Exper. Biol. & Med., *49:*662, 1942.
8. Howe, P. R.: Further studies of the effect of diet upon the teeth and bones. J.A.D.A., *10:*201, 1923.
9. Irving, J. T.: The influence of diets low in magnesium upon the histological appearance of the incisor tooth of the rat. J. Physiol., *99:*8, 1940.
10. Kaushonsky, L. I.: The chemical analyses of teeth, roots, and crowns affected by pyorrhea alveolaris and dental caries. Dent. Cos., *74:*468, 1932.
11. Klein, H., Orent, E. R., and McCollum, E. V.: Effects of magnesium deficiency on teeth and their supporting structures in rats. Am. J. Physiol., *112:*256, 1935.
12. McClure, F. J.: Observations on induced caries in rats. VI. Summary results of various modifications of food and drinking water. J. D. Res., *27:*34, 1948.
13. McCollum, E. V., and Orent, E. R.: Effects on the rate of deprivation of magnesium. J. Biol. Chem., *92:*XXX (Soc. Proc.), 1931.
14. Murray, M. M., and Bowes, J. H.: The composition of enamel, dentin and root in caries and pyorrhea. Brit. D. J., *61:*473, 1936.
15. Ockerse, T.: The chemical composition of enamel and dentin in high and low caries areas in South Africa. J. D. Res., *22:*441, 1943.
16. Ulrich, J. L.: Chemical analyses of teeth affected by dental caries and pyorrhea alveolaris, Dent. Cos., *67:*1204, 1925.
17. Yamane, G. M., and Singer, L.: The effect of subminimal magnesium on the syrian hamster. J. D. Res., *32:*708, 1953. Abstract.

WATER

The nutritional requirement for water is paramount. One cannot tolerate water deprivation for so long a period of time as abstinence from food. Structurally, about 70 per cent of the lean body mass of man is water.

Distribution

Water is found in the body in three fluid compartments.[2] These are classified as follows: (1) the intravascular compartment (blood plasma), (2) the extravascular compartment (interstitial fluid),

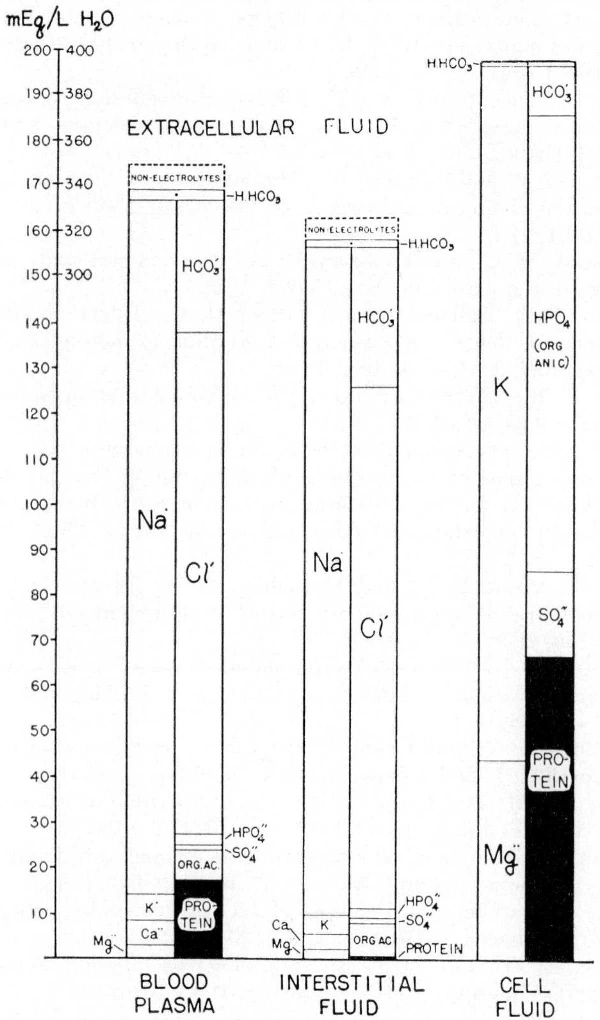

FIGURE **40.** The chemical composition of extracellular fluids and cell fluid. Note that the values are given as milliequivalents per liter of water contained in the fluid instead of per liter of plasma. It will be seen that the patterns of blood plasma and interstitial fluid are almost identical; the greatest single item of difference is in the amounts of protein. This makes necessary adjustment of the concentrations of the diffusible ions which will preserve the total cation-anion equivalence (Donnan equilibrium). The nonelectrolyte concentration (glucose, urea, etc.) is seen to be very small in comparison with that of the electrolytes although the total quantity carried to the tissue cells and into the urine over a unit of time is several times larger. Note the predominance of potassium and the high protein content of cell fluid. (Adapted from Gamble, J. L.: Chemical Anatomy, Physiology and Pathology of Extracellular Fluid. 5th ed. Cambridge, Mass., Harvard University Press, 1950.)

and (3) the intracellular compartment, which contains the bulk of the body water (Fig. 40).

Each of the compartments contains electrolytes. In the extracellular fluids, which consist of blood plasma and interstitial fluid, sodium is the major cation and chlorine the major anion. The chemical compositions of plasma and interstitial fluid are almost identical; they differ primarily in the absence or low concentration of protein in the latter. Potassium and magnesium are the major cations of the intracellular fluid, while phosphate is the major anion. This compartment contains three times the protein concentration of the vascular compartment.

Function

In addition to its role as an important structural component of the body, water serves as the vehicle for transporting organic and inorganic nutrients via the blood plasma and interstitial fluids into the cells and conveying secretions and excretions from the body. The water in the interstitial compartment is called upon first to counteract any dehydration process, thereby helping to maintain the volume of water in the plasma and cellular fluid compartment vitally constant. Water also serves to maintain a constant *p*H and osmotic pressure in each of the compartments. Water plays another important role, that of contributing to temperature regulation by virtue of its evaporation from the skin and elimination from the lungs.

Water Balance

Water balance involves the following: (1) maintaining a constant total amount of water in the body, (2) maintaining the proper distribution of water between cells and extracellular fluid, and (3) maintaining a constant volume of circulating blood. Sodium and potassium play important roles in maintaining the proper distribution of water between cells and extracellular fluid.

If, for example, the daily water intake and output of an individual amounted to 2,000 ml., the intake might be subdivided as follows: 1,000 ml. of liquid food (water, milk, soup, coffee, etc.), 700 ml. of water present in solid foods as moisture, and 300 ml. of metabolic water or water of oxidation. The output might be subdivided as follows: over 1,000 ml. of urine, 500 ml. from skin as sweat, 400 ml. from lungs as moist air, and 100 ml. in stools.

Requirements

Water requirement in man is determined by body heat production, renal solute load, the concentrating capacity of the kidney and losses due to sweat. There is a direct relationship between water and salt requirements.

The average daily intake should be between 2300 and 3100 ml. Actually, under normal conditions the thirst sensation assures an adequate fluid intake. However, under conditions of extreme heat and excessive sweating when the water intake must be appreciably increased, one cannot rely entirely upon the thirst sensation alone to regulate the amount of fluid intake.

SODIUM

Sources

Common table salt which is used to season and flavor both uncooked and cooked foods represents the single largest source of sodium. In the body, sodium is the major cation associated with the chloride and bicarbonate anions found in the blood plasma and the extracellular fluid. The largest amounts are found in skin and bone.

Function

The principal function of sodium is the regulation of osmotic pressure between extracellular and intracellular fluid compartments. It maintains the acid-base balance of blood and body fluids. It is also concerned with the contraction of muscle and the conduction of nerve impulses.

Pathology

The adrenal cortex controls sodium metabolism. In Addison's disease, resulting from adrenocortical insufficiency, there is an increased excretion of sodium in the urine. The classic clinical picture of this disease is anorexia, nausea, weariness, lassitude, sunken eyes, hollow cheeks, muscle cramps and falling blood pressure.[3] In extreme sodium deficiency shock can occur.

On the other hand, sodium retention has been observed to occur in hypertension, congestive heart failure and ascites.

Dental Pathology. Moore[4] suggested that diets poor in sodium chloride diminished dental caries and improved the assimilation of calcium. He reasoned that "living cells already saturated with electropositive sodium ions find the utilization of calcium difficult." Therefore, excess sodium chloride will have a decalcifying effect. Furthermore, he stated, civilized people may have teeth that are inferior to those of primitive folk because of their excessive use of salt.

Requirements

The average daily intake of NaCl is 10 to 15 grams, which is much above the body's normal requirement.

Excessive water loss, either through perspiration, diarrhea or vomiting, requires an increased intake of salt. In accordance with the Recommended Daily Dietary Allowance for sodium, "One additional gram of salt should be consumed for each liter of water in excess of 4 liters daily."

CHLORINE

In food the chloride anion is usually associated with sodium, as in common table salt. The normal diet usually contains sufficient amounts of this ion to meet the needs of the body except during periods of excessive loss as a result of perspiration, diarrhea, vomiting or adrenocortical disease.

In the body, the chloride ion constitutes the chief anion of the extracellular fluid compartment of the body. Chlorides are found in the cerebrospinal fluid, interstitial fluids, blood plasma and gastrointestinal secretions.

POTASSIUM

Sources

Potassium is found in appreciable amounts in dried fruits such as prunes and raisins. In the body, potassium is the principal cation of the intracellular fluid.

Function

Potassium plays a most important role in the contraction of cardiac, smooth and skeletal muscle as well as in the excitation of nerve tissue. It is essential for the growth of normal young tissue and of abnormal cancerous tissue. It plays an important part in intracellular osmotic pressure and is concerned with maintaining acid-base balance in the cell.

Pathology

A potassium deficiency can be produced by (1) loss of fluids through vomiting or diarrhea, (2) adrenocortical insufficiency, (3) increased alkalosis of extracellular fluid, and (4) excessive sodium intake. Excessive administration of insulin in diabetes control may shift potassium from the extracellular fluid into the cells, thus producing a hypokalemia.

A potassium deficiency will adversely affect carbohydrate metabolism by inhibiting glycogen deposition and by interfering with the normal functions of enzyme systems.

In animals the tissues most readily affected by a potassium deficiency are the myocardium, striated muscle and kidney.

Dental Caries. Both the Emory and Harvard diets had equal amounts of sucrose, yet there was a difference in cariogenicity when they were fed to experimental animals.[5] The Emory group noted that the Harvard diet contained 75 per cent more K and they reasoned that this might be responsible for the difference in cariogenicity. Therefore, they designed an experimental diet in which they altered the Na:K ratio from 1:2 to 2:1. This change in ratio had no effect on its cariogenicity.

Requirement

The results of a limited experiment[1] indicate that 0.8 to 1.3 grams potassium per day appears to approach the minimum requirement for maintaining equilibrium.

A 1500 calorie diet, consisting of animal and vegetable foods, will contain approximately 2.5 grams of potassium. Therefore, an extremely low calorie diet would be required to produce less than the desirable 1.5 grams of potassium. No daily allowance for potassium has been recommended.

REFERENCES

1. Food and Nutrition Board: Recommended Dietary Allowances, Revised. Nat'l. Acad. Sci.-Nat'l. Res. Council, Pub. No. 589, 1958.
2. Gamble, J. L.: Chemical Anatomy, Physiology and Pathology of Extracellular Fluid. 6th edition. Cambridge, Harvard University Press, 1954.

3. McCance, R. A.: Medical problems in mineral metabolism. Lancet, *230:* 823, 1936.
4. Moore, C. U.: Mineral metabolism in relation to dentition. II. Base-forming and salt poor diet. J.A.D.A., *20:*1591, 1933.
5. Wynn, W., Haldi, J., Bentley, K. D., and Law, M. W.: Further studies on the difference in cariogenicity of two diets comparable in sucrose. J. Nut., *67:*569, 1959.

Chapter VII

Trace Elements

GENERAL INFORMATION

The discovery of trace elements and their recognition as important factors in maintaining life and health of animals dates back to 1807[2] when it was found that sheep afflicted with "pining" disease could be cured by shifting them from restricted grazing areas to different pastures. Later it was found that the soil in the new grazing fields was richer in cobalt than the old areas. In 1900[6] sheep in New Zealand were beset with "bush sickness," which was also shown to result from a cobalt deficiency, although it was first thought that iron was the missing element. Iodine had been used empirically for the treatment of goiter as far back as 1820,[25] but it was seventy-five years later that it was first found in the thyroid gland.

It is evident from these few examples that the importance of trace elements was recognized one hundred and fifty years ago. However, it has only been in the last decade or so that progress has been made in understanding the role of these metallic ions in biological systems and in the prevention of deficiency diseases. With his present knowledge of trace elements, the biochemist now can explain some of the catalytic processes associated with the intermediary metabolism of foods. The physician is also becoming aware of possible relationships between trace metals and chronic diseases,[21] and the dentist has recently added the trace element, fluorine, to his dental armamentarium in his fight against dental caries.

Definition

Trace elements are inorganic micronutrients which affect biological systems at concentrations as low as 10^{-6} to 10^{-12} gram/gram of wet tissue. They have also been called oligo-elements ("oligo" from the Greek, meaning scanty).[24] In 1946,[1] iron, copper, manganese, zinc, iodine and cobalt were considered the indispensable trace elements. Ten years later, Schroeder[21] stated that only "five trace elements are believed essential for mammalian metabolism: manganese, cobalt, copper, zinc and molybdenum." It is evident that all investigators are not in complete accord on the number of trace elements which are essential. For example, fluorine has been suggested as an essential trace element in view of its limited ability at optimal levels to prevent dental caries.[16] However, because it is difficult to prepare an absolutely fluorine-free experimental diet, a true test of its indispensability for normal growth and reproduction has not been adequately established. Furthermore, it is questionable whether growth should be considered the sole criterion for essentiality.[15]

Other trace elements have been found in animal and vegetable tissues; these are aluminum, antimony, arsenic, barium, boron, bromine, cadmium, chromium, gallium, lead, lithium, mercury, molybdenum, nickel, rubidium, scandium, silver, strontium, tin, titanium, and vanadium.[4,21]

PHYSIOLOGY

Trace elements, much like vitamins, act primarily by participating in enzyme reactions. Indeed, they have been termed "inorganic vitamins." They participate in these reactions in two forms, (a) as metallo-enzymes or (b) as metal/enzymes.[25]

Metallo-enzymes are organic compounds which have specific, fixed, inseparable metal ions incorporated within the protein molecule. These metals are not easily dialyzable nor can other metals substitute for them. If, however, the element is split from the molecule by some vigorous manipulation, all measurable biological activity is lost, e.g., iron in cytochrome and catalase enzymes, magnesium in chlorophyll.

Metal/enzymes are more common in nature. They are compounds in which the metal ions are not integral parts of the enzyme molecule but are held in loose association with the enzymes; they are easily dialyzable. Their most important function is to activate catalytic reactions. For example, manganese activates the enzyme arginase, which splits arginine into ornithine and urea.

It is evident that the trace element, either as an integral part of an enzymal molecule or as a "loose enzyme metal complex," functions primarily as a catalyst. Iodine, which is a component of the thyroglobulin molecule, and cobalt, which is part of the vitamin B_{12} molecule, are exceptions.

GENERAL SYSTEMIC PATHOLOGY OF METAL IMBALANCE

No true metal deficiency other than that of iron has been demonstrated in man. In animals, however, manganese deficiency has been shown to affect the bones and joints of pigs and rabbits. A deficiency of cobalt has already been mentioned as the cause for "bush sickness" or enzootic marasmus.

There is some evidence that a metal imbalance may be associated with such conditions as arterial hypertension, atherosclerosis, disseminated lupus erythematosus, neurologic disorders and other chronic diseases. Arterial hypertension may result from competition among trace metals. An excess of cadmium and lead and a deficiency in vanadium may contribute to permanent renal hypertension. In atherosclerosis, a metal may be involved in cholesterol and fatty acid synthesis. Schroeder[21] concludes that many chronic diseases may be influenced by either a deficiency or an excessive amount of essential trace metals.

ORAL PATHOLOGY OF METAL IMBALANCE

Separate sections are to be devoted to iron, fluorine, iodine and copper and will include a discussion of their influence on the incidence of dental caries and other oral pathology. The relationship between other trace elements and the incidence of dental caries will be discussed here.

Dental Caries

The discovery that a natural ash has minerals other than fluorine, or mineral ratios that show caries inhibitory properties, has served as a stimulus for investigations in the area of the relation of trace elements in general to caries incidence.[22] Furthermore, a hypothesis has been advanced that the regional differences observed in human caries experience may be attributed to the different trace minerals present in the soil of these areas.[10,19] It has been demonstrated that corn grown in high caries areas differs significantly from that grown in low caries areas in the amounts of such trace elements as copper, aluminum, iron and molybdenum.[17] Several papers will be reviewed here in which have been reported the results of investigations on the effects of single or multiple trace minerals to inhibit or to accelerate dental caries.

Caries Accelerators. Cadmium, despite its ability to act like fluorine as an enzyme poison, was found to be cariogenic rather than cariostatic.[7] It did not initiate caries but acted as a spreading factor.[14]

When excessive amounts of zinc, barium or thallium were given to animals in a purified diet, free of all trace elements but, unfortunately, also deficient in other essential nutrients, the incidence of caries increased.[20] Because nutrients other than the test ones were omitted, it is difficult to interpret the results of this work.

Children showing a higher selenium concentration in the urine also had a higher rate of caries attacks.[8]

A mixture consisting of oxides of four trace minerals (zinc, aluminum, manganese and iron) and a magnesium salt was cariogenic.[9]

Wisotzky and Hein[26] found that platinum was very cariogenic.

Caries Inhibitors. Rygh[20] found no tooth decay in rats fed an excess of strontium and vanadium. This property of vanadium has been confirmed by Geyer,[5] who found that the significant inhibition of caries by vanadium pentoxide was independent of the route of administration or the amount offered. The caries inhibitory properties of vanadium have also been reported by Kruger.[12]

This latter investigator found that a salt mixture of boron, molybdenum and fluorine, as well as these individual elements, caused a reduction in caries when fed to hamsters during the period of enamel mineralization.[11]

Gold in the form of auric chloride, when added to the drinking water of the Syrian hamster, produced a significantly lower caries score than in control animals.[26]

Elements without Effect on Caries. A mixture of boron, copper, manganese and molybdenum,[11] as well as the individual elements, boron[13] and aluminum,[28] did not produce any significant effect in the incidence of caries when added to a cariogenic diet.

Periodontal Disease

Since gingival tissues are affected by the chronic ingestion of heavy metals such as lead, silver and mercury, Wisotzky and Hein[27] investigated the effect of metallic ion ingestion on alveolar crest resorption. Salts of the principal metals, magnesium and lead, as well as those of such trace elements as lithium, vanadium, platinum, palladium and gold, were tested. Only the platinic ion markedly accelerated alveolar crest resorption; these same animals also showed bone porosity in the skull. Precipitated metal lines were seen in the gingival tissues of animals exposed to palladium, cadmium and lead; however, there was no alveolar bone resorption in these animals.

REFERENCES

1. Anon: Present knowledge of the minerals in nutrition. Nut. Rev., *4:*195, 227, 1946.
2. Baudisch, O.: The importance of trace elements in biologic activity. J.A.M.A., *123:*959, 1943.
3. Baumann, E.: Ueber das normale Vorkommen von Jod in Tierkoerper. Ztschr. f. physiol. Chem., *21:*319, 1895, in J.A.M.A., *120:*609, 1942.
4. Dingle, H., and Sheldon, J.: A spectrographic examination of the mineral content of human and other milk. Biochem. J., *32:*1078, 1938.
5. Geyer, C. F.: Vanadium: a caries-inhibiting trace element in the Syrian hamster. J. D. Res., *32:*590, 1953.
6. Gilruth, T. A.: Bush and Taurange disease in cattle and sheep. Annual Report No. 8, New Zealand Dept. of Agriculture, p. 187, 1900.
7. Ginn, J. T., and Volker, J. F.: Effect of cadmium and fluorine on the rat dentition. Proc. Soc. Exper. Biol. & Med., *57:*189, 1944.
8. Hadjimarkos, D. M., Storvick, C. A., and Remmert, L. F.: Selenium and dental caries: an investigation among school children of Oregon. J. of Pediatrics, *40:*451, 1952.
9. Harris, R., Nizel, A. E., and Gardner, D. S.: Effects of food ash and trace minerals upon dental caries in hamsters. 4th. Int. Cong. Nut., Paris, France, p. 195, 1957.
10. Hewart, R. E. T., and Eastcott, D. F.: Dental caries in New Zealand. Med. Res. Council of New Zealand, 1956.
11. Kruger, B. J.: The effect of "trace elements" on experimental dental caries in the albino rat. I. A study of boron, copper, fluorine, manganese and molybdenum. Australian Dent. J., *3:*236, 1958.
12. Kruger, B. J.: The effect of "trace elements" on experimental dental caries in the albino rat. II. A study of aluminium, boron, fluorine, iodine and vanadium. Australian Dent. J., *3:*298, 1958.
13. Kruger, B. J.: The effect of "trace elements" on experimental dental caries in the albino rat. III. A study of boron and copper. Australian Dent. J., *3:*374, 1958.
14. Leicester, H. M.: The effect of cadmium on the production of caries in the rat. J. D. Res., *25:*337, 1946.

15. McElroy, W. M.: Trace elements in biology and agriculture. Pub. Health Rep., *73:*747, 1958.
16. Moore, C. V., Innes, J., and Innes, E. M.: The essential trace elements; in Joliffe, E., Tisdall, M. D., and Cannon P. R.: Clinical Nutrition. New York, Paul B. Hoeber, Inc., 1950.
17. Nizel, A. E., and Harris, R. S.: The caries producing effect of similar foods grown in different soil areas. N. E. J. of Med., *244:*361, 1951.
18. Nizel, A. E., and Harris, R. S.: Effects of ashed foodstuffs on dental decay in hamsters. J. D. Res., *34:*513, 1955.
19. Nizel, A. E., and Bibby, B. G.: Geographic variations in caries prevalence in soldiers. J.A.D.A., *31:*1619, 1944.
20. Rygh, O.: Narkse tennlacfne tid. *60:*1, 1950; in Nut. Rev., *8:*178, 1950.
21. Schroeder, H. A.: Trace metals and chronic disease. Advances in Int. Med., *8:*259, 1956.
22. Shaw, J. H., and Sognnaes, R.: Experimental rat caries. V. Effect of fluorine on the caries conduciveness of a purified ration. J. Nut., *53:*207, 1954.
23. Sheldon, J. H., and Ramage, H.: A spectrographic analysis of human tissues. Biochem. J., *25:*1608, 1931.
24. Vallee, B. L.: The function of trace elements in biology. Sci. Monthly, *72:*368, 1951.
25. Vallee, B. L.: Trace elements in biochemistry and nutrition. Nut. Rev., *10:*65, 1952.
27. Wisotzky, J., and Hein, J. W.: Effects of drinking metallic salt solutions metallic ions above and below hydrogen in the electromotive series on dental caries in the Syrian hamster. J.A.D.A., *57:*796, 1958.
27. Wisotzky, J., and Hein, J. W.: Effects of drinking metallic salt solutions on alveolar crest resorption in the Syrian hamster. J. Perio., *29:*205, 1958.
28. Wynn, W., and Haldi, J.: Dental caries in the albino rat on high sucrose diets containing different amounts of aluminium. J. Nut. *54:*285, 1954.

IRON

Historically, the use of iron for the treatment of disease dates back to the mid-seventeenth century when first Sydenham, and later Willis,[4] used iron for the treatment of chlorosis (a form of iron-deficiency anemia that imparted a characteristic greenish pallor to the skin and was prevalent in adolescent girls). The early Greeks treated anemia with drinking water in which a sword had been allowed to rust.[1] However, the discovery of Manghini, in 1746, that iron was present in human blood emphasized the nutritional importance of iron.

Chemistry

Occurrence. The average adult body contains a very small amount of iron, only 3 to 5 grams. Yet this small amount is found in such important body chemicals as hemoglobin, myoglobin and oxidative enzyme systems.

Hemoglobin, which is composed of four ferroprotoporphyrin molecules conjugated to a single globulin molecule, contains about 55 to 60 per cent of the body iron. The chief function of hemoglobin is to transport oxygen from the lungs to tissues and to remove carbon dioxide from the tissues to the lungs.

Iron is part of such oxidative enzymes as cytochrome, peroxidase and catalase, and in this form it constitutes about 30 to 35 per cent of the total body iron.

The rest of the body iron, about 10 per cent, is found primarily in muscles as myoglobin.

The best food sources of iron are eggs, molasses, liver, beef muscle and dried fruits.

Physiology

Absorption. The amount of iron absorbed depends upon the form in which it reaches the small intestine and the conditions prevailing there. Water-soluble, ionizable and ultrafiltrable compounds are best absorbed; reduced iron (ferrous rather than ferric) and acid-soluble iron salts fall into this category. In food, iron exists primarily in the ferric (Fe^{+++}) form. The presence of adequate amounts of hydrochloric acid in the stomach and the presence of reducing agents, such as ascorbic acid, in foods, help to convert the iron into the more utilizable ferrous (Fe^{++}) form. However, phosphates and phytic acid form insoluble complexes with iron which cannot be absorbed.

Iron is absorbed into the intestinal mucosal cells, which contain the iron-binding protein, apoferritin. The rate of iron absorption depends to some extent upon the degree of unsaturation of this compound with respect to iron. The amount of apoferritin that is available to combine with iron is the factor which determines the amount that will be absorbed. When apoferritin combines with iron, it forms ferritin. Therefore, iron absorption by the intestinal mucosa is mediated through ferritin. This is sometimes referred to as the "mucosal block theory."[5] When hemoglobin is low, iron is transferred from the ferritin molecule in the intestinal mucosa to the serum protein fraction (siderophilin) to rebuild the hemoglobin. As this iron is released from the intestinal mucosa, the apoferritin is free to absorb more food iron. Actually, the need for new iron from food is not very great, because iron derived from the heme portion of hemoglobin can constantly be reused.

Storage. Iron is stored chiefly in the reticuloendothelial cells of the liver, from which it can be released when needed. It is also stored in the spleen, kidney and bone marrow.

The iron that is stored in the liver and can be withdrawn whenever needed is known as the "labile pool of iron." In contrast, the "parenchymal iron," which is present in the oxidative enzymes and myoglobin, is inviolate; it cannot be withdrawn even under the most severe iron deficiency.

Utilization. Minute amounts of copper will materially aid the transformation of assimilated iron into hemoglobin. The copper does not enter into the reaction but acts as a catalyst.

Calcium will also enhance the utilization of iron because it exerts a "sparing" action.

Excretion. The amount of iron excreted daily is very small because iron is constantly reused. If an amount is ingested in excess of that needed, it is excreted primarily via the feces and, sometimes, through the skin.

Requirements

The average adult loses, through all routes, between 0.5 and 1.5 mg. of iron per day. A balance can be maintained with a dietary intake of about 8 mg. However, a daily intake of 12 mg. is recommended in order to provide for individual variations. During the first year of life, when the demand for iron is highest, the recommended daily intake is 0.8 mg./kg. of body weight. From 3 to 6 years of age, 0.3 to 0.4 mg./kg. is desirable. In adolescents (13 to 15 years of age) and in pregnancy and lactation, 15 mg. is recommended.

General Systemic Pathology of Iron Deficiency

Iron deficiency anemia occurs most often as a result of increased body requirements during growth and pregnancy or as a result of excessive blood loss during menses or from an accident. This deficiency disease can also result from an inadequate intake of iron, such as occurs among older people who live on a "tea and toast" diet. Factors which interfere with iron absorption, such as achlorhydria, intestinal hypermotility, diarrhea or vomiting, may also contribute to an iron deficiency anemia.

This anemia is characterized by the formation of small, poorly pigmented, red cells, otherwise known as hypochromic microcytes. It is effected by an inadequacy in erythropoiesis and hemoglobin formation resulting from a deficiency of iron.

Hypochromic anemia may develop in infants after 4 months of age for three reasons: (1) the depletion of the reserve iron of

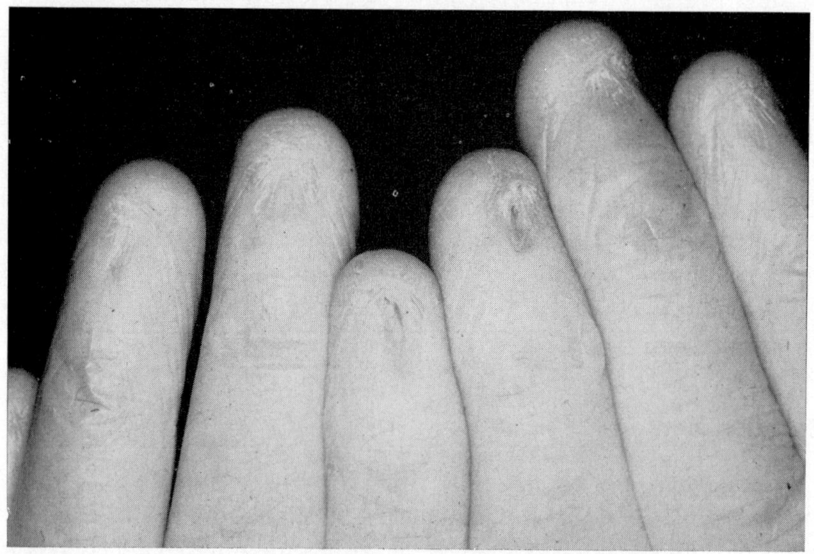

FIGURE 41. Plummer-Vinson syndrome. Spoon-shaped appearance of finger nails (Koilonychia) due to iron deficiency anemia.

the infant, which had been supplied by the mother, (2) the increasing demand of rapid growth, which involves increased blood volume, and (3) the exclusive use of milk during the first few months of infancy and a long delay in introducing iron-rich foods, such as eggs and meat, into the diet.

Stresses encountered during spurt growth and pregnancy may produce a physiological anemia because the total plasma volume is increased in both these conditions. For example, chlorosis is an iron deficiency anemia which occurs primarily in adolescent girls and is characterized by a greenish skin pallor. The combined demands of the spurt growth period and menstruation are factors contributing to the deficiency.

Iron needs during pregnancy are higher than normal because

of fetal needs, post-partum hemorrhage and iron loss in lactation.

"Idiopathic" hypochromic anemia occurs in middle-aged women because of depleted iron stores resulting from menorrhagia or achlorhydria.

Uncontrolled hemorrhage, which can occur in such conditions as peptic ulcer, hemorrhoids and open wounds, may cause an iron deficiency anemia. This is the most common cause of anemia in males. The male is not so susceptible to anemia as the female because he suffers only pathologic blood loss, whereas the female can incur not only pathologic loss but also physiologic blood loss during menstruation and pregnancy.

When patients have a hypochromic anemia that is accompanied by dysphagia (difficulty in swallowing), which may be due to web formation in the esophagus, the condition is referred to as the Plummer-Vinson syndrome. In addition, the patient tires easily and experiences many gastrointestinal upsets. The complexion is pallid and longitudinal ridges develop on the fingernails, which assume a spoon-shaped appearance. This is called koilonychia (Fig. 41).

Oral Pathology of Iron Deficiency

Tongue and Mucous Membranes. Iron deficiency anemia or Plummer-Vinson disease is characterized by such oral signs as fissures in the labial commissures and superficial glossitis (Fig. 42). The papillae of the tongue are atrophied, thus giving the tongue a smooth, shiny and red appearance. All oral mucous membranes are atrophied and appear ashen-gray. It is believed that oral tissues thus affected are more susceptible to carcinoma.

The clinical appearance of the tongue in an iron deficiency resembles very closely that seen in a niacin, riboflavin or other B complex deficiency. The tongue has been variously described as a "blotching irregular denudation of the papillae," as having an "absence of epithelial tufts" of the filiform papillae, or as containing "dusky red irregular spots." Darby[2] feels that the clinician should be aware that angular cheilosis and glossitis can be caused by an iron deficiency as well as by a B vitamin complex deficiency.

Dental Caries. McClure[6] found that iron did not have any pronounced effect on the induction of caries in the rat. Iron had both a stimulatory and inhibitory effect upon the growth of oral bacteria when tested by an "auxoanographic" culture plate method.[8]

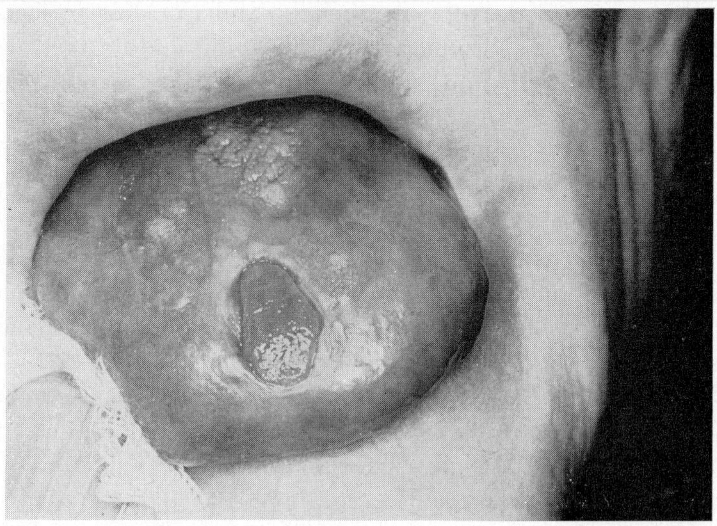

FIGURE 42. Plummer-Vinson syndrome. Glossitis and ulceration due to iron deficiency anemia. (Courtesy Dr. P. McCarthy.)

The addition of iron salts to saliva containing sucrose had no effect on acid production.[3]

Toxicity

The deposition of excessive iron in the body is associated with such conditions as hemosiderosis, hemochromatosis and aplastic anemia.[7]

Hemosiderosis is a disease which is characterized by the continuous deposition of hemosiderin, a granular, yellow-brown iron pigment, within tissues and cells. This accumulation may result from the excessive hemolysis (destruction of red cells) that accompanies sickle cell anemias and from multiple transfusions. Excess iron may also accumulate in patients who, to treat their anemia, have received large amounts of iron over long periods of time. The normal mechanism that controls the absorption of iron from the intestine (ferritin) is either not functioning properly or is by-passed if the iron is given parenterally.

Hemochromatosis, sometimes called bronze diabetes, is characterized by the accumulation of hemosiderin in tissue, cirrhosis of the liver, bronzing of the skin and diabetes. Endogenous hemochromatosis results from a genetic defect in hemoglobin metabolism; the incidence of this disease appears to be greater in males over the age of forty. Exogenous hemochromatosis is not characterized by a sex or age factor; it results primarily from the intake of excessive iron effected by numerous transfusions or by parenteral or prolonged oral administration in the treatment of anemia.

Aplastic anemia results from an inhibition of hematopoiesis. Toxic agents, such as benzol, arsenicals, chloramphenicol, aminopyrine and acetophenetidin, as well as radiant energy, bacterial infections and uremic poisoning depress bone marrow function. Clinically, the patient develops a pallor and tires easily. The red cell count may be depressed to 2 million or less. If the leukocyte count drops to 1,000 to 2,000 and the platelets are depressed, a condition called pancytopenia ensues. The bleeding time is prolonged and blood clot formation is poor.

REFERENCES

1. Anon.: Trace elements in nutrition. III. Iron. Borden's Rev. of Nut. Res., *5:*1, 1944.
2. Darby, W. J.: The oral manifestations of iron deficiency. J.A.M.A., *130:*830, 1946.
3. Forbes, J. C., and Smith, J. D.: Studies on the effect of metallic salts on acid production in saliva. J. D. Res., *31:*129, 1952.
4. Fowler, W. M.: Chlorosis—an obituary. Ann. Med. History, *8:*168, 1936.
5. Granick, S.: Ferritin. IX. Increase of the protein apoferritin in the gastrointestinal mucosa as a direct response to iron feedings; the function of ferritin in the regulation of iron absorption. J. Biol. Chem., *164:*737, 1946.
6. McClure, F. J.: Observations on induced caries in rats. VI. Summary results of various modifications of food and drinking water. J. D. Res., *27:*34, 1948.
7. Robbins, S. L.: Textbook of Pathology with Clinical Applications. Philadelphia, W. B. Saunders Co., 1957.
8. Stephan, R. M.: In vitro studies of the effects of some chemical substances on the growth of oral microorganisms and on their ability to dissolve tooth salts. J. D. Res., *28:*652, 1949. Abstract.

FLUORINE

Chemistry

Fluorine is the lightest and most reactive member of the halogen family, which also includes chlorine, bromine and iodine. It is a ubiquitous element found as a fluoride salt in plants, soil and water.

Source. Fluorides such as calcium fluoride (fluorspar) and sodium aluminum fluoride (cryolite) and fluorapatite are found in the earth's crust. However, this widely occurring element is very unevenly distributed in natural water supplies. There are three million people in the United States who have been consuming natural fluoride-bearing water in excess of 1 ppm. for decades and about five million more people whose water supplies contain from 0.5 to 1.0 ppm. fluorine.[20] At present, as a result of the artificial fluoridation of water supplies to a level of 1.0 ppm., another thirty-five million people are ingesting this micronutrient daily.

Food-borne fluorides are as assimilable as water-borne fluorides but constitute a very small part of the total daily fluoride intake. Foodstuffs such as meat, eggs, vegetables, cereals and fruits have an average fluoride content of 0.02 to 0.70 ppm. On the other hand, canned salmon, sardines and mackerel contain 7 to 12 ppm. fluoride. Milk has a very negligible amount of fluoride, 0.1 to 0.5 ppm. If tea, which has 75 to 100 ppm. fluoride, were to become more popular as a beverage, it could conceivably contribute considerable fluoride to the dietary, for each cup contains approximately 0.12 mg. In areas where water supplies contain negligible amounts of fluoride, approximately 0.18 to 0.56 mg. of fluoride is consumed daily from food.[2,30]

Physiology

Absorption, Excretion and Storage. The results of balance experiments with human subjects demonstrated that soluble fluorides, such as sodium fluoride, were almost completely absorbed and that sparingly soluble fluorides, such as bone meal and calcium fluoride, were less completely absorbed.[34] The rapid excretion of fluorine in the urine and perspiration is one of the most important safeguards that the body possesses against the storage of toxic levels of this element. Experimental subjects, drinking water containing up to 4.5 ppm. fluorine, excreted over 90 per cent of the element in the urine.[27] Bones and teeth contain the highest amounts of fluorine in the body, whereas tissues that are low in calcium do not store fluorine.

General Systemic Pathology of Fluorine Ingestion

There is much clinical, statistical and x-ray evidence that the ingestion of 1.0 ppm. fluoride is safe.[19,21,25,26,28,32] Even with an intake of 8.0 ppm., no general systemic pathology was found. An investigation[26] was conducted in which a general physical examination as well as an x-ray examination of bones was initially done on over 100 individuals in each of two neighboring communities; one community (Bartlett) had 8.0 ppm. fluoride in its water supply, while the water supply of the other community (Cameron) had only 0.5 ppm. fluoride. Ten years later, the same individuals who were still living in these communities were given physical and x-ray examinations similar to those performed originally. The results indicated that the presence of 8.0 ppm. fluoride in the Bartlett water supply had produced only one disease, namely severely mottled teeth. A slightly higher incidence of cardiovascular disease was found in Cameron. Complementary evidence[17] has recently been obtained from a survey of over 700 necropsy findings on residents of Colorado Springs where the fluoride level of the drinking water is 2.5 ppm. The study contained four groups of individuals who had lived in this city for the following lengths of time: (1) less than five years, (2) 5 to 20 years, (3) over 20 years, and (4) unknown length of time. Statistical data were assembled on the major causes of death, such as cancer, cardiovascular diseases, etc., as well as on such incidental findings as thyroid diseases, gallstones, renal diseases, etc. It was concluded that the various residency groups showed no significant difference in the development of any particular type of pathosis. Moreover, long-time residents did not contract any diseases different from those observed in short-term residents.

In a second report by the same pathologists,[18] a comparison was made between the bone pathology of individuals who ingested fluoride-containing waters for a long time and that of a control group; there was no difference in the gross or histologic architecture. The calcified structures that were studied included compact cortical bone, periosteum, spongy bone of the medulla, bone marrow and intervertebral lumbar body joint. Zipkin et al.[49] did an ash and fluorine analysis on the same bones that had previously been studied histologically. They found that the fluoride content of these bones increased proportionately with increasing concentrations of fluoride in the drinking water, up to 4.0 ppm. However, the highest measurable fluoride content of bone was much below the theoretical maximum.

McClure[35] stated as a result of a study on the chemistry of bone from a woman who had ingested water containing 8.0 ppm. fluoride for thirty-four years that 0.5 to 0.6 per cent fluoride in human bones did not affect them adversely. Human skeletal tissue appeared to have a high degree of physiological tolerance to fluoride accumulation.

Exposure for a prolonged period of time to the fumes of fluoride which are evolved in the manufacture of aluminum cans from cryolite may produce poisoning. Gastrointestinal, cardiac and respiratory disturbances have been noted.[40] A rigid spine, resulting from hypercalcification of the back ligaments and general osteosclerosis, is the pathognomonic sign of the poisoning.

Oral Effects of Fluoride Ingestion

Mottled Enamel. Epidemiological surveys[12] have shown that 90 per cent of the children who ingested 1.0 ppm. of fluoride daily

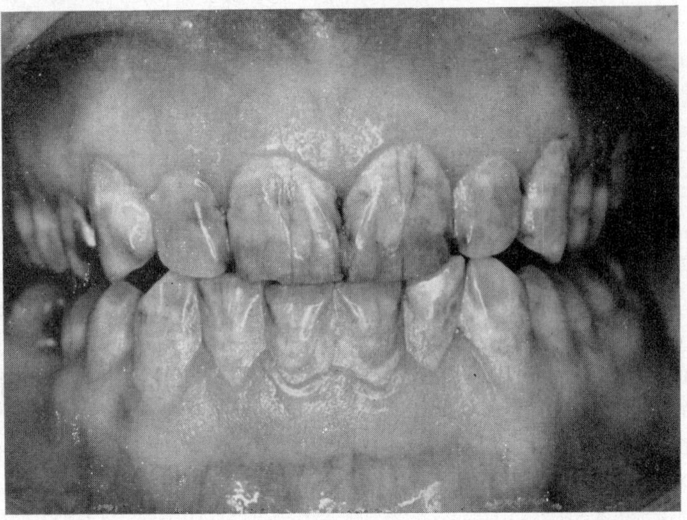

FIGURE 43. Mottled enamel due to fluorosis.

had no dental abnormality. Approximately 10 per cent had such slight enamel change that it could only be detected by an experienced dental examiner. The lay person would not be able to see this questionable or mild degree of mottling. However, daily ingestion of 2.0 to 8.0 ppm. of fluoride will produce varying degrees of dental hypoplasia.

Mottled enamel is usually found in permanent anterior teeth on the labial surfaces, although it has also been observed in deciduous teeth.[43] The teeth lose their normal translucency and appear dull and opaque. Chalky white blotches are irregularly distributed over the surface. In more severe cases yellowish and even brown discoloration (Fig. 43) appears which can darken to a brownish black, depending on the amount of fluoride ingestion. Usually the surface is smooth, but in severe cases it can become pitted, as in enamel hypoplasia.

Microscopically, the enamel is characterized by the absence of, or by poorly developed, interprismatic cementing substance; also the rods are incompletely calcified.[1] Schour and Smith[41] described the histologic dental changes that occurred in the incisor teeth of rats injected with or fed sodium fluoride (Fig. 44). The dentin, which was affected first, had an abnormal interglobular texture. It had wider than usual light and dark layers, corresponding to normal and abnormal calcification. The enamel showed brown rings. The ameloblasts were short, and the epithelial papillae became irregular in number and arrangement. There was a rhythmic disturbance in the appositional activity of the ameloblasts, which produced a "v"-shaped defect in the enamel corresponding to localized areas of arrested enamel formation.

Studies on the Mottled Enamel–Fluoride Relationship. Black teeth (denti neri) were noted in natives of Italy by Dr. Eager who reported the observation in 1902. Black and McKay, at the behest of the Colorado Springs Dental Society, investigated the "Colorado brown stain" in teeth and wrote several papers[4] describing the syndrome, which was called mottled enamel.

Stains and defects were found to be limited to the teeth of individuals who, as children, lived in communities in which the water supply came from deep artesian wells. However, no mottling developed in the teeth of a person who had moved to one of these endemic areas after his enamel had completely calcified.

McKay[37] found that mottled enamel was endemic in other western states besides Colorado, namely Arizona, Arkansas and California. Moreover, descriptions of mottling similar to McKay's findings were reported from other areas such as the Bahama Islands, Holland, Italy, Mexico, North Africa, South America and Spain.

Although McKay had suspected that something in the water supply was the factor responsible for mottled enamel, repeated standard analyses showed no difference between samples of water from endemic and immune areas.

Churchill,[6] a chemist for the Aluminum Company of America, first demonstrated during a routine analysis that there was more

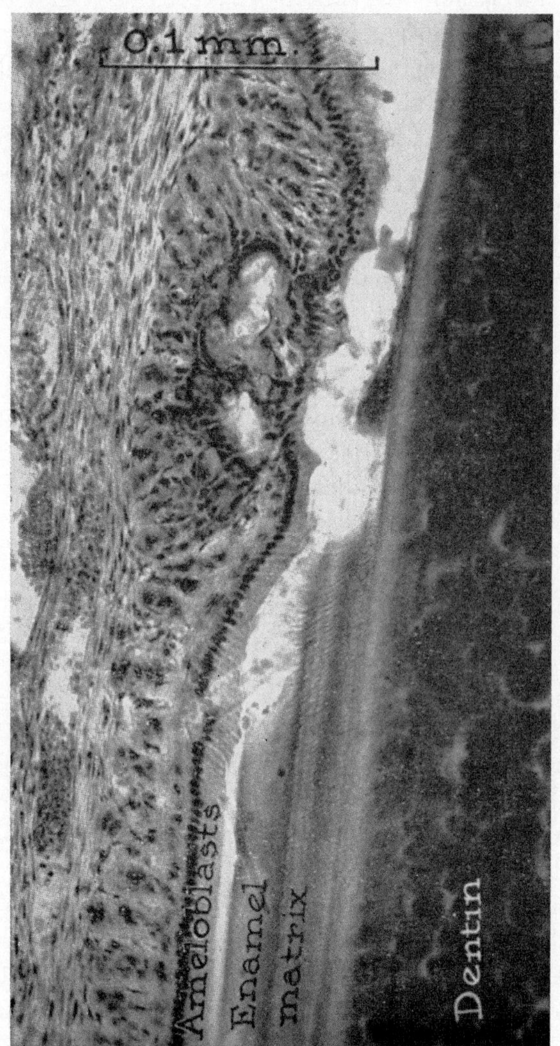

FIGURE 44. Histological dental changes in rat incisor after injection with NaF. Note the persistence of enamel matrix, the stratification in the enamel and the hypoplastic defect under disturbed enamel epithelium. (From Schour and Smith, Bull. No. 52, U. of Ariz. Col. of Agriculture, June, 1934.)

than the usual amount of fluorine present in the water supply of Bauxite, Arkansas. He wrote to McKay about his findings and requested him to obtain samples of water from other endemic mottled-enamel areas. Samples of water from six endemic areas and thirty normal areas were submitted. Fluorine was found in comparatively large amounts in the water samples from each of the six endemic areas but was practically absent from the water samples of the thirty other communities.

At the same time two other laboratories[44,47] found fluorine to be the etiological factor of mottled enamel. Smith et al.[44] conducted a feeding experiment in which the drinking water of St. David, Arizona, was fed to one group of rats while littermates were given drinking water with a known amount of sodium fluoride. Both groups of rats developed the same type of mottled effect on the incisor teeth. It was, therefore, concluded that fluorine was the cause of mottled enamel.

Additional proof that fluorine was the cause of mottled enamel came when the water supplies of two communities, Oakley, Idaho, and Bauxite, Arkansas, were changed. The residents of Oakley obtained their water from a cold spring instead of a warm spring, while the residents of Bauxite obtained their water from adjacent areas where the teeth of the residents had been free from mottled enamel. Eight and ten years later, the children of Oakley and Bauxite who had been raised in these communities during this period did not show the enamel defect which had been prevalent in their older brothers and sisters. Analyses of the new water supplies in each town showed an absence of fluorine.[37]

The Dental Caries–Fluoride Relationship. *Human Studies.* In the latter part of the nineteenth century, both Erhardt[16] and Crichton-Browne[10] suggested that dental caries might be due to a fluoride deficiency. According to Crichton-Browne, this fluoride deficiency resulted from the excessive intake of overrefined foods. However, nothing was done to prove Crichton-Browne's hypothesis.

Although McKay's main interest was to find and ultimately eliminate the causative factor of mottled enamel, he made an interesting observation about the incidence of dental caries in these patients. He stated that both he and Dr. G. V. Black noted a "curious absence of decay" in the teeth of children with mottled enamel.[36] Certainly, the "incidence of caries in the mottled enamel was no greater than in 'normal' enamel."

In 1928 Bunting and co-workers[5] observed that children born and raised in Minook, Illinois, had considerably less caries than (1) the children in other communities, or (2) children who moved to Minook after tooth development was complete. Lowered lactobacilli counts also accompanied the reduction in caries incidence. Interestingly, at the time of the examination, the reason for this difference was not known. However, a few years later when the drinking water was found to have 2.5 ppm. fluoride, it was postulated that the lowered caries experience must have been due to the presence of fluoride.

This relative freedom of decay in individuals with dental fluorosis was also noted in the southwestern part of the Japanese

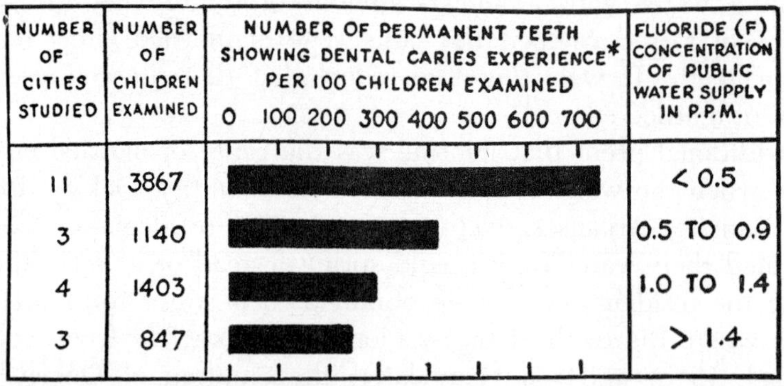

NUMBER OF CITIES STUDIED	NUMBER OF CHILDREN EXAMINED	NUMBER OF PERMANENT TEETH SHOWING DENTAL CARIES EXPERIENCE* PER 100 CHILDREN EXAMINED 0 100 200 300 400 500 600 700	FLUORIDE (F) CONCENTRATION OF PUBLIC WATER SUPPLY IN P.P.M.
11	3867		< 0.5
3	1140		0.5 TO 0.9
4	1403		1.0 TO 1.4
3	847		> 1.4

FIGURE 45. Amount of dental caries (permanent teeth) observed in 7257 selected 12–14 year old white schoolchildren of 21 cities of 4 states classified according to the fluoride concentration of the public water supply. (Dean, H. T. et al.: Public Health Reports, 57: 1155, 1942.)

Archipelago by Masiki and in Argentina by Erausquin, Pasquilini and Celli.[12]

Three epidemiological studies were designed by Dean[11,12,13,14,15] to investigate the relationship between fluoride in water supplies and low caries incidence.

In 1938 Dean found that from a selected sample of 236 nine year old children, the number that were caries-free was much higher among those exposed to water that had 1.7 to 2.5 ppm. fluoride compared to those who used water with 0.6 to 1.5 ppm. fluoride.

The following year Dean et al. reported the results of comparative dental studies conducted on the inhabitants of four cities: Galesbury and Monmouth, with a water supply containing 1.7 to 1.8 ppm. fluoride, and Macomb and Quincy, with 0.2 to 0.1 ppm. fluoride in the water. The caries rate was much higher in the cities with low fluoride water; the incidence of proximal caries of the upper incisor teeth was 16 times greater in the inhabitants of the low fluoride cities compared to those living in the high fluoride cities.

A third epidemiological survey of dental caries and lactobacilli counts was conducted on 7257 white schoolchildren, aged 12 to 14 years, from twenty-one cities having different fluoride concentrations, namely: (1) >1.4 ppm.; (2) 1.0 to 1.4 ppm.; (3) 0.5 to 0.9 ppm.; and (4) <0.5 ppm. The caries experiences, in terms of DMF

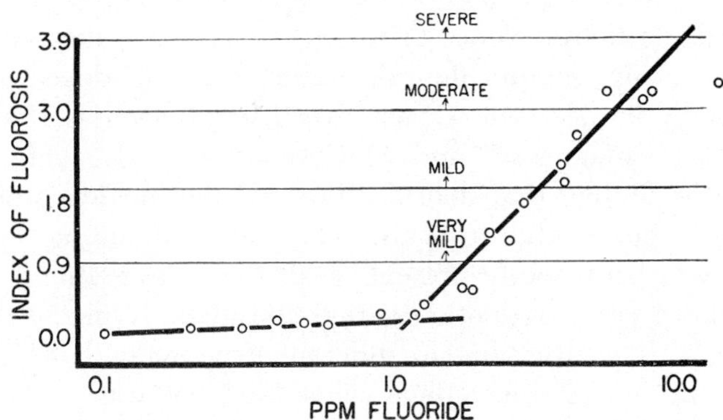

FIGURE 46. Average indexes of fluorosis plotted against the water content of fluoride (logarithmic scale). (Hodge, H. C., in J.A.D.A., Vol. 40, April, 1950.)

teeth, were 245, 291, 400 and 745 respectively (Fig. 45). Lactobacilli counts were reduced in proportion to the reduction in dental caries experience.

The results of these three epidemiological surveys have been corroborated by other investigations on the incidence of decay in deciduous teeth in other areas of the United States. Adult inhabitants of Argentina, England and Hungary, who were exposed to fluorides during their tooth development, also had a low caries incidence. (Artificial fluoridation is discussed in Chapter XVI.)

Utilizing the results of the several epidemiological studies, Hodge[22] related the level of water-borne fluorides with the amount of mottling and caries incidence. In Figure 46 it can be seen that the "index of fluorosis" line intersects with the "DMF rate" line at 1.0 ppm. fluoride. Therefore, 1.0 ppm. fluoride is the concentration which gives maximal tooth health with minimal hazard.

Fluoride Content of Teeth. At the beginning of the nineteenth century, chemists like Morichini, Gay-Lussac and Berzelius found fluoride in human teeth.[9] Later, Magitot[29] related the integrity of enamel to the "minute quantities of fluoride of calcium it contains."

More recently, Armstrong and Brekhus[3] conducted fluoride analyses on a very small number of caries-susceptible and caries-immune teeth. They found that fluoride content was higher in the less caries-susceptible teeth. However, this finding was not confirmed by McClure and Likens[33] who conducted fluoride analyses on large numbers of teeth and found no significant difference between the fluoride content of sound and carious enamel or dentin.

Animal Caries. In 1938 Miller[38] reported the effects of fluoride compounds on the incidence of caries in animals. A dietary supplement of 250 mg. sodium fluoride reduced the incidence of caries in the rat by 90 per cent. Other investigators, such as Hodge and Finn,[23] Cox,[8] Sognnaes,[45] and McClure,[31] were also able to corroborate the finding that fluorides lowered the incidence of dental caries in experimental animals. The caries-inhibiting effect of fluorides was consistently present in all the investigations, but the magnitude of caries reduction varied considerably in the different experiments. This was due to different experimental designs that involved the age of the animal when the diet was initiated, the manner of supplementation, the amount of fluoride and the length of the experimental period.

Mechanism of Fluoride Actions. Once a fluoride-dental caries relationship had been established, it became important to know and understand the mechanism whereby fluorides protected teeth from decay. From this a practical technique could be developed for the use of this trace element as a dental-caries preventive.

The local effect of fluorides on tooth substance was demonstrated by an in vitro study[48] in which fluorides containing the radioactive isotope of fluorine, F^{18}, were allowed to interact with powdered enamel. It was shown that powdered enamel, like the calcium phosphate and hydroxyapatite of bone, could adsorb fluoride in accordance with Freundlich's adsorption isotherm. Even with intact enamel, small but detectable amounts of fluoride ion (0.02 mg.) were found adsorbed to the surface. The hydroxyl ion of hydroxyapatite exchanges with the fluoride ion, thus forming fluorapatite; the latter compound is less soluble than hydroxyapatite. Volker[48] found that teeth treated with sodium fluoride were more acid resistant than untreated teeth (Fig. 47).

Other investigators[39] found that when rat molars were treated with fluorides, they were comparatively more resistant to erosion from fluids containing citrate and lactate than untreated molars.

It is also possible that fluoride ion acts as an enzyme poison by interfering with carbohydrate metabolism, thus blocking lactic acid formation. Fluoride ion can also interfere with the metabolic activity of *Lactobacillus acidophilus.*

Hodge and Sognnaes[24] have offered the following hypothesis for the mechanism of fluoride action: "Fluorine is adsorbed or bound in combination in enamel or in dentin, and probably of most

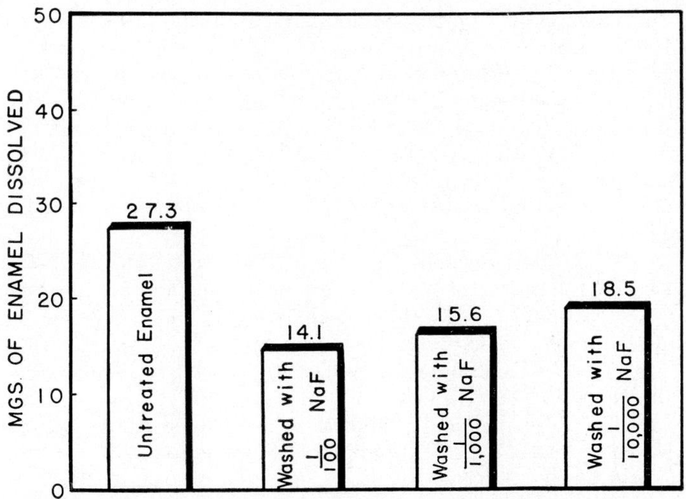

FIGURE 47. Acid solubility of fluoride-treated enamel. (From Volker, J. F. and Bibby, B. G., Medicine *20*:211, 1941.)

importance, on the surface of the tooth, thereby (1) lowering the solubility of the calcified part; (2) giving a relatively high local concentration of fluoride which inhibits those bacterial or enzymatic processes that are otherwise believed to dissolve the protein and the calcified material; (3) changing the salivary milieu as shown by the lower *L. acidophilus* counts."

Toxicity

Twenty-five hundred mg. of fluorine is possibly a fatal dose.[46] Therefore, it can be seen that the presence of 1.0 ppm. fluoride in water supplies leaves a considerable safety margin against fatal poisoning.

REFERENCES

1. Applebaum, E.: Mottled enamel. D. Cosmos, *78:*969, 1936.
2. Armstrong, W. D., and Knowlton, M.: Fluorine derived from food. J. D. Res., *21:*326, 1942.
3. Armstrong, W. D., and Brekhus, P. J.: Possible relationship between the fluorine content of enamel and resistance to dental caries. J. D. Res., *17:*393, 1938.
4. Black, G. V., and McKay, F. S.: Mottled teeth: an endemic developmental imperfection of the enamel of the teeth heretofore unknown in the literature of dentistry. D. Cosmos, *58:*129, 477, 627, 781, 894, 1916.
5. Bunting, R. W., Crowley, M., Hard, D. G., and Keller, M.: Further studies on the relation of bacillus acidophilus to dental caries. D. Cosmos, *70:*1002, 1928.
6. Churchill, H. V.: Occurrence of fluoride in some waters of the United States. Ind. Eng. Chem., *23:*996, 1931.
7. Committee on Dental Health, Food and Nutrition Board: Control of tooth decay. Washington, Nat. Acad. of Sciences-Nat. Res. Council, 1953.
8. Cox, G. J.: Experimental dental caries. IV. Fluorine and its relation to dental caries. J. D. Res., *18:*481, 1939.
9. Cox, G. J.: Fluorine and dental caries; in Food and Nutrition Board, ed.: Survey of Literature of Dental Caries, Publication 225. Washington, Nat. Acad. of Sciences-Nat. Res. Council, 1952.
10. Crichton-Browne, J.: Tooth culture. Lancet, *2:*6, 1892.
11. Dean, H. T.: Endemic fluorosis and its relation to dental caries. Pub. Health Rep., *53:*1443, 1938.
12. Dean, H. T.: Epidemiological studies in the United States; in Moulton, F. R., ed.: Dental Caries and Fluorine. Washington, Am. Assoc. for the Adv. of Science, 1946.
13. Dean, H. T., Arnold, F. A., Jr., and Elvove, E.: Domestic waters and dental caries. V. Additional studies of the relation of fluoride domestic waters to dental caries experience in 4425 white children age 12–14 years, of thirteen cities in four states. Pub. Health Rep., *57:*1155, 1942.
14. Dean, H. T., Jay, P., Arnold, F. A., Jr., McClure, F. J., and Elvove, E.: Domestic waters and dental caries, including certain epidemiological aspects of oral *Lactobacillus acidophilus.* Pub. Health Rep., *54:*862, 1939.
15. Dean, H. T., Jay, P., Arnold, F. A., Jr., and Elvove, E.: Domestic water and dental caries. II. A study of 2832 white children, aged 12–14 years, of eight suburban Chicago communities, including *Lactobacillus acidophilus* studies of 1761 children. Pub. Health Rep., *56:*761, 1941.
16. Erhardt, Dr. (II): Kali fluoratium zür erhaltung der Zahne. Memorabilien. Monatsh. rationelle Aerzte, *19:*359, 1874.
17. Geever, E. F., Leone, N. C., Geiser, P., and Lieberman, J.: Pathologic studies in man after prolonged ingestion of fluoride in drinking water. I. Necropsy findings in a community with a water level of 2.5 ppm. J.A.D.A., *56:*499, 1958.
18. Geever, E. F., Leone, N. C., Geiser, P., and Lieberman, J. E.: Pathological studies in man after prolonged ingestion of fluoride in drinking water. Pub. Health Rep., *73:*721, 1958.
19. Hagan, T. L., Pasternack, M., and Scholz, G. C.: Waterborne fluorides and mortality. Pub. Health Rep., *69:*450, 1954.
20. Hill, I. N., Jelinek, O. E., and Blayney, J. R.: The Evanston dental caries

study. III. A preliminary study on the distribution of fluorine in communal water supplies in the United States. J. D. Res., *28:*398, 1949.

21. Hilleboe, H. E.: History of the Newburgh-Kingston caries-fluorine study: final report. J.A.D.A., *52:*291, 1956.
22. Hodge, H. C.: Concentration of fluoride in drinking water to give the point of minimum caries with maximum safety. J.A.D.A., *40:*436, 1950.
23. Hodge, H. C., and Finn, S. B.: Reduction in experimental rat caries by fluorine. Proc. Soc. Exp. Biol. & Med., *42:*318, 1939.
24. Hodge, H. C., and Sognnaes, R. F.: Experimental caries and a discussion of the mechanism of caries inhibition by fluorine; in Moulton, R. F., ed.: Dental Caries and Fluorine. Washington, Am. Assoc. for Adv. of Science, 1946.
25. Leone, N. C., Shimkin, M. B., Arnold, F. A., Stevenson, C. A., Zimmerman, E. R., Geiser, P. B., and Lieberman, J. E.: Medical aspects of excessive fluoride in a water supply. Pub. Health Rep., *69:*925, 1954.
26. Leone, N. C., Stevenson, C. A., Hilbish, T. F., Sosman, M. C.: A roentgenologic study of a human population exposed to high-fluoride domestic water; a ten-year study. Am. J. Roentgenol., *74:*874, 1955.
27. Machle, W., and Largent, E. J.: The absorption and excretion of fluorides. II. The metabolism at high levels of intake. J. Indust. Hyg. and Toxicol., *25:*112, 1943.
28. Machle, W., Scott, E. W., and Largent, E. J.: Absorption and excretion of fluorides: normal fluoride balance. J. Indust. Hyg. and Toxicol., *24:* 199, 1942.
29. Magitot, E.: Treatise on Dental Caries. Translated by Thomas H. Chandler, Boston. Cambridge, Houghton, Osgood and Co., 1878.
30. McClure, F. J.: Fluorine in foods; survey of recent data. Pub. Health Rep., *64:*1061, 1949.
31. McClure, F. J.: Observations on induced caries in rats. III. Effect of fluoride on rat caries and on the composition of rat's teeth. J. Nut., *22:* 391, 1941.
32. McClure, F. J.: Nondental physiologic effects on trace quantities of fluorine; in Moulton, R. F., ed.: Dental Caries and Fluorine, A Symposium. Washington, Amer. Assoc. for Adv. of Science, 1946.
33. McClure, F. J., and Likens, R. C.: Fluorine in human teeth studied in relation to fluorine in the drinking water. J. D. Res., *30:*172, 1951.
34. McClure, F. J., Mitchell, H. H., Hamilton, T. S., and Kinser, C. A.: Balances of fluorine ingested from various sources in food and water by five young men; excretion of fluorine through the skin. J. Indust. Hyg. and Toxicol., *27:*159, 170, 1945.
35. McClure, F. J., McCann, H. G., and Leone, N. C.: Excessive fluoride in water and bone chemistry: comparison of two cases. Pub. Health Rep., *73:*741, 1958.
36. McKay, F. S.: The establishment of a definite relation between enamel that is defective in its structure as mottled enamel; and the liability to decay. II. D. Cosmos, *71:*747, 1929.
37. McKay, F. S.: Mottled enamel: early history and its unique features; in Moulton, F. R., ed.: Fluorine and Dental Health. Washington, Amer. Assoc. for Adv. of Science, 1942.
38. Miller, B. F.: Inhibition of experimental dental caries in the rat by fluoride and iodoacetic acid. Proc. Soc. Exp. Biol. & Med. *39:*389, 1938.
39. Restarski, J., Gortner, R., and McCay, C.: Effect of acid beverages containing fluorides upon teeth of rats and puppies. J.A.D.A., *32:*668, 1945.

40. Roholm, K.: Fluorine Intoxication: A Clinical-hygienic Study. London, H. K. Lewis & Co., 1937.
41. Schour, F., and Smith, M. C.: Mottled teeth: an experimental and histologic analysis. J.A.D.A., *22:*796, 1935.
42. Shaw, J. H.: Should fluorides be added to water supplies? The Scientific Monthly, *79:*232, 1954.
43. Smith, M. C., and Smith, H. V.: The occurrence of mottled enamel on the temporary teeth. J.A.D.A., *22:*814, 1935.
44. Smith, M. C., Lantz, D. M., and Smith, H. V.: The cause of mottled enamel; a defect of human teeth. Tuscon, Univ. of Arizona Press, Agr. Exp. Station Tech. Bull., *32:*253, 1931.
45. Sognnaes, R. F.: Effect of topical fluorine application on experimental rat caries. Brit. D. J., *70:*433, 1941.
46. Sognnaes, R. F.: Relative merits of various fluoridation vehicles; in Shaw, J., ed.: Fluoridation as a Public Health Measure. Washington, Amer. Assoc. for Adv. of Science, 1954.
47. Velu, H.: Compt. rend. Soc. de biol., *108:*750, 1931.
48. Volker, J. F.: The effect of fluorine on the solubility of enamel and dentin. Proc. Soc. Exp. Biol. & Med., *42:*725, 1939.
49. Zipkin, I., McClure, F. J., Leone, N. C., and Lee, W. A.: Fluoride deposition in human bones after prolonged ingestion of fluoride in drinking water. Pub. Health Rep., *73:*732, 1958.

IODINE

Chemistry

Source. Iodine is found in varying amounts in foods and condiments, depending upon the soils and waters from which they are derived. In areas like the Great Lakes the soils and waters are deficient in iodine; therefore, the foods grown in these areas, as well as the drinking water, are deficient in this element. Iodine deficiency can also be caused by the excessive use of foods like cabbage. This family of vegetables contains compounds which are goitrogenic.

In the body, iodine is stored in the colloid of the alveoli of the thyroid gland. The hormone secreted by this endocrine gland has two iodine-containing amino acids, thyroxine and diiodotyrosine. The iodine present in these amino acids is derived from inorganic iodide salts.

Physiology

Iodine is rapidly absorbed from the gastrointestinal tract and enters the circulation. There appears to be a mechanism in the thyroid gland which concentrates iodine there. The thyroid-to-serum iodide ratio is approximately 250:1 in man.

The thyroid gland controls energy metabolism, undoubtedly the most basic function occurring in the body. Under normal conditions, the thyroid gland contains approximately 40 mg. of iodine per 100 gm. of tissue. If the concentration of iodine drops to below 10 mg. per 100 gm. of tissue, the thyroid gland undergoes compensatory activity; this is manifest by hyperplasia of the epithelium or by excess colloidal deposition.

Requirements

The average recommended daily intake of iodine is between 100 and 200 micrograms, or about 1 to 3 micrograms per kg. of body weight. During periods of stress such as adolescence and pregnancy increased amounts are required.

General Systemic Pathology of Iodine Imbalance

Hypothyroidism. Cretinism and myxedema are pathologic conditions resulting from low thyroid metabolism. These diseases are characterized by retarded physical and mental development. The body tissues have a pseudo-edematous appearance, the basal metabolic rate and blood flow are low, and the pulse is slow.

Hyperthyroidism. In this disease, which is characterized by excessive activity of the thyroid gland, there is frequently an enlargement of the gland, which may be so extreme as to produce a visible goiter. Hyperplastic goiter is firm, elastic and quite clearly demarcated, and the thyroid gland rises and falls with deglutition. It is associated with clinical symptoms of thyrotoxicosis, such as loss of weight despite increased appetite, exophthalmos, tremor, palpitations and elevated basal metabolic rate.

Oral Pathology of Iodine Imbalance

In hypothyroidism, the jaws are small and the rate of tooth eruption is retarded.[8] Hypothyroid patients have a predisposition to dental caries,[2,5] enamel erosion and root resorption.[3,4]

In experimental hypothyroidism, produced by thyroidectomy, a retardation in eruption time, dentin formation and root development was observed.[9,10] Connective tissue of the supporting structures of the teeth showed reduced amounts of cellular and vascular elements. Oral epithelial tissues, epithelial attachment and other ectodermal derivatives are aplastic in a thyroid deficiency; this may be responsible for scaly oral mucosa, diminished salivation, retarded tooth eruption and degenerated epithelial attachment.

Glickman and Pruzansky[6] reported that in hypothyroidism induced by propyl-thiourocil there was no observable gingival disease, but there was a retardation in the apposition of the alveolar bone.

Adults affected with hyperthyroidism show no unusual irregularities in the teeth and jaws, but the alveolar bone may appear somewhat rarefied. There also may be some hypersalivation.

When desiccated thyroid was incorporated in the diet of experimental animals, Muhler and Shafer[7] found that the incidence of caries was decreased. This preparation was just as effective as sodium fluoride in inhibiting dental caries. It was even more effective when combined with sodium fluoride.

REFERENCES

1. Baume, L. J., and Becks, H.: The effect of thyroid hormone on dental and paradental structures. Paradentologie, *6:*89, 1952.
2. Becks, H.: Carbohydrate restriction in the prevention of dental caries using the L.a. count as one index. J. Cal. D. A., *26:*753, 1950.
3. Becks, H.: Root resorptions and their relation to pathologic bone formation. Part I. Statistical data and roentgenographic aspect. Int. J. Orth. and Oral Surg., *22:*445, 1936.
4. Becks, H., and Cowden, R. C.: Root resorptions and their relation to pathologic bone formation. Part II. Classification, degrees, prognosis, and frequency. Am. J. Orth. and Oral Surg., *28:*513, 1942.
5. Burkett, L. W.: Oral Medicine. Philadelphia, J. B. Lippincott Co., 1946.
6. Glickman, I., and Pruzansky, S.: Propyl-thiouracil-hypothyroidism in the albino rat. J. D. Res., *26:*471, 1947.
7. Muhler, J. C., and Shafer, W. G.: Experimental dental caries. IV. The effect of feeding desiccated thyroid and thiouracil on dental caries in rats. Science, *119:*687, 1954.
8. Schour, I., and Massler, M.: Endocrines and dentistry. J.A.D.A., *30:*595, 763, 943, 1943.
9. Ziskin, D., Salmon, T., and Applebaum, E.: The effect of thyro-parathyroidectomy at birth and at 7 days on dental and skeletal development of rats. J. D. Res., *19:*93, 1940.
10. Ziskin, D., and Applebaum, E.: The effect of thyroidectomy upon growing teeth of monkeys. J. D. Res., *19:*304, 1940.

COPPER

Chemistry

Copper is an element that is essential for hemoglobin synthesis and erythropoiesis.

Source. In the average varied American diet, copper is usually present in adequate amounts. Oysters, calves liver and beef liver are notably high in this trace mineral.

Physiology

Copper functions as a catalyst in iron metabolism and hemoglobin synthesis. It is not part of the hemoglobin molecule like iron, but it is present in the blood.

In addition, copper has an important role in the activity of such enzymes as ascorbic acid oxidase, cytochrome oxidase, catalase and tyrosinase. The latter enzyme is necessary for the formation of pigment in the body.

Requirements

Copper is excreted by the body very slowly. Studies in adult man show that 2 mg. per day will maintain him in balance. Infants and children require about 0.05 mg. per kg. of body weight. A copper deficiency in infants is less likely if they are fed breast milk rather than cow's milk, for the former has a higher copper content.

General Systemic Pathology of Copper Imbalance

It was once believed that milk diets produced anemia because they were deficient in iron alone. However, it was observed that hemoglobin could not be regenerated by the addition of pure inorganic iron salt to the milk diet. Hemoglobin regeneration took place only when a copper salt was administered simultaneously with the iron.[6] Therefore, a copper deficiency can produce anemia.

A copper deficiency may cause achromotrichia, which is loss of pigment in the hair.

A copper deficiency may induce a loss of calcium and phosphorus from bone, thus producing a fragile structure.

Abnormal copper metabolism has been shown to occur in Wilson's disease, which involves the central nervous system.

Pathology of Copper Imbalance

Dental Caries. Copper has consistently been found in human saliva,[1] but no relationship has been established between its salivary level and dental caries. However, copper concentrations in excess of the normal amounts found in human saliva appear to inhibit acid production.[1,2]

McClure[5] and Kruger[4] found that copper salts added as a supplement to a cariogenic diet did not exert any significant cariostatic action in experimental animals.

Stephan[7] found that copper inhibited the growth of oral organisms. Hein[3] reported that both copper chlorophyllin and copper sulfate were caries preventive in experimental animals. Furthermore, copper sulfate seemed to affect the initiation rather than the progression of dental decay.

REFERENCES

1. Dreizen, S., Spies, H. A., and Spies, T. D.: The copper and cobalt levels of human saliva and dental caries activity. J. D. Res., *31*:137, 1952.
2. Forbes, J. C., and Smith, J. D.: Studies on the effect of metallic salts on acid production in saliva. J. D. Res., *31*:129, 1952.
3. Hein, J. W.: Effect of copper sulfate on initiation and progression of dental caries in the Syrian hamster. J. D. Res., *32*:654, 1953. Abstract.
4. Kruger, B. J.: The effect of "trace elements" on experimental dental caries in the albino rat. III. A study of boron and copper. Australian D. J., *3*:374, 1958.
5. McClure, F. J.: Observations on induced caries in rats. VI. Summary results of various modifications of food and drinking water. J. D. Res., *27*:34, 1948.
6. Stein, H. B., and Lewis, R. C.: The stimulating action of copper on erythropoiesis. J. Nut., *6*:465, 1933.
7. Stephan, R. M.: In vitro studies of the effects of some chemical substances on the growth of oral microorganisms and on their ability to dissolve tooth salts. J. D. Res., *28*:652, 1949. Abstract.

Chapter VIII

Vitamins; Fat-Soluble Vitamins

Vitamins

DEFINITION

Vitamins are organic substances that possess enzyme-like properties. They act similarly to hormones and, like them, are required in minute amounts. But hormones are manufactured by the ductless glands, whereas vitamins are derived primarily from food. (In some instances vitamins may be derived from sources other than food; e.g., vitamin D may be formed in the skin; vitamin C may be made in the adrenal glands.) From a functional standpoint vitamins do not contribute to the structure of the body nor do they themselves supply energy; instead, they help to release energy from foodstuffs and to regulate body functions.

HISTORY

Vitamins were discovered, not as a result of their positive functions, but rather by study of the diseases that are associated with diets that lack some of these substances. For example, a Japanese doctor, Takaki,[5] attributed beriberi to the lack of such foodstuffs as meat, barley and fruit. The classic work of Lind, reported in the second edition of his *Treatise on Scurvy* in 1757, is another example of this approach, in which the curative effects of "salads and summer fruits" were established.

McCollum, in his book *A History of Nutrition,*[3] relates several fascinating stories on how vitamins were discovered. Several of them are recorded here.

During the Siege of Paris in the latter part of the nineteenth century, because of the shortage of milk and other foods, a substitute formula for babies was devised in which fat was emulsified in a sweetened, albuminous solution. The infants who were fed this formula became very ill, according to Dumas. He concluded from this that something essential to life was lacking in the artificial milk.

In 1880 Lunin fed mice a purified diet of casein, milk fat, milk sugar and a salt mixture which imitated the ash of milk. He deduced, "Mice can live well under these conditions when receiving suitable foods (e.g., milk), but as the experiments show that they cannot subsist on proteins, fats, and carbohydrates, salts and water, it follows that other substances indispensable for nutrition must be present in milk besides casein, fat, lactose, and salts."

Eijkman, a Dutch physician working in Java, recognized beriberi in humans. In 1896 he produced, by accident, typical neurologic signs of beriberi in chickens and pigeons by feeding them cooked, polished rice, scraps from the wards of a military hospital. This procedure was stopped and *gaba* (rice still in the husk) was substituted with the result that the fowl were cured of their paralysis. From this he reasoned that in bran there was a medicine or antitoxin that could counteract the beriberi "germ" or nerve poison. Grijns, who continued Eijkman's work, proved that there was no toxin in polished rice and that the so-called antitoxin effect of the polishings was actually a curative effect resulting from some unidentified essential nutrient.

In 1905 Pekelharing found that mice did not survive if fed a baked mixture of casein, egg albumin, rice flour, lard and physiologically important salts plus water. However, if milk or whey was substituted for the water in these experimental diets, the animals grew well. He wrote, "There is still an unknown substance in milk which even in very small quantities is of paramount importance to nourishment. Undoubtedly, this substance not only occurs in milk, but in all sorts of foodstuffs, both of vegetable and animal origin."

Casimir Funk, a Polish biochemist, in 1912 isolated from rice polishings a crystalline substance which cured pigeons of polyneuritis. Since he found, on chemical analysis, a nitrogen radical present in the curative compound, he surmised that this was an "amine." Because this "amine" was vital to life, he further described this anti-beriberi factor as a "vitamine." Funk advanced the theory that there were four different "vitamines" which were active in preventing beriberi, scurvy, pellagra and rickets. Although these diseases were once considered to result from an intoxication or an infection, he suggested that the deficiency of an essential nutrient rather than the presence of a poisonous substance should be considered the etiologic factor.

NOMENCLATURE

Vitamins were first called "accessory factors" by Hopkins[6] in 1906. Then, in 1912, Funk[2] suggested the name "vitamines" to emphasize that these factors were not only accessory to the other major nutrients but were, indeed, vital to life. McCollum and Davis,[4] in 1915, suggested that letters of the alphabet be assigned to each of the "vitamines" and that, in addition, the descriptive physicochemical phrase, water-soluble or fat-soluble, precede the alphabetic letter. Thus, the "vitamine" that prevented eye disease was called fat-soluble A since it was identified first, and the nutrient that prevented beriberi, which was discovered next, was called water-soluble B. These vitamins were also known by the diseases they cured, e.g., anti-beriberi, anti-scurvy, anti-pellagra, anti-rickets.

Because these accessory factors did not contain an amine group as the term implies, Drummond suggested that the letter "e" be dropped from "vitamine" and the word "vitamin" be used in its place. This was readily adopted by the workers in nutrition.

As new vitamins were discovered, successive letters of the alphabet were assigned to them. However, some letters were used because they were the first letter of a word that described the principal characteristic of the vitamin. For example, vitamin K, which is concerned with the coagulation of blood, was derived from the Scandinavian and German "Koagulation."[1]

In addition to letters, numerical and even alphabetic subscripts were added to identify separate factors in a vitamin group. The confusion was compounded by using subscripts for different purposes. In the water-soluble B complex group, the subscripts were used to differentiate vitamins that had different chemical and physiologic activity. In the fat-soluble vitamin group, the subscripts were used to label closely related chemical compounds having the same physiologic activity.

In order to overcome the general confusion that seemed to be developing on the nomenclature of vitamins, the presently more acceptable procedure is to use the chemical name; for example, thiamine and riboflavin instead of B_1 and B_2.

To the biochemist, all vitamins are chemically and physiologically different. Therefore, there appears to be no justification for any grouping procedure. To the clinician, however, it is helpful to discuss the fat-soluble vitamins as one group and the water-soluble as another, because, in clinical practice, it is customary to prescribe either a water-soluble or a fat-soluble multivitamin preparation. Since this text is clinically oriented, the discussion of vitamins will be in terms of fat-soluble and water-soluble groupings.

REFERENCES

1. Dam, H.: The antihemorrhagic vitamin of the chick. Biochem. J., *29:*1273, 1935.
2. Funk, C.: The etiology of the deficiency diseases: beriberi, polyneuritis in birds, epidemic dropsy, scurvy, experimental scurvy in animals, infantile scurvy, ship beriberi, pellagra. J. State Med., *20:*341, 1912.
3. McCollum, E. V.: A History of Nutrition. Boston, Houghton Mifflin Co., 1957.
4. McCollum, E. V., and Davis, M.: The nature of the dietary deficiencies of rice. J. Biol. Chem., *23:*181, 1915.
5. Takaki, K.: Health of the Japanese Navy. Lancet, *2:*86, 1887.
6. Willcock, E. G., and Hopkins, F. G.: The importance of individual amino acids in metabolism: observations on the effect of adding tryptophane to a dietary in which zein is the sole nitrogenous constituent. J. Physiol., *35:*88, 1906.

Fat-Soluble Vitamins

VITAMIN A

History

The classic studies of McCollum and Davis, and Osborne and Mendel from 1913 to 1915, dealing with the effects of butterfat on general growth and eye disease, led to the discovery of vitamin A.[14] To relieve eye disorders three types of fat were used, namely vegetable fat, butterfat and cod liver oil. Because only the latter two fats had a beneficial effect, the scientists deduced that this disease did not stem from a deficiency of fat but rather from some nutrient in the fat.

Cod liver oil was originally considered to contain a single vitamin, fat-soluble A. McCollum[11] was able to demonstrate that cod liver oil had both an antixerophthalmic vitamin (vitamin A) and an antirachitic vitamin (vitamin D). These he could separate and isolate by heating the cod liver oil and passing a stream of air through it.

Steenbock and Gross[19] made the observation that, in addition to cod liver oil, yellow foods like carrots and sweet potatoes were good sources of vitamin A.

Chemistry

Vitamin A is a pale, viscous, yellow, fat-soluble, unsaturated cyclic alcohol. Under ordinary cooking procedures it is fairly stable, but it is destroyed when exposed to ultraviolet light. In the presence of antimony trichloride, vitamin A solutions form an intensely blue color. This characteristic reaction is used as a means to measure the amount of vitamin A in foods.

Vitamin A has the empiric formula $C_{20}H_{29}OH$ and contains the β-ionone ring. Its structural formula is

```
CH3     CH3
   \   /
    C                 CH3                     CH3
   / \                 |                       |
H2C   C—CH═CH—C═CH—CH═CH—C═CH—CH2OH
 |    ‖
H2C   C—CH3
   \ /
    C
    H2
```

Sources. The liver oils of fish and mammals are good sources of vitamin A. It occurs in two forms, vitamin A_1 and vitamin A_2; the former is found in salt-water fish and mammals while the latter occurs in fresh-water fish. Although both forms have the same physiologic activity, vitamin A_2 is not so vigorous a growth promoter in rats as vitamin A_1. Vitamin A_1 is also found in such animal products as butter, milk and eggs.

Many of the pigments of green and yellow vegetables, the so-called carotenoid pigments or carotenes, are provitamins or precursors to vitamin A. Nine different carotenoid substances have been found to have vitamin A activity, but the four most active are alpha-, beta-, and gamma-carotene, and cryptoxanthin. Beta-carotene is most important because it exhibits the greatest activity. However, it is approximately one-half as biologically active as vitamin A.

Physiology

Absorption and Utilization. Vitamin A can be utilized by man, but plant carotenoid, as such, cannot. The provitamins A such as β-carotene are converted into vitamin A in the wall of the small intestine, esterified, and then transported via the lymph to the blood. In order to assure complete absorption, adequate amounts of bile salts and pancreatic juice are essential. Diseases which interfere with fat metabolism, such as sprue or celiac disease, or abnormal fat storage, as in cirrhosis of the liver, will cause a deficiency of vitamin A through faulty absorption. Other conditioning factors, such as diarrhea and excessive mineral oil intake, will also interfere with its absorption.

Storage. Because of the nature of its chemical and physical properties, vitamin A is neither quickly acquired nor is it readily lost. This vitamin can be stored by the body in sufficient quantities to meet nutritional needs for long periods. In experimental animals it has been demonstrated that the liver is the organ where maximum storage of vitamin A takes place.[17]

Function. The chief function of vitamin A is to preserve the integrity of epithelial tissue. In prolonged avitaminosis A columnar and cuboidal epithelial cells degenerate to stratified squamous cells which become cornified.

Vitamin A stimulates new growth. In fact, it was originally designated as the "growth-promoting vitamin," but this type of descriptive label was judged inadequate in view of the newer knowledge of nutrition; other vitamins besides vitamin A were shown to be concerned with growth.

In the eye, vitamin A is required for the proper functioning of the retinal rods. These rods contain a pigment called visual purple, or rhodopsin, a carotenoid-protein complex. In the presence of light the visual purple is converted in a series of steps to lumi-rhodopsin to meta-rhodopsin to scotopsin, a protein, and a vitamin A aldehyde having a specific configuration, called retinene. In the dark, retinene combines with scotopsin to form rhodopsin, which restores the sensitivity of the retina. This is called dark adaptation, and occurs only if adequate vitamin A is present. If the regeneration of visual

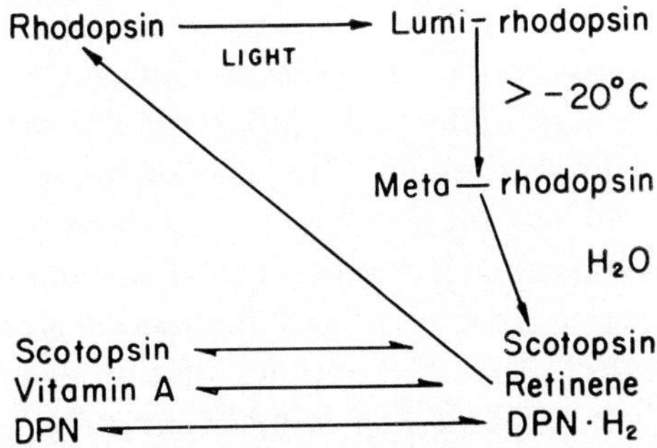

FIGURE 48. Diagram of visual cycle. (From: Nutritional Data, published by H. T. Heinz Co., Inc.)

purple is incomplete, a condition known as night blindness will ensue. This whole process is called the "visual purple cycle."[21,22] (See Fig. 48.)

Requirements

The minimum daily recommended allowance of vitamin A is 5,000 units for adults and growing children. Six thousand to 8,000 units are recommended for the third trimester of pregnancy and the lactation period.

General Systemic Pathology of Vitamin A Deficiency

Skin. Vitamin A deficiency is manifested in the skin as a dryness or xerosis, which gives it a rough, toadlike appearance. There is a hyperplasia and hyperkeratinization of the epidermis and a plugging of the hair follicles, producing a papular eruption; this is called follicular hyperkeratosis. Changes are seen in epithelial cells that have a secretory function; e.g., the mucosa of the digestive system, the respiratory tract and the genito-urinary system, and cells of the sensory organs and the endocrine system may undergo hyperkeratinization. Microscopically, there is an atrophy of the columnar or cuboidal cells with gradual replacement by stratified, squamous, keratinized epithelium.

Eye. Keratinization takes place not only in the skin but also in the eye. The mucous membranes of the sclera and cornea become keratinized, giving the surface a rough, granular appearance. This is xerophthalmia of the conjunctival membrane.

Another common sign of vitamin A deficiency is the appearance of Bitot's spots, which are white, elevated, sharply outlined patches not wetted by tears and covered with material resembling dried foam. The cornea may undergo keratomalacia, a process characterized by ulceration and softening, often accompanied by infection.

Bone. In a review of the effect of avitaminosis A in bone, Irving[7] states that Wolbach found normal intramembranous bone formation with a cessation of remodeling sequences. On the other hand, Irving suggests that the activity of the osteoblasts was uncontrolled and disorganized. This would retard the growth of endochondral bone and even produce a complete cessation of long bone growth.

Nervous System. Because bony growth is limited, the brain and spinal cord continue to grow in a confined skeletal area which produces pressure changes in the central nervous system.

Oral Pathology of Vitamin A Deficiency

Teeth. Wolbach and Howe[25] and others[12,16] have shown that a vitamin A deficiency in rats profoundly diminishes, or completely arrests, the growth of their incisor teeth. Both the enamel organ and odontoblasts undergo atrophy. Irregular activities of the labial and lingual odontoblasts take place which result in a thick labial dentin and a thin lingual dentin. Enamel hypoplasia and reduction in enamel deposition can also result from poor ameloblastic differentiation in the hamster[15] (Fig. 49) as well as in the rat.

Smith and Lantz,[18] as well as Irving and Richards,[8] have noted that the growing enamel of the rat incisor loses its orange pigment, which is the final product of ameloblasts, and turns dull white and opaque.

In children, Dinnerman[4] found, vitamin A deficiency produced atrophy of the enamel organ and metaplasia of the ameloblasts to nonspecialized stratified epithelium in the developing tooth germ. This resulted in hypoplasia. The changes in the dentin, consisting of poor calcification and wider than normal predentin areas, were not pathognomonic of this disease.

Boyle[2] described the following histologic changes in the tooth germs of a 3½ month old infant with vitamin A deficiency: atrophy of enamel and cessation of enamel formation, replacement of ameloblasts and stellate reticulum by squamous epithelium, defectively calcified dentin, and wide predentin with capillary cell inclusions.

There were no dental changes in a number of children who had the characteristic clinical signs of vitamin A deficiency,[1] nor does this avitaminosis have an effect on dental caries incidence.[10]

Periodontium. Several investigators[3,9,13] have noted gingival hyperplasia and hyperkeratosis in vitamin A deficiency induced in rats.

Glickman and Stoller[5] reported that vitamin A-deficient albino rats had deeper periodontal pockets than control animals, but only

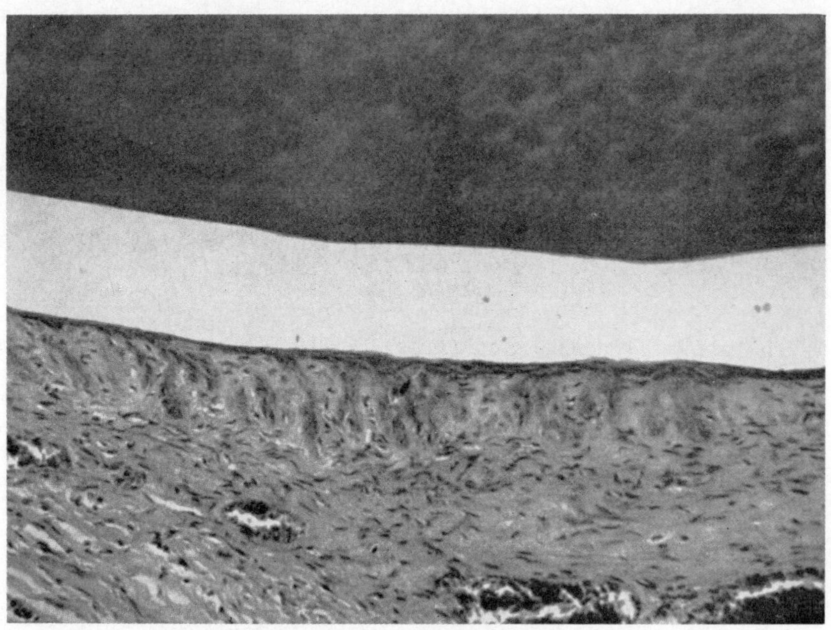

FIGURE 49. Section of enamel organ of the lower incisor of a deficient animal. The columnar ameloblasts have been replaced by a thin, nonkeratinized squamous epithelium which shows peglike proliferations into the subjacent tissue. Interglobular dentin is also present. (hematoxylin and eosin: ×260). (Salley, J. J., and Bryson, W. F., in J. of Dental Research, Vol. 36, 1957.

in the presence of a local irritating factor. These deeper pockets were the result of a proliferation of the basal cells of the epithelium of the gingival sulcus (Fig. 50). However, they did not see any evidence of periodontal membrane or alveolar bone involvement as a result of vitamin A deficiency without local irritants.

Hamsters made deficient in vitamin A showed in their alveolar bone an extensive proliferation of bone marrow cells with an infiltration of acute and chronic inflammatory cells.[6] There also was a decrease in quantity of old and new bone.

In humans, a case[20] of advanced suppurative periodontitis has

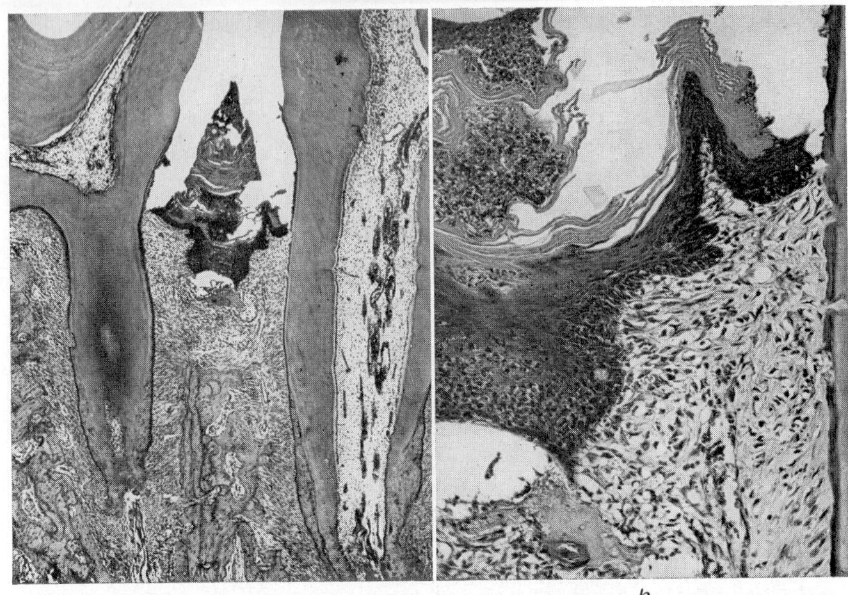

FIGURE 50*a*. Epithelial proliferation, pocket formation and abscess formation associated with irritation from food debris in vitamin A-deficient albino rat. Fig. 50*b*. Mesiodistal survey section of interdental region in area of local irritation induced by inserting amalgam between the molar teeth of a vitamin A-deficient albino rat. Detailed study of gingiva shown in Fig. 50*a*. Note pronounced hyperkeratosis associated with local irritation in vitamin A-deficient albino rat. (Glickman: Clinical Periodontology, first edition.)

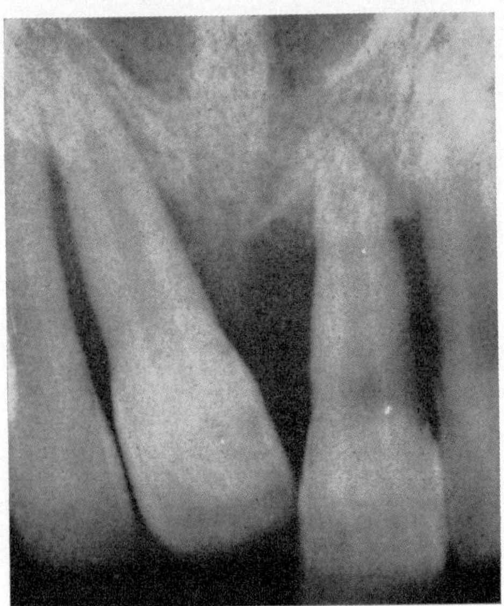

FIGURE 51. Upper anteriors. (Sud, V., in J. of Dentistry for Children, Vol. XXV, No. 1, First quarter, 1958.)

been reported in an 11 year old girl who presented the following clinical signs and symptoms: (1) "toad skin" type of hyperkeratosis on both legs, (2) stunted growth with pallor, (3) Bitot's spots in both conjunctivae, (4) ulceration of nasal mucous membrane, and (5) night blindness for one year. The oral mucosa was inflamed and all teeth showed some periodontal involvement, but the upper anterior teeth had 5 to 8 mm. pocket depths with suppuration. The dental x-rays showed marked alveolar crest resorption, especially between the upper anterior teeth (Fig. 51). By the use of large doses of both vitamins A and D and an adequate diet, plus some antibiotic therapy and thorough prophylaxis, the gingivae improved and the teeth tightened.

Toxicity

The ingestion of 50 to 100 times the normal daily recommended intake of 5,000 I.U. of vitamin A has produced clinical signs of toxicity manifested by drowsiness, headache and vomiting.

One of the more serious complications of excessive vitamin A intake is the possibility of producing hypoprothrombinemia. Carotenemia, manifested by a yellow discoloration of the skin, has been shown to develop as a result of the daily ingestion of 100,000 units or more of vitamin A over a prolonged period of time.

Hypervitaminosis A has been shown to produce excessive bone fragility in the experimental animal. The following microscopic findings have been noted: thickening of the cortex of the long bones, increased osteoclasia, decreased mineralization of the osteoid matrix and decreased osteoblastic activity. Under the influence of toxic doses of this vitamin, bone growth is as great in a 10 to 15 day period as would be expected in a year.[24] In addition, there may be loss of hair, excessively dry, scaly skin and enlargement of liver and spleen. The liver is enlarged because it stores over nine-tenths of the body's vitamin A.

REFERENCES

1. Block, C. E.: Vitamin A deficiency and dental anomalies in man. Acta Paediat., *11*:536, 1930.
2. Boyle, P. E.: Manifestations of vitamin A deficiency in a human tooth germ. Case report. J. D. Res., *13*:39, 1933.
3. Boyle, P. E., and Bessey, O. A.: The effect of acute vitamin A deficiency on the molar teeth and paradental tissues with a comment on deformed incisor teeth in this deficiency. J. D. Res., *20*:236, 1941.

4. Dinnerman, M.: Vitamin A deficiency in unerupted teeth of infants. Oral Surg., Oral Med. and Oral Path., *4:*1024–38, 1951.
5. Glickman, I., and Stoller, M.: The periodontal tissues of the albino rat in vitamin A deficiency. J. D. Res., *27:*758, 1948.
6. Hirschi, R. G.: Postextraction healing in vitamin A deficient hamsters. J. Oral Surg., *8:*3, 1950.
7. Irving, J. T.: A comparison of the influence of hormones, vitamins and other dietary factors upon the formation of bone, dentine and enamel. Vitamins and Hormones, *15:*291, 1957.
8. Irving, J. T., and Richards, M. B.: Influence of age upon requirements of vitamin A. Nature, *144:*908, 1939.
9. King, J. D.: Abnormalities in gingival and subgingival tissues due to diets deficient in vitamin A and carotene. Brit. D. J., *68:*349, 1940.
10. Marshall-Day, C. D.: Nutritional deficiencies and dental caries in Northern India. Brit. D. J., *76:*115, 1944.
11. McCollum, E. V., Simmonds, N., Becker, J. E., and Shipley, P. G.: Studies on experimental rickets. XXI. An experimental demonstration of the existence of a vitamin which promotes calcium deposition. J. Biol. Chem., *53:*293, 1922.
12. Mellanby, H.: Preliminary note on defective tooth structure in young albino rats as a result of vitamin A deficiency in maternal diet. Brit. D. J., *67:*187, 1939.
13. Mellanby, H.: Effect of maternal dietary deficiency of vitamin A on dental tissues in rats. J. D. Res., *20:*489, 1941.
14. Moore, T.: Vitamin A in the normal individual. A Symposium on Nutrition. Baltimore, Johns Hopkins Press, 1953.
15. Salley, J. J., and Bryson, W. F.: Vitamin A deficiency in the hamster. J. D. Res., *36:*935, 1957.
16. Schour, I., Hoffman, M. M., and Smith, M. C.: Changes in incisor teeth of albino rats with vitamin A deficiency and effects of replacement therapy. Am. J. Path., *17:*529, 1941.
17. Sherman, H. C., and Boynton, L. C.: Quantitative experiments upon the occurrence and distribution of vitamin A in the body, and the influence of the food. J. Am. Chem. Soc., *47:*1646, 1925.
18. Smith, M. G., and Lantz, E. M.: Changes in incisors of albino rats accompanying deficiency of vitamin A. J. Home Econ., *25:*411, 1933.
19. Steenbock, H., and Gross, E. G.: Fat soluble vitamins. IV. The fat soluble vitamin content of green plant tissues together with some observations on their water soluble vitamin content. J. Biol. Chem., *41:*149, 1920.
20. Sud, V.: Advanced suppurative periodontitis associated with avitaminosis "A." J. Dent. Child., *25:*45, 1958.
21. Wald, G. J.: On rhodopsin in solution. J. Gen. Physiol. *21:*795, 1937–1938.
22. Wald, G. J., Durell, J., and St. George, R. C. C.: The light reaction in the bleaching of rhodopsin. Science *111:*179, 1950.
23. Wolbach, S. B., and Bessey, O. A.: Tissue changes in vitamin deficiencies. Physiol. Rev., *22:*233, 1942.
24. Wolbach, S. B.: Pathology in relation to nutritional research. Nut. Rev., *3:*193, 1945.
25. Wolbach, S. B., and Howe, P. R.: The incisor teeth of albino rats and guinea pigs in vitamin A deficiency and repair. Am. J. Path., *9:*275, 1933.

VITAMIN D

History

Even in the time of Herodotus (525 B.C.), sunlight was regarded as the reason for bone formation being heavier in the skulls of Egyptians than in those of the Persians. The former wore no head covering and benefited from the sun's ultraviolet light, whereas the Persians wore turbans. With our present knowledge of the role of sunlight in the formation of vitamin D and its influence upon calcification, a plausible explanation of this early observation is obvious.

Since the beginning of the nineteenth century, it has been recognized that children living in dark, crowded quarters and children exposed to the long, dark days of winter showed an increased susceptibility to rickets. In 1919 rickets was cured by Huldschinsky[8] with ultraviolet rays. Steenbock and Black[25] as well as Hess and Weinstock[7] simultaneously showed that by irradiating sterol fraction of foods with sunlight, antirachitic properties would appear.

In 1922 McCollum[14] found that when cod liver oil, which he thought contained only vitamin A, was heated and oxygenated, it lost its antixerophthalmic properties but retained its antirachitic properties. This new vitamin was named vitamin D.

Chemistry

Compounds with vitamin D activity are white, odorless, crystalline substances, soluble in such fat solvents as ether, chloroform, acetone, and alcohol but insoluble in water. They are stable to oxidation, heat, acid or alkalis and can be stored for extended periods in the body.

There are no sensitive chemical methods for measuring vitamin D. Vitamin D assays are done by determining the amount of mineralization in the cartilagenous material between the diaphysis and epiphysis of the tibia of rats fed test materials containing vitamin D. This type of assay can measure as little as one-half of one international unit.

Sources. Thus far ten antirachitic substances having the sterol structure have been isolated. Ergosterol, which occurs naturally in green plants and mushrooms, is one of these provitamins. By activating it with sunlight or other sources of ultraviolet light, the compound D_2 (calciferol or viosterol) is formed. In a similar way, vitamin D_3 is made in the animal body by the action of ultraviolet light on the provitamin in the skin, 7-dehydrocholesterol. Both D_2 and D_3 have equal biologic value for the human.

The structural formulae for D_2 and D_3 are:

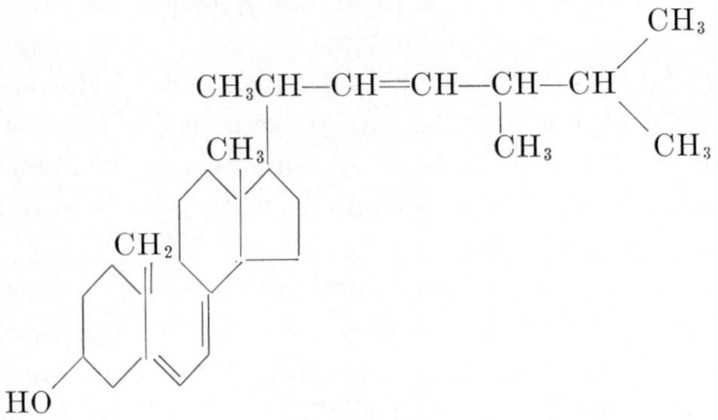

CH_3
$CH_3CH{-}CH{=}CH{-}CH{-}CH$
CH_3 CH_3 CH_3
CH_2
HO

Vitamin D_2

CH_3
$CH_3CHCH_2CH_2CH_2CH$
CH_3 CH_3
CH_2
HO

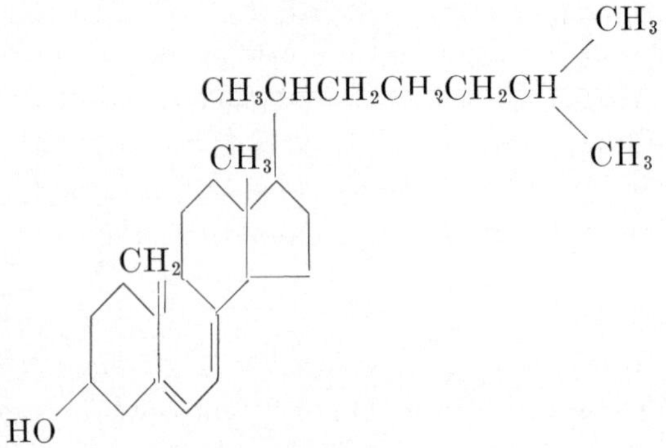

Vitamin D_3

Animal sources of vitamin D such as fish liver oils are preferred because they are usually accompanied by vitamin A.

Vitamin D enriched milk is the most common source of vitamin D. This enrichment process is effected in one of three ways: (1) by adding either a natural or a synthetic vitamin D concentrate to milk, (2) by irradiating the milk, or (3) by feeding irradiated yeast to the cow. The first is the preferred method.

Physiology

Absorption and Function. Adequate bile is required for the absorption of vitamin D. Therefore, conditioning factors such as disease of the gallbladder, pancreas or liver will interfere with absorption.

Excessive ingestion of mineral oil will prevent the absorption of vitamin D because the vitamin dissolves in the oil and is excreted before it has time to be absorbed.

One of the prime functions of vitamin D is to enhance the absorption of calcium and phosphorus from the intestinal tract. It also elevates the serum calcium and phosphorus levels and is related to parathyroid function. It aids the retention of the already absorbed calcium and phosphorus provides for proper bone mineralization, and thus prevents rickets. Vitamin D is also interrelated with the citrate level of the serum. Therefore, bone mineralization, and in fact normal growth, depends on adequate vitamin D, citrate and proper calcium:phosphorus ratio.

It activates alkaline phosphatases from the kidneys, intestines and bones; an increase in alkaline serum phosphatase can be used to detect avitaminosis D.

Requirements

The daily recommended allowance for vitamin D depends upon the amount of exposure to sunlight. It is of prime importance that when outdoor activities are restricted for prolonged periods of time, daily vitamin D supplements of 800 I.U. be given to infants and to women in the latter half of pregnancy. Under ordinary circumstances, 400 I.U. per day satisfies the requirement for vitamin D.

General Systemic Pathology of Vitamin D Deficiency

The classic clinical signs of vitamin D deficiency are rickets in children and osteomalacia in adults. Although the etiology of rickets was not then understood, the clinical signs and symptoms of the disease were described in 1650 by Glisson. It is believed that he coined the name rickets from the Anglo-Saxon word "wrickken," meaning bend or twist. In 1885 Pommer[19] described the pathologic changes in human rickets and in 1890 Palm[18] showed that the prevalence of rickets was correlated with a lack of sunlight. It was not until 1906 that Willcock and Hopkins[29] recognized this disease as a nutritional deficiency. They thought that it was caused by the absence of "accessory foodstuffs."

Experimental rickets, proven by x-ray, chemical and histologic procedures, was produced in dogs by Edward Mellanby[15] in 1918 by several diets. But the addition of cod liver oil could both cure and prevent this condition. In 1922 McCollum et al.[14] demonstrated that vitamin D was the second fat-soluble accessory food factor found in cod liver oil.

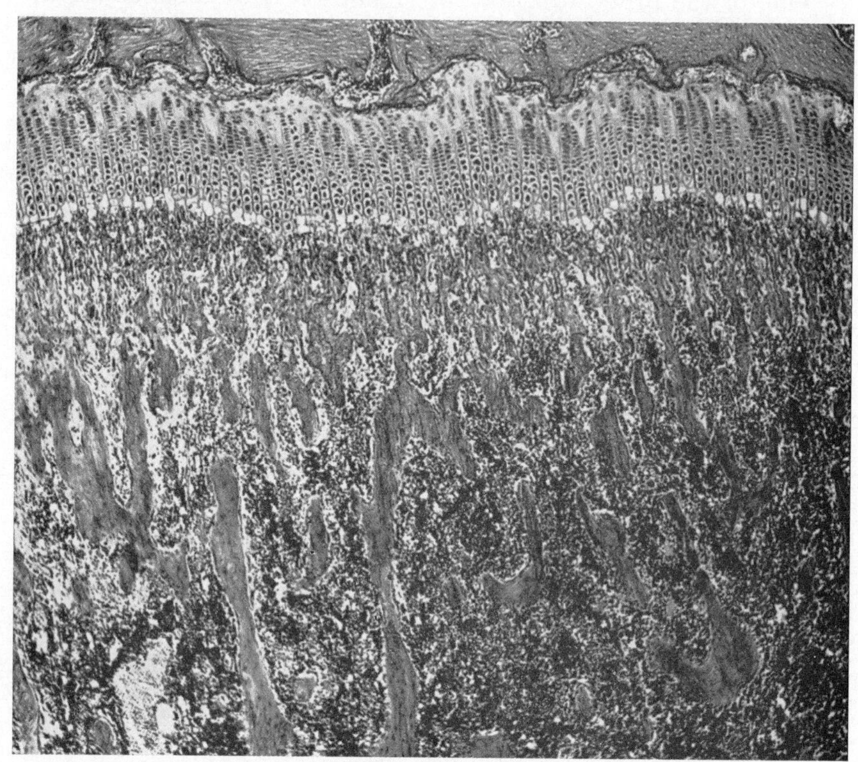

FIGURE 52. Tibia, guinea pig. This shows the upper tibial epiphyseal cartilage and underlying bone. Note straight rows of cartilage cells and trabeculae of bone beneath. The marrow cells are abundant and are found up close to the cartilage. H. and E. (×60). (Follis, R. H., Jr.: Deficiency Disease. Charles C Thomas, 1958.)

To understand the microscopic changes that characterize rickets, it is necessary to understand the normal growth and structural pattern of long bones. In endochondral bone formation the epiphyseal cartilage grows continuously both toward the diaphysis, which is the shaft, and toward the distal end of the bone. At the epiphyseal plate (metaphysis), the cartilage cells line up in a palisade-like arrangement to form vertical columns (Fig. 52). The provisional zone of calcification is made up of these cartilagenous spicules with capillaries and osteoblasts growing between them.

Osteoid tissue, formed by the osteoblasts, replaces the cartilage, and the deposition of calcium and phosphate in the osteoid forms bone.

In rickets the palisade-like arrangement of cartilage cells is replaced by irregular haphazard rows. There is a lack of orderly change from cartilagenous material to calcified bone which is the basic alteration that characterizes rickets (Fig. 53). Mineralization

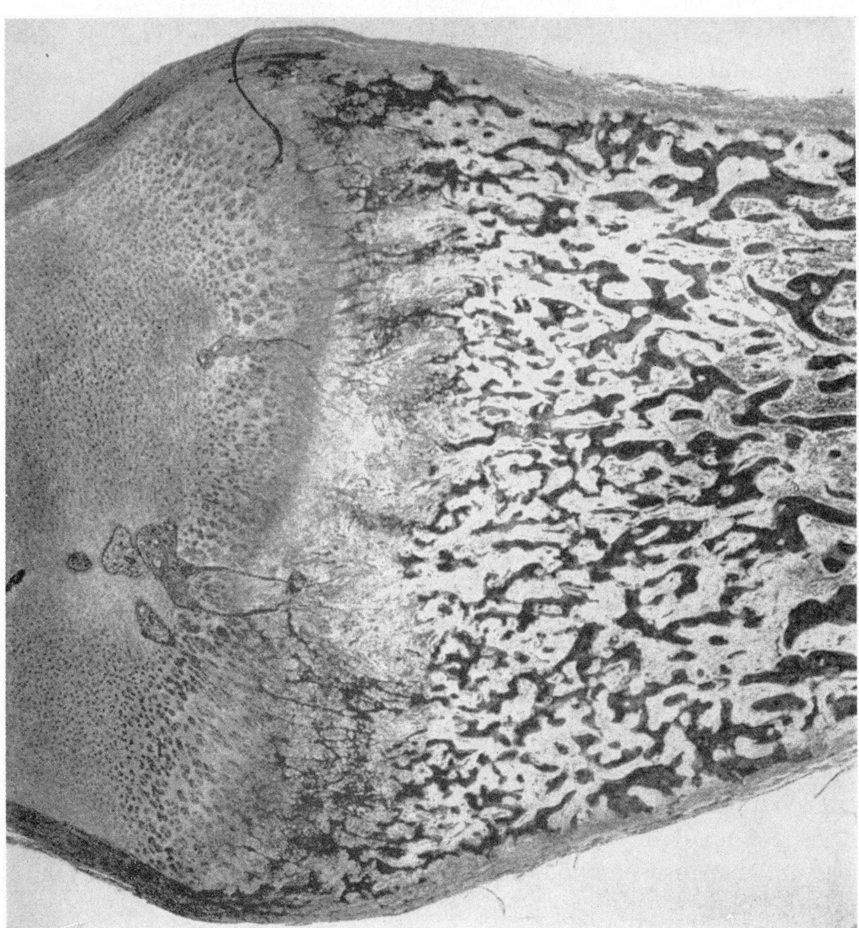

FIGURE 53. Rib. Moderate rickets. Costochondral junction from a seven-month-old colored male dying acutely in three days of lobular pneumonia. Note increase in width of cartilage shaft junction. Especially prominent in the increase is width of zone of proliferative cartilage cells and irregularities in the calcification of the region. Note also tongues of cartilage projecting down toward the shaft surrounded on either side by invading vessels. The trabeculae beneath the cartilage are more numerous than usual. There is a great deal of osteoid on such trabeculae. (Follis, R. H., Jr.: Pathology of Nutritional Disease, Charles C Thomas, 1948.)

of the osteoid matrix does not occur and the matrix is seen microscopically as a broad zone of pink-staining tissue surrounding bone trabeculae. As a result, in the metaphyseal area at the osteochondral junction there is an overgrown and disorganized zone of cartilage, capillaries and fibroblasts.

Owing to the weight of the body and the softness of the osteoid and cartilagenous material, skeletal deformities result. The vitamin D-deficient infant who places greatest stress upon his head as he lies in the crib develops soft spots in the skull called craniotabes. The frontal and parietal bones undergo a thickening or bossing, giving the head a squared appearance. Closing of sutures and anterior fontanelles may be delayed. There is an overgrowth of cartilage at the costochondral junction of the chest, giving rise to the rachitic rosary. The sternum protrudes and the sides of the rib cage are depressed, producing a "pigeon breast" deformity. At the lower margin of the rib cage the diaphragm causes a sharp depression known as Harrison's groove. When the child begins to walk, there may be changes in the vertebral column and long bones. There may be a lumbar lordosis, which is a forward curvature of the spine, as well as the typical bowing of the legs, or even knock-knees.

This disturbed calcification of the epiphyseal cartilage is visualized on x-ray as irregular and broad epiphyseal disks. Decalcification is seen as a thinning and laminating of the cortical bone.

Laboratory analyses indicate the absence of calcium in the urine but increased amounts in the stools. There is increased serum alkaline phosphatase activity because of the increased osteoblastic activity. The serum calcium value may be low normal, and the serum phosphorus is generally slightly decreased.

Osteomalacia is adult rickets in which the costochondral joints are characterized by an accumulation of uncalcified osteoid tissue. It is prevalent in women of the Orient, who have been drained of calcium because of numerous pregnancies and the prolonged nursing of babies.

Oral Pathology of Vitamin D Deficiency

Eruption of Teeth. In children, a vitamin D deficiency retards the eruption of teeth.[24] A similar delay in tooth eruption time has been demonstrated in vitamin D-deficient rats.[27]

Enamel Hypoplasia. The developing enamel in a child's tooth may become hypoplastic as a result of rickets. The ameloblasts are unable to function as a result of a lack of vitamin D and the enamel calcifies poorly and may in some areas fail to form (Fig. 54). The mechanism for the formation of enamel hypoplasia has been explained by two theories: (1) the folding and collapse of uncalcified enamel matrix, and (2) ameloblastic degeneration. It should be pointed out that not all rachitic children develop hypoplastic teeth. In fact, Eliot et al.[5] showed that only about one-third of all the children with rickets developed enamel hypoplasia. Likewise, Sarnat and Schour[20] found that only 1 out of 6 children with rickets

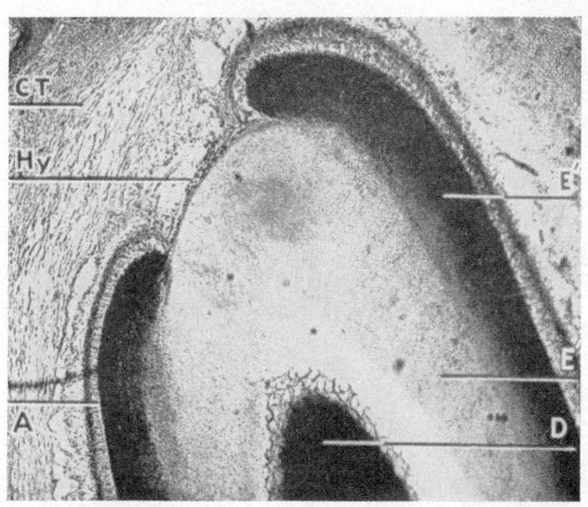

FIGURE 54. Enamel hypoplasia near the incisal edge of a permanent tooth germ of a rachitic child. D, dentin; E′, inner zone of enamel; E″, outer zone of enamel; A, ameloblasts, Hy, enamel hypoplasia; CT, connective tissue surrounding the germ. (Courtesy of J. R. Blayney from Kronfeld and Boyle: Histopathology of the Teeth. 4th edition. Lea & Febiger, 1959.)

had enamel hypoplasia. However, this hypoplasia resulting from vitamin D deficiency is made more severe by concurrent calcium deficiency.[10,23]

Dentin Hypoplasia. Normally the dentin matrix (predentin), which is usually a narrow layer next to the pulp, becomes mineralized by calcium salts. These salts are deposited in globules which grow by concentric deposition and finally unite to form fully calcified dentin. Any disturbance in calcification such as appears in rickets will leave interglobular spaces in the dentin which represent uncalcified dentin matrix (Fig. 55).

The large amount of dentin matrix in the rachitic tooth, like the osteoid in rachitic bone, is the result of delayed calcification and hypertrophy of the matrix. The predentinal layers are widened

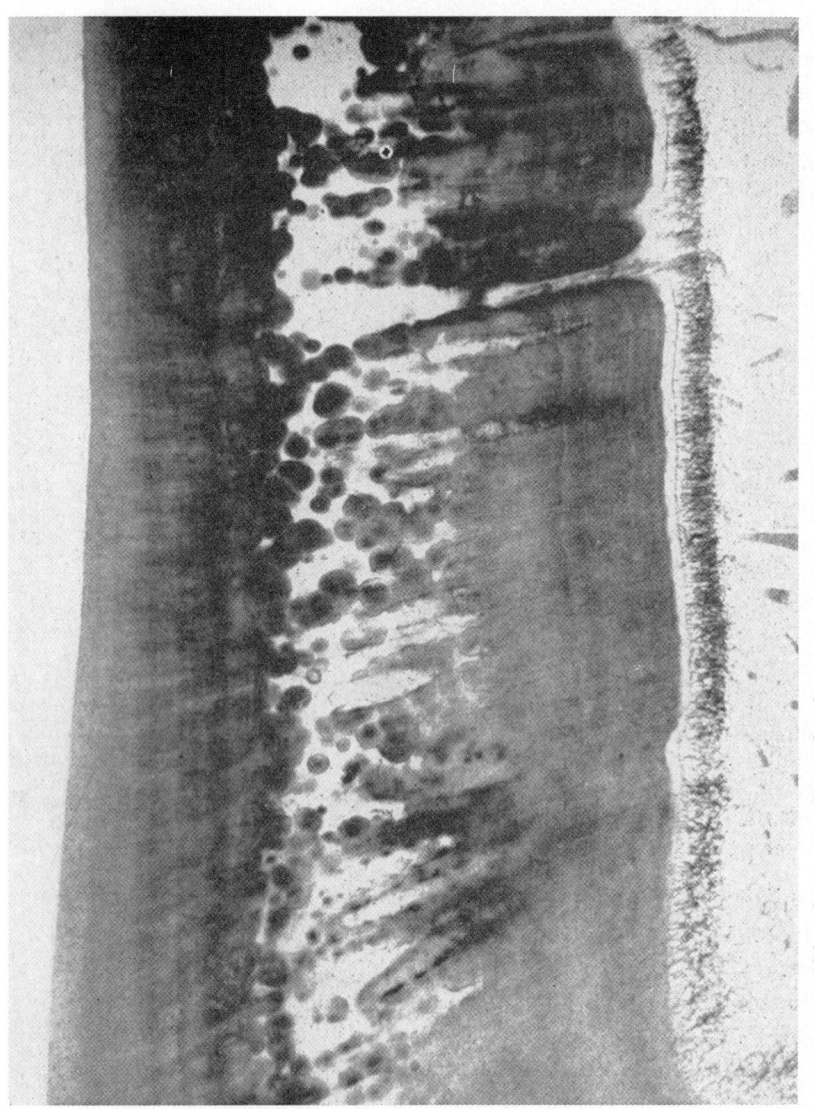

FIGURE 55. Section of tooth showing poor calcification of dentin in dog fed diet low in calcium without vitamin D. Interglobular spaces and odontoblasts enclosed in dentin are to be noted. (Becks, H., and Weber, M., in J.A.D.A., Vol. 18, No. 1, 1931.)

and there is interglobular dentin. In a severe deficiency this widening was found to be as much as 90 microns, compared to the normal value of 10 to 20 microns.[9,26] The appearance of a calciotraumatic line in the dentin is the earliest sign of an acute deficiency in vitamin D.[26]

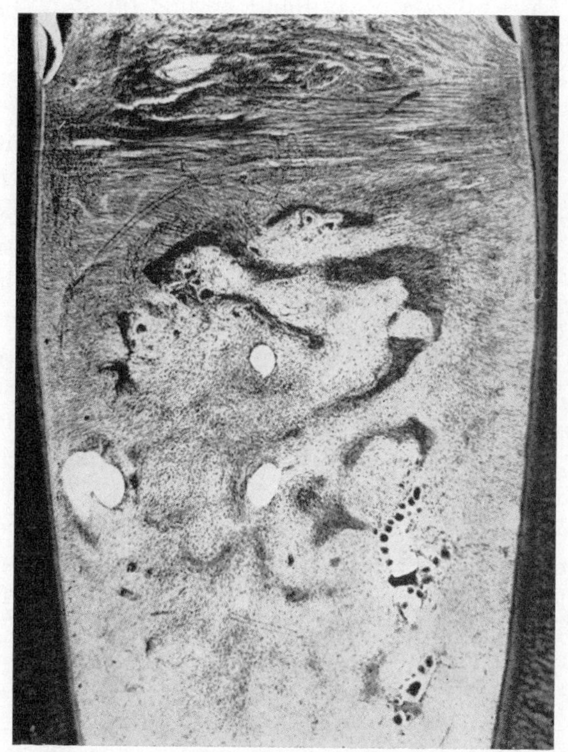

FIGURE 56. Crest of interalveolar bone in dog fed diet low in calcium without vitamin D, showing typical picture of osteodystrophia fibrosa: nearly complete resorption of original alveolar process, new formation of fibroblastic osteoid tissue and poorly calcified fiber bone, giant cells, fibrous marrow. There is loss of attachment of Sharpey's fibers supporting the teeth. Such a picture might explain clinical loosening of teeth (paradentosis). (Becks, H., and Weber, M., in J.A.D.A., Vol. 18, No. 1, 1931.)

Hypoplasia-Dental Caries Relationship. Mellanby[16] demonstrated hypoplastic tooth changes in rachitic rats, but not caries. In spite of this inability to produce rat caries on a vitamin D deficient diet, she still suggested that, in humans, abnormalities of the surface enamel, which were called M-hypoplasia, predisposed the tooth to increased caries susceptibility. Some[1,4] have confirmed this hypothesis, and others[22] have found no correlation between rachitic hypoplasia and caries susceptibility.

Most investigators agree on the basic principle that the initiation of dental caries is no more frequent in a hypoplastic tooth than in a normal tooth. However, once the caries has started in the hypoplastic tooth, it grows and spreads more rapidly. Mellanby and Coumoulos[17] as well as McBeath and Verlin[13] observed that vitamin D supplements fed to children reduced the incidence of dental caries. However, neither Malan and Ockerse[11] or Marshall-Day and Sedwick[12] found vitamin D supplements in children's diets an effective means of caries prevention. In a review of the literature on the relationship between vitamin D supplements and incidence of dental caries, Shaw[21] pointed out that proponents for supplementation have never claimed that "normal vitamin D metabolism was the only factor required for the maintenance of normal teeth." His conclusion was that a beneficial effect will result with regard to the control and prevention of dental caries if adequate amounts of vitamin D are given to children with an otherwise adequate diet.

Periodontium. Animals that are vitamin D deficient will show uncalcified alveolar bone with wide demineralized osteoid borders which resist resorption.[27]

In dogs, Becks and Weber[3] found, vitamin D deficiency produced osteoporosis of the alveolar bone, a replacement of the bone by fibro-osteoid tissue, and an obliteration of the lamina dura and the periodontal membrane (Fig. 56).

Toxicity

Undesirable side effects have been observed in adults receiving 100,000 or more I.U. of vitamin D daily for several months and in children receiving 40,000 I.U. daily. A few years ago it was found that large amounts of vitamin D gave relief to people suffering from arthritis, and many took one million units a day over a period of months. Later it was found that these people developed side effects, not unlike those found in atherosclerosis, which were more serious than the arthritic condition that was being treated.

Huge amounts of vitamin D will induce a very intense calcification of the bone by assisting in the absorption and deposition of calcium in excessive amounts. Hypercalcemia, hyperphosphatemia, deposition of calcium in many of the organs, especially in the arteries, and dense calcification of the bone along the metaphysis are characteristic of overcalcification resulting from excess vitamin D intake. In addition, the formation of renal calculi and adrenal dysfunction are often seen. Vitamin D is, undoubtedly, the most toxic of all the vitamins when ingested in excess of one's needs.

Effects of Hypervitaminosis D on Teeth and Periodontium. Excessive intake of vitamin D will produce irregular dentin formation

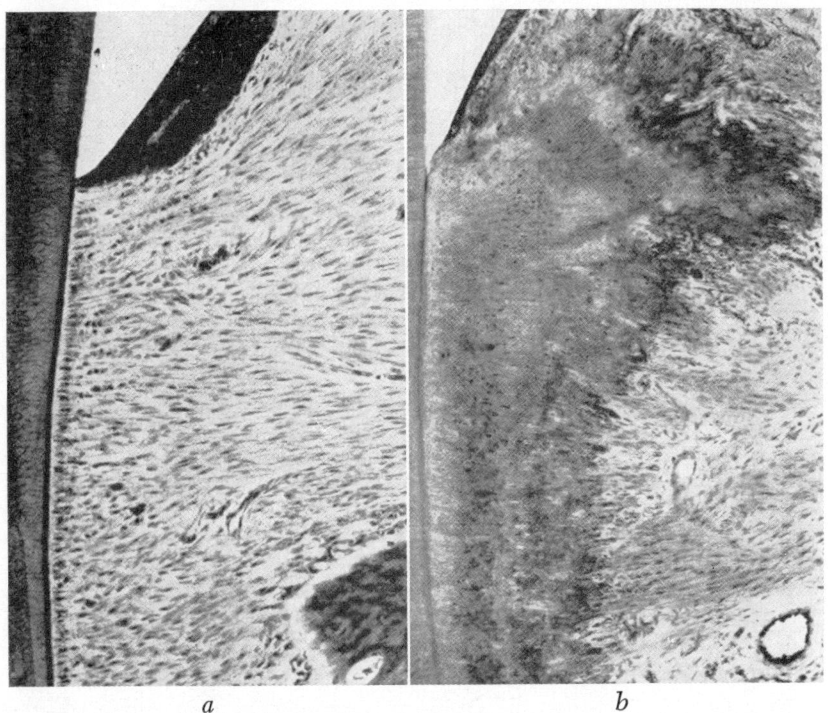

a *b*

FIGURE 57. High magnification of section showing pathologic calcification of subepithelial connective tissue and peridental membrane of experimental dog (*b*) in contrast to control dog (*a*). (Becks, H., in J.A.D.A., Vol. 29, No. 17, 1942.)

and pulp stones in the teeth.[6] The alveolar bone, periodontal membrane and gingiva become hypercalcified (Fig. 57).[2] The cementum increases so that ankylosis between tooth and bone may result. Extensive amounts of calculus may also be present.

REFERENCES

1. Anderson, P. B., Williams, C. H. M., Halderson, H., Summerfeldt, C., and Agnew, R. S.: The influence of vitamin D in the prevention of dental caries. J.A.D.A., *21*:1349, 1934.

2. Becks, H.: Dangerous effects of vitamin D overdosage on dental and paradental structures. J.A.D.A., *29:*1947, 1942.
3. Becks, H., and Weber, M.: Influences of diet on bone system with special reference to alveolar process and labyrinthine capsule. J.A.D.A., *18:* 197, 1931.
4. Bibby, B. G.: The relationship between microscopic hypoplasia (Mellanby) and dental caries. J. D. Res., *22:*218, 1943. Abstract.
5. Eliot, M. M., Souther, S. P., Anderson, B. G., and Arnim, S. S.: A study of the teeth of a group of school children previously examined for rickets. Am. J. Diseases Child., *48:*713, 1934.
6. Harris, L. J., and Innes, J. R. M.: Mode of action of vitamin D; studies on hypervitaminosis D; influence of calcium-phosphate intake. Biochem. J., *25:*367, 1931.
7. Hess, A. F., and Weinstock, M.: The antirachitic value of irradiated cholesterol and phytosterol. II. Further evidence of change in biological activity. J. Biol. Chem., *64:*181, 1925.
8. Huldschinsky, K.: Heilung von Rachitis durch kunstliche Hohensonne. Dent. Med. Wchnschr, *45:*712, 1919.
9. Karshan, M.: Calcification of teeth and bones on rachitic and non-rachitic diets. J. D. Res., *13:*301, 1933.
10. Klein, H.: Etiology of enamel hypoplasia in rickets as determined by studies on rats and swine. J.A.D.A., *18:*866, 1931.
11. Malan, A. E., and Ockerse, T.: Effect of calcium and phosphorus intake of school children upon dental caries, body weight, and heights. S. Afr. D. J., *15:*153, 1941.
12. Marshall-Day, C. D., and Sedwick, H. J.: Fat-soluble vitamins and dental caries in children. J. Nut., *8:*309, 1934.
13. McBeath, E. C., and Verlin, W. A.: Further studies on role of vitamin D in nutritional control of dental caries in children. J.A.D.A., *29:*1393, 1942.
14. McCollum, E. V., Simmonds, N., Becker, J. E., and Shipley, P. G.: Studies on experimental rickets. XXI. An experimental demonstration of the existence of a vitamin which promotes calcium deposition. J. Biol. Chem., *53:*293, 1922.
15. Mellanby, E.: The part played by an "accessory factor" in the production of experimental rickets. J. Physiol., *52:*IX, 1918.
16. Mellanby, M.: Diet and teeth; an experimental study. London, Med. Res. Council, Special Reports Series, No. 140.
17. Mellanby, M., and Coumoulos, H.: Improved dentition of 5 year old London school children: comparison between 1943 and 1929. Br. Med. J., *1:*837, 1944.
18. Palm, T. A.: The geographical distribution and aetiology of rickets. Practitioner, *45:*270, 321, 1890.
19. Pommer, G.: Untersuchungen ueber Osteomalacie und Rachitis. Liepzig, F. C. W. Vogel, 1885.
20. Sarnat, B. G., and Schour, I.: Enamel hypoplasia (chronologic enamel aplasia) in relation to systemic disease: chronologic, morphologic and etiologic classification. I. J.A.D.A., *28:*1989, 1941; II. J.A.D.A. *29:*67, 1942.
21. Shaw, J. H.: Nutrition and dental caries; in Jeans, P. C., ed.: Survey of the Literature on Dental Caries. Washington, Nat. Acad. of Sc.-Nat. Res. Council, Publication 225, 1952.

22. Shelling, D. H., and Anderson, G. M.: Relation of rickets and vitamin D to the incidence of dental caries, enamel hypoplasia and malocclusion in children. J.A.D.A., *23:*840, 1936.
23. Sjoquist, P. E.: Microscopic formation of enamel deformation caused by rickets or spasmophilia and theory of their mechanism of evolution. Acta Pediat. (Supp. 2), *19:*281, 1957.
24. Spiedel, T. D., and Stearns, G.: Relation of vitamin D intake to age of infant at time of eruption of first deciduous incisor. J. Pediat., *17:*506, 1940.
25. Steenbock, H., and Black, A.: Fat-soluble vitamins. XVII. The induction of growth promoting and calcifying properties in a ration by exposure to ultraviolet light. J. Biol. Chem., *61:*405, 1924.
26. Weinmann, J. P., and Schour, I.: Experimental studies in calcification. I. Effect of rachitogenic diet on dental tissues of white rat. Am. J. Path., *21:*821, 1945.
27. Weinmann, J. P., and Schour, I.: Experimental studies in calcification. II. Effects of rachitogenic diet on alveolar bones of white rat. Am. J. Path., *21:*833, 1945.
28. Weinmann, J. P., and Schour, I.: Experimental studies in calcification. III. Effect of parathyroid hormone on alveolar bone and teeth of normal and rachitic rat. Am. J. Path., *21:*857, 1945.
29. Willcock, E. G., and Hopkins, F. G.: The importance of individual amino acids in metabolism: observations on the effect of adding tryptophane to a dietary in which zein is the sole nitrogenous constituent. J. Physiol., *35:*88, 1906.

VITAMIN E

History

In 1922 Evans and Bishop[1] discovered that there was a factor missing in a purified ration that was necessary for normal reproduction in rats. The addition of vegetables to the diet rectified this condition, and they called this factor vitamin E, the antisterility vitamin. In 1936 Evans and his group[2] isolated an alcohol from wheat germ oil having vitamin E activity and called it alpha-tocopherol. The name was derived from the Greek words *tokos,* meaning childbirth, and *pherein,* meaning to carry, i.e., an alcohol which helps the bearing of young.

Chemistry

Vitamin E is a fat-soluble, light-yellow viscous oil. It is stable to heat and acids in the absence of oxygen but unstable to alkalis, ultraviolet light and oxygen. However, it is only very slowly oxidized. It is a naturally occurring, strong anti-oxidant, and its presence in oils delays their becoming rancid.

There are a number of tocopherols which differ from one another chemically only in the number and position of methyl groups on the ring moiety. Of the four most common tocopherols, called alpha, beta, gamma and delta, alpha-tocopherol is the most active. The empiric formula of alpha-tocopherol is $C_{29}H_{50}O_2$, and its structural formula is

```
          CH3
           |
           C       CH2
         // \     /   \
HO—C        C          CH2            CH3            CH3            CH3
   |        ||         |              |              |              |
   C        C          C—(CH2)3—C—(CH2)3—C—(CH2)3—C—CH3
  / \\     / \        /|              |              |              |
CH3    C        O     CH3             H              H              H
       |
      CH3
```

α-Tocopherol

Source. Tocopherols are present in large amounts in the germ portion of cereals which are used for human consumption, as, for example, wheat germ oil. It is also found in cottonseed oil, corn oil and peanut oil, but not in olive oil. The green-leaved plants, meat, butter, milk, eggs and fish liver oils are additional sources of vitamin E. Because vitamin E is so widely distributed in these common foods and because it is stored in fat depots and the liver for long periods of time, a frank deficiency state in human beings is unlikely.

Physiology

Absorption and Function. As in the case of other fat-soluble vitamins, the presence of bile salts and fats is desirable for absorption.

One of the chief positive biochemical functions of vitamin E is to serve as an antioxidant. The tocopherols, by accepting oxygen, protect other unsaturated compounds in the body against destruction. For example, they protect unsaturated fatty acids, ascorbic acid and vitamin A against destruction in the body.

It has been shown recently that the synthesis of some of the adrenocortical hormones requires vitamin E. In this case it acts as a coenzyme.

There are several other functions of vitamin E that might be mentioned: (1) it promotes normal reproduction in many animals; (2) it is involved in cell maturation; and (3) it can protect foods against certain noxious agents, e.g., carbon tetrachloride.

Requirements

The daily adult per capita consumption of vitamin E has been estimated to be about 14 mg. However, the present knowledge of the human requirements for vitamin E is not sufficiently adequate to suggest a recommended allowance.

General Systemic Pathology of Vitamin E Deficiency

Vitamin E has been called an antisterility factor because its absence adversely affects the reproductive organs of animals. In the male there is an irreversible degeneration of the testicle, producing a permanent sterility. In the female this sterility is temporary because the germinal epithelium can be restored by vitamin E treatment.

Rats that are on a prolonged vitamin E-deficient diet show a muscular dystrophy and an extensive pigmentation of the muscle. This pigment is formed by the auto-oxidation of unsaturated fat, a process which normally is prevented by the antioxidant properties of vitamin E.

There has been no evidence of a vitamin E deficiency in man. There are no definite indications for its use in clinical medicine, and its prescription for the treatment of any human disease needs to await further experimental and corroborative evidence.

Oral Pathology of Vitamin E Deficiency

Pindborg[4] described the histologic changes in the enamel organ of animals that had been subjected to a vitamin E deficiency as consisting of damage to the capillaries, edema and disorganization of both the stratum intermedium and outer enamel epithelium (the papillary layer). The ameloblasts were disarranged and, because they piled up and folded, they formed cystic cavities (Fig. 58).

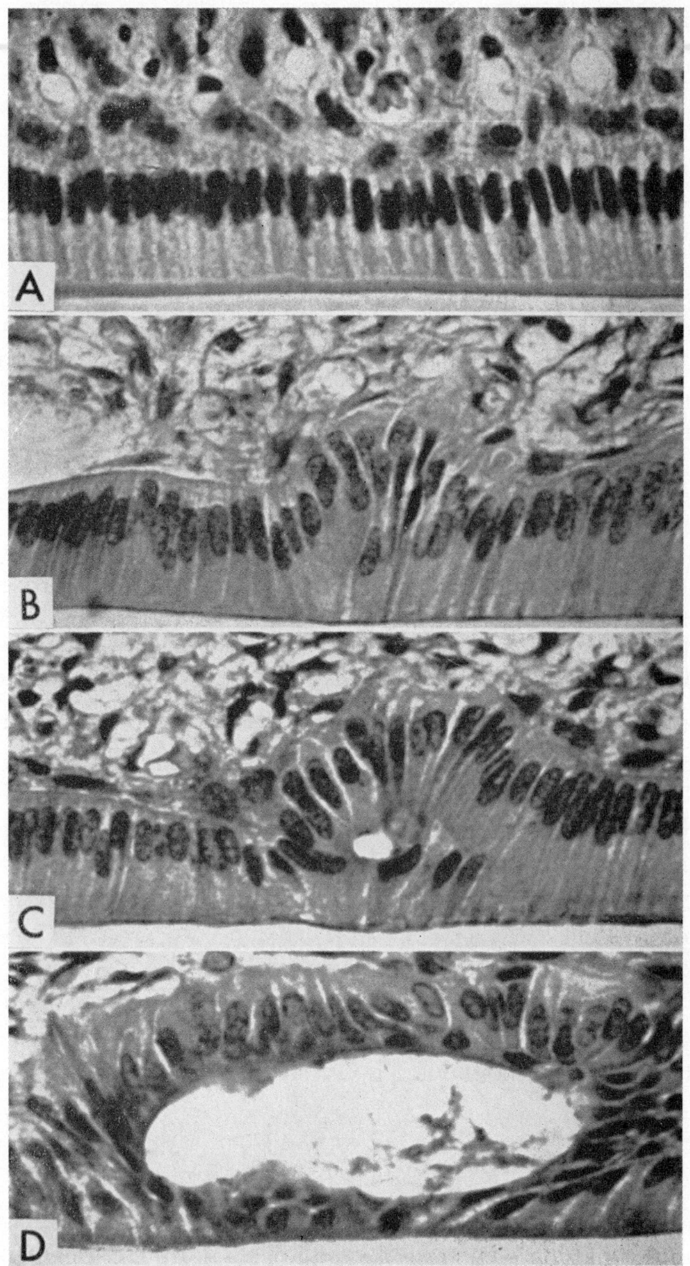

FIGURE 58. Photomicrographs of the middle third of the enamel organ of upper incisors. Orig. mag. ×600.

A. Control rat receiving stock diet.

B. Rat (No. 437) receiving vitamin E-deficient diet (Group A) for 213 days. Note piling up of ameloblasts into edamatous tissue.

C. Rat (No. 437) receiving vitamin E-deficient diet (Group A) for 213 days. Note that folding of ameloblasts has progressed.

D. Rat (No. 437) receiving vitamin E-deficient diet (Group A) for 213 days. Note cavity formed by folding ameloblasts.

(Pindborg, J. J., in J. D. Res., Vol. 31, No. 6, 1952.)

Grossly, a chalky white depigmentation appeared on the continuously growing incisor of the rat.[3]

The significance of these chemical and histopathologic manifestations of vitamin E deficiency in tooth structure is not clearly associated with its resistance or susceptibility to dental caries.

REFERENCES

1. Evans, H. M., and Bishop, K. S.: On the existence of a hitherto unrecognized dietary factor essential for reproduction. Science, *56:*650, 1922.
2. Evans, H. M., Emerson, O. H., and Emerson, G. A.: The isolation from wheat germ oil of an alcohol, x-tocopherol, having the properties of vitamin E. J. Biol. Chem., *113:*319, 1936.
3. Granados, H., and Dam, H.: Inhibition of pigment deposition in incisor teeth of rats deficient in vitamin E from birth. Proc. Soc. Exp. Biol. & Med., *59:*295, 1945.
4. Pindborg, J. J.: The effect of vitamin E deficiency on the rat incisor. J. D. Res., *31:*805, 1952.

VITAMIN K

History

As a result of investigations of a deficiency disease which produced hemorrhagic symptoms in chicks, Dam, a Danish investigator, discovered vitamin K.[2] This vitamin, according to Dam[3] was concerned with coagulation or, more accurately, prothrombin time There are two natural sources of vitamin K; vitamin K_1 is found in food, whereas vitamin K_2 is produced by bacterial synthesis in the intestinal tract.

Chemistry

Vitamin K is fat-soluble, stable to heat and reducing agents but sensitive to light, alkalis, strong acids and oxidizing agents.

Sources. Vitamin K is found in alfalfa, cabbage, spinach and other green vegetables, as well as tomato, cheese, egg yolk and liver.

The most potent source of vitamin K_1 is alfalfa meal, from which the vitamin was extracted and chemically identified as 2-methyl-3-phytyl-1, 4-naphthoquinone. Its empiric formula is $C_{13}H_{46}O_2$. In clinical practice menadione (2-methyl-1, 4-naphthoquinone), a synthetic preparation, is widely used.

The structural formulae are:

```
        H     O
        |     ‖
        C     C
      //  \  /  \
  H—C      C      C—CH₃     CH₃        CH₃           CH₃           CH₃
    |      ‖      ‖         |          |             |             |
  H—C      C      C—CH₂—CH=C—(CH₂)₃—CH—(CH₂)₃—CH—(CH₂)₃—CH—CH₃
      \\  /  \  /
        C     C
        |     ‖
        H     O
```

Vitamin K
(2-methyl-3-phytyl-1, 4-naphthoquinone)

```
        H     O
        |     ‖
        C     C
      //  \  /  \
  H—C      C      C—CH₃
    |      ‖      ‖
  H—C      C      C—H
      \\  /  \  /
        C     C
        |     ‖
        H     O
```

Menadione
(2-methyl-1, 4-naphthoquinone)

Physiology

Absorption. As with other fat-soluble vitamins, bile is required for absorption of vitamin K. Biliary tract diseases will condition a vitamin K deficiency. The presence of adequate bile is so vital that the oral ingestion of the synthetic preparation must be accompanied by bile salts. However, when water-soluble analogues of vitamin K are prescribed, this is not necessary.

Function. Vitamin K is essential for the maintenance of a normal prothrombin level in the blood plasma even though it is not part of the prothrombin molecule. Because prothrombin is necessary for the production of thrombin which, in turn, reacts with fibrinogen to produce fibrin, a vitamin K deficiency will reduce blood coagulability with consequent increased bleeding.

The process of formation of a fibrin clot may be expressed as follows:

1. Prothrombin + thromboplastin + calcium → thrombin
2. Thrombin + fibrinogen → fibrin clot

Another function of vitamin K is to stimulate gastric secretion which will counteract achlorhydria or hypoacidity of the stomach.

Requirements

The practice of routine maternal or neonatal administration of vitamin K is now being questioned. If there is no liver disease, supplements to maternal diets are unnecessary. In prematurity, however, anoxia or erythroblastosis (which are both conducive to neonatal hemorrhage) may arise. Under these circumstances, 2 to 5 mg. of synthetic water-soluble K may be administered to the mother and 1 to 2 mg. to the baby.

General Systemic Pathology of Vitamin K Deficiency

Since the intestinal bacterial flora can synthesize vitamin K_2, an exogenous source of this vitamin is not absolutely essential. A deficiency, which indeed is rare, could occur if there was some secondary conditioning factor that interfered with absorption of the vitamin. Overuse of antibiotics, sulfa drugs or vitamin K antagonists can arrest the bacterial synthesis of this vitamin.

Clinically, a deficiency of this vitamin might conceivably be seen in the newborn infant whose intestinal bacterial flora had not yet developed sufficiently to synthesize its own vitamins. This can be overcome by administering a vitamin K preparation to the infant.

Oral Pathology

It has been reported[4] that saliva produces less acid when incubated with vitamin K. Vitamin K probably acts as an enzyme inhibitor.

The relationship between vitamin K in chewing gum and the incidence of dental caries in young adults has been studied. After an 18 month experimental period, Burrill[1] reported that gum containing vitamin K was somewhat cariostatic. However, the results were not subjected to a statistical evaluation. In a second experiment performed by others,[5] the chewing of gum containing 1 mg. of synthetic vitamin K for 10 minutes after a snack or meal had no effect on the incidence of dental caries.

REFERENCES

1. Burrill, D. G., Calandra, J. C., Tilden, E. B., and Fosdick, L. S.: The effect of 2-methyl-1, 4-naphthoquinone on the incidence of dental caries. J. D. Res., *24*:273, 1945.

2. Dam, H.: The antihemorrhagic vitamin of the chick. Biochem. J., *29:*1273, 1935.
3. Dam, H., and Schonheyder, F.: A deficiency disease in chicks resembling scurvy. Biochem. J., *28:*1355, 1934.
4. Fosdick, L. S., Fancher, O. E., and Calandra, J. C.: The effect of synthetic vitamin K on the rate of acid formation in the mouth. Science, *96:*45, 1942.
5. Medical Department Professional Service Schools. Bull. Y. S., Army Med. Dept., *5:*265, 1946.

Chapter IX

Water-Soluble Vitamins

VITAMIN C (L-ASCORBIC ACID)

History

From the fifteenth to the eighteenth century new lands were being discovered and explorers like Vasco da Gamma and Jacques Cartier were sailing into new waters. The storage of perishable foods for these long voyages was impossible; fresh fruits and vegetables were not included in the usual ration with the result that scurvy became prevalent amongst crew members. One of the first successful attempts to cure this disease was made by Jacques Cartier during his explorations in Canada. The local Indians suggested that he treat his sick expeditioners with a brew of pine needles and pine bark, which proved to be very helpful.

In the middle of the eighteenth century, James Lind, an English surgeon, gave lemons and oranges to two scorbutic sailors. To ten others who had succumbed to the disease, he fed either cider, cream of tartar or other drugs. He noted that those who received the citrus fruit made a complete recovery, and those offered the cider made only a slight improvement, whereas the men treated with other drugs became worse. Lind was scientific enough not only to conduct such a controlled experiment but also to write a treatise on it, which was published in 1753.[14] The importance of Lind's findings were so far-reaching that the British government decreed that limes be included in the daily ration of every British sailor. This is the reason that British sailors, even today, are referred to as "limeys."

Chemistry

Ascorbic acid is a colorless crystalline solid which is freely soluble in water but insoluble in fat solvents. In solution, its *p*H is between 1 and 2; it behaves, and even tastes, like an acid. When slight amounts of alkali are added to vitamin C solution, the vitamin becomes unstable. The most outstanding physical characteristic of this vitamin is its extreme sensitivity to oxidation, particularly in the presence of copper or iron. It is changed so rapidly in the presence of air, light and heat that much of it is usually found in the oxidized form, dehydroascorbic acid. The employment of the most rigidly supervised processing and storage techniques is required to maintain vitamin C in its biologically active form in foods. Freezing has no deleterious effect on this vitamin. When foods containing ascorbic acid are cooked, it is recommended that closed vessels such as a pressure cooker be used and that water be slightly acidified. The use of open vessels or copper utensils, or the addition of soda to the cooking water, promotes the oxidation and subsequent loss of vitamin C.

Source. Parsley and green peppers are two of the richest sources of vitamin C on a gram per gram basis, but they are not too widely consumed. The more popular good sources of ascorbic acid are the citrus fruits (oranges, grapefruit, lemons and limes) tomatoes, cantaloupe and strawberries. Cooked vegetables such as spinach, cabbage, turnips, potatoes, peas and asparagus also contain this vitamin but in smaller amounts.

Human milk contains a fair supply of vitamin C if the mother eats an abundance of raw fruits and vegetables. On the other hand, cow's milk usually contains very little vitamin C. This means that babies who receive a milk formula require another source of vitamin C. Orange juice is usually offered the baby by the time it is a month old.

Structure. Chemically, ascorbic acid is 2, 3-dienol-1-gulonic acid lactone, a hexose derivative. In the presence of indophenol dyes, iodine, oxygen and other oxidizing agents, two hydrogen atoms are given up and the acid is oxidized to dehydroascorbic acid. This is a reversible reaction because dehydroascorbic acid can be reduced by H_2S and other reducing substances and changed back to ascorbic acid. In fact, to determine the vitamin C activity of a food, the sum of both the ascorbic and dehydroascorbic acid contents is measured.

The structural formulae for L-ascorbic acid and dehydro-L-ascorbic acid are:

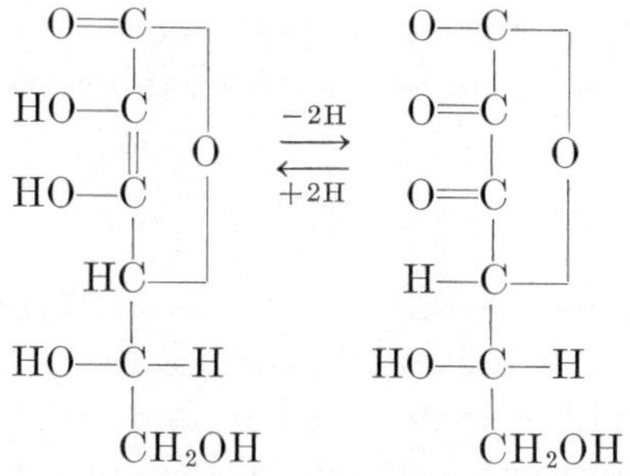

```
     O=C──┐                 O─C──┐
       |  |                   |  |
   HO─C   |      -2H        O=C  |
      ||  O     ──→             |  O
   HO─C   |     ←──         O=C  |
       |  |      +2H            |  |
     HC──┘                  H─C──┘
       |                        |
   HO─C─H                  HO─C─H
       |                        |
     CH2OH                    CH2OH
 L-ascorbic acid     Dehydro-L-ascorbic acid
```

Physiology

Ascorbic acid is rapidly absorbed from the small intestines and passed through the portal system into the general circulation. It is stored in the pituitary, adrenal cortex and many other organs. The signs of a deficiency take many months to become clinically visible.

The most important function of vitamin C is to produce and maintain tissues of mesenchymal origin such as collagen, osteoid, dentin and intercellular cement substance. Vitamin C in some unknown manner participates in the transformation of soluble procollagen to insoluble collagen, a protein which forms the framework for dentin and bone formation. It is also essential for the repair of bone fractures.

In adequate amounts ascorbic acid increases the resistance of traumatized and injured tissues to infection and decreases the fragility and permeability of the capillaries. It is involved in phagocytosis and acts as a detoxifying agent for bacterially and chemically toxic substances.

Vitamin C plays an important role in the metabolism of amino acids, other vitamins and hormones. For example, tissues deficient in ascorbic acid cannot oxidize the amino acid tyrosine, which is excreted in urine that darkens upon standing.

There is also an interrelationship between vitamin A and ascorbic acid. Vitamin C can moderate the toxic signs of huge doses of vitamin A in experimental animals; conversely, vitamin A-deficient animals that have hemorrhagic tendencies can be helped by ascorbic acid. (Other interrelationships are discussed in Chapter X.)

It can partially replace the vitamin B_{12} requirement of some lactic acid bacteria and stimulate the formation of the citrovorum factor from folic acid. The conversion of folic acid to folinic acid is mediated by vitamin C.

Vitamin C, by preventing the destruction of oxysteroids, plays a role in the production of the adrenocortical hormones.

Requirements

Most animal species produce ascorbic acid from other materials and, therefore, are not dependent upon a dietary source. However, the primates, including man, monkey and the guinea pig, do not have the ability to produce vitamin C at a rate commensurate with their requirement; they, therefore, depend upon food to meet their vitamin C requirements.

As little as 10 mg. per day is sufficient to prevent scurvy in man. However, the recommended daily dietary allowance for the infant is 30 mg., for the adult 75 to 100 mg.

General Systemic Pathology of Vitamin C Deficiency

Ascorbic acid deficiency usually results from a primary nutritional inadequacy due to the insufficient intake of foods rich in this vitamin.

Frank acute scurvy is rare nowadays because it takes four to six months of a complete absence of dietary vitamin C to produce an actual tissue deficiency. The signs of deficiency include loss of appetite, lethargy and irritability. The hair loses its luster, and the skin becomes rough and coarse due to increased layers of keratin. There is follicular keratosis. Under the skin, due to increased capillary fragility, there are numerous petechiae and ecchymotic spots (Figs. 59 and 60). The complexion is sallow due to a normocytic normochromic anemia and the loss of blood from hemorrhage.

The primary feature of scurvy is the inability of fibroblasts to form intercellular substances.[21] The rate of wound healing is retarded due to the lack of a collagenous matrix; this impedes the formation of mature fibrous tissue.[1,12] Abscesses are not confined by the usual collagenous connective tissue barrier, and thus there is opportunity for greater susceptibility to infection.[17]

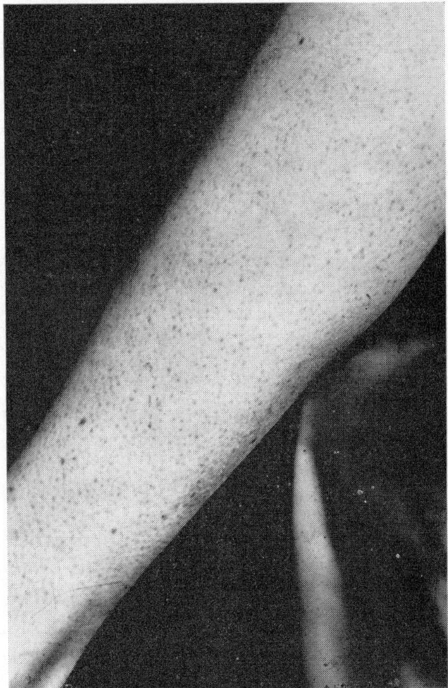

FIGURE 59. Perifollicular hemorrhages on the leg of a boy, age 16, with scurvy. (From the Merck Report, May, 1956. Merck and Co. Inc., Rahway, N. J.)

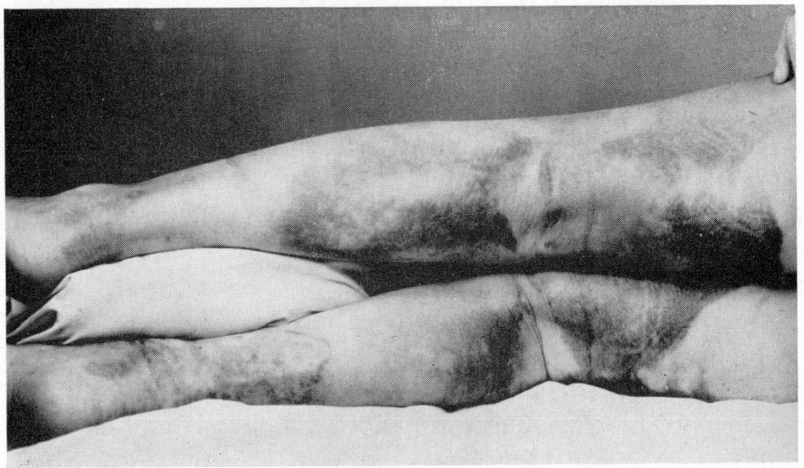

FIGURE 60. Extensive confluent ecchymoses on the legs of a patient with scurvy. The ecchymotic areas were brawny and indurated. (From the Merck Report, May, 1956. Merck and Co. Inc., Rahway, N. J.)

Bone formation is impeded because osteoblasts cannot form a bone matrix. Thus any stress upon the bones will cause them to bend or fracture. Furthermore, the absence of intercellular substance between endothelial cells results in capillary walls that allow the escape of blood cells and serum into the subcutaneous tissues. If this blood extravasation burrows under the periostium, it will produce subperiosteal hematomas. This is manifest clinically by pain and swelling in the femur and humerus. Infants will show enlargement of the costochondral junction.

The following x-ray findings are seen in infantile scurvy: thickening of the epiphyseal plate or "white line" at the ends of long bones; a "halo" appearance of the epiphyses; a zone of rarefaction immediately shaftward of the "white line"; a separation of the epiphyses; spur formation; a ground glass appearance of the shaft; and a thinning of the cortex.

Often no clinical signs of scurvy accompany laboratory findings which show that the ascorbic acid plasma level is zero. A truer index of ascorbic acid deficiency may be obtained by determining the concentration of the vitamin in the white cell-platelet layer of centrifuged blood; levels below 0.1 mg. per cent usually indicate scurvy. As a rule, other blood findings are normal, with the possible exception that the bleeding and the coagulation times may be prolonged.

Oral Pathology of Vitamin C Deficiency

Teeth. Because the guinea pig incisor tooth grows so rapidly (2 mm. each week), it is most suitable for studying the effects of reduced ascorbic intake. The amount of dentin formation as shown by the alizarin technique is a measure of the adequacy of ascorbic acid intake.[5] A scorbutic diet will cause the odontoblasts to atrophy so that their orderly palisade arrangement is replaced by a haphazard irregularity.[16] (See Fig. 61.) The malfunctioning of the odontoblasts produces an irregular dentin or no dentin at all. The replacement dentin is of the osteodentin type. The pulp is usually engorged and dilated from the increased blood. A few of the odontoblasts form some isolated dentin which becomes entrapped in the pulp. The ameloblasts are affected adversely and eventually atrophy.[4]

Boyle[3] examined histologic sections of teeth from a scorbutic infant and reported the presence of some small cysts and slight hemorrhage in the enamel organ.

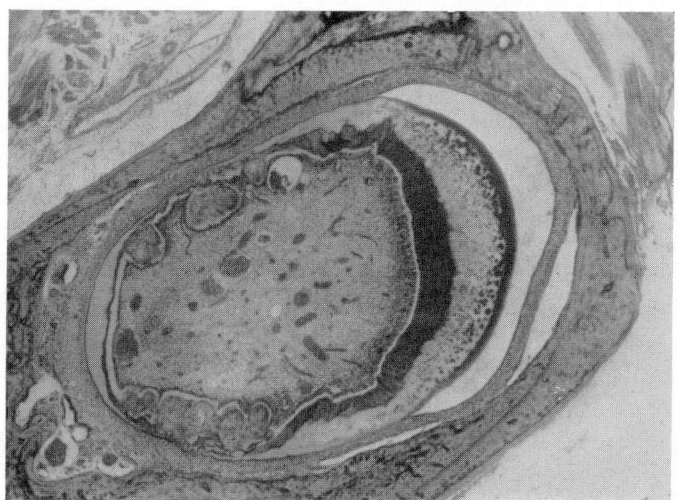

FIGURE 61. Incisor tooth of scorbutic guinea pig. Dentin formation during the period of scurvy is marked by the zone beneath the irregular gray line in the dentin. Small dentin masses are present within the pulp. Odontoblasts are very numerous, palisaded and irregular. (Courtesy Boston Children's Hospital, from Dr. Wolbach's collection.)

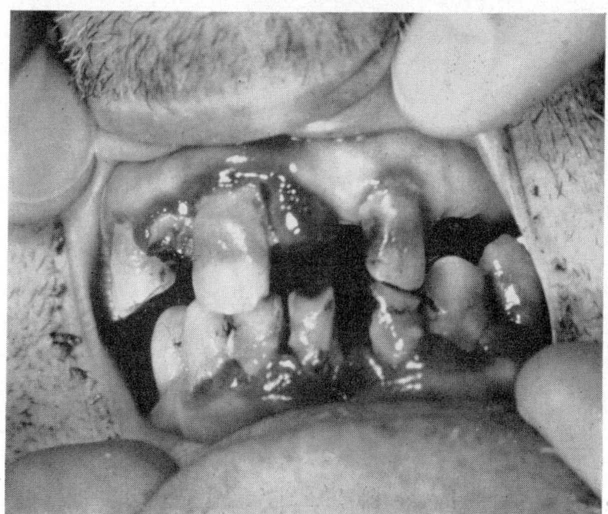

FIGURE 62. Swollen blue-red gingival lesions in a patient with severe scurvy. (Note edentulous areas are free of lesions.)

There is no direct convincing evidence that dental caries is in any way initiated or extended by ascorbic acid deficiency. Hanke[11] has advocated liberal ingestion of orange juice as a possible deterrent to decay and has presented some clinical evidence for this viewpoint. McBeath[16] has not been able to confirm this.

Periodontium. The characteristic oral lesions of scurvy are swollen and bleeding gingivae which envelop and almost completely conceal the teeth. In edentulous areas there are no mucosal changes (Fig. 62). The edematous, freely bleeding gingivae become secondarily infected by anaerobic organisms, producing an acute necrotizing gingivitis with its characteristic punched-out, membranous, interdental papillae and fetid breath.

Histologically, in avitaminosis C there are disturbance in alveolar bone formation, destruction of the collagenous fibers, increased osteoclastic resorption and engorged capillaries[6] (Fig. 63). Both Glickman[9,10] and Waerhaug[21] found that in vitamin C-deficient

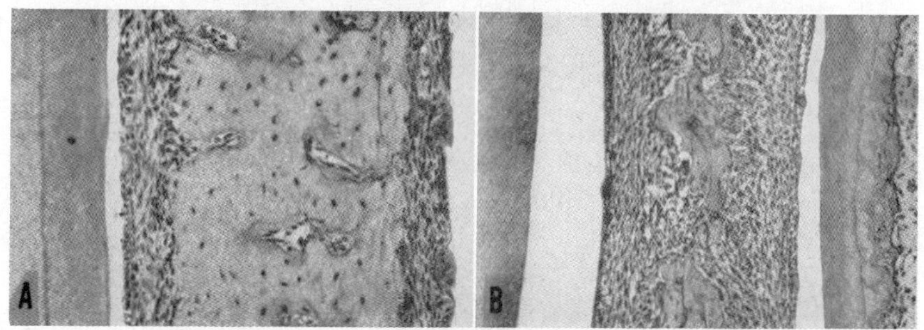

FIGURE 63. *A,* control animal; *B,* vitamin C-deficient animal. Note erosion of bone margins, no new bone formation, edema and degeneration of periodontal membrane fibers, and enlarged vessels in animal *B* compared to animal *A.* (Glickman, I.: Acute vitamin C deficiency and periodontal disease. I. The periodontal tissues of the guinea pig in acute vitamin C deficiency. J. D. Res., 27:9, 1948.)

animals the destruction of the periodontal fibers is more advanced on the alveolar wall side and to a much lesser extent on the cemental side. The periodontal destruction in avitaminosis C differs from that of periodontitis complex in that in the former condition there is a generalized breakdown of the periodontal fibers, but the fibers that are least affected are those just below the epithelial cuff. On the other hand, in periodontitis complex the primary site of destruction of the periodontal fibers is localized in areas below the deepened pockets.[21]

This lack of periodontal support may make the tooth loose to the point of exfoliation. Definite interruptions in the lamina dura due to atrophy of the alveolar bone were noted six months after Crandon[8] had put himself on a vitamin C-deficient diet. This, incidentally, was the first tissue change noted, even preceding any gingival or dermal changes.

There are two schools of thought on vitamin C deficiency as the etiologic factor in gingivitis. Burrill reported that even 6 to 7 months of vitamin C deprivation in human beings under controlled conditions did not produce the typical edematous purplish red and freely bleeding gingiva, unless accompanied by a lack of oral cleanliness. Others, like Radusch[18] and Restarski,[19] have also found no correlation between low vitamin C levels in the blood and the incidence of gingivitis. The opposite viewpoint has been expressed by Kruse[13] as well as Stuhl,[20] who have independently suggested that gingivitis is a manifestation of a latent or subclinical vitamin C deficiency. Blockley and Baenziger[2] also state that "in cases of periodontal disturbances associated with low vitamin C levels the gingival inflammation cannot be removed completely by local treatment however vigorous unless ascorbic acid therapy is employed."

Toxicity

Massive intakes of ascorbic acid either by injection or by mouth have not produced any toxicity. This is undoubtedly due to its apparently limited storage and its very rapid excretion.

REFERENCES

1. Bartlett, M. K., Jones, C. M., and Ryan, A. E.: Vitamin C and wound healing. I. Experimental wounds in guinea pigs. N. E. J. Med., *226:*469, 1942.
2. Blockley, C. H., and Baenziger, P. E.: Investigation into the connection between the vitamin C content of the blood and periodontal disturbances. Brit. D. J., *73:*57, 1942.
3. Boyle, P. E.: Tooth germ in acute scurvy. J. D. Res., *14:*172, 1934.
4. Boyle, P. E.: The effect of ascorbic acid deficiency on enamel formation in the teeth of guinea pigs. Am. J. Path., *14:*843, 1938.
5. Boyle, P. E., Bessey, O. A., and Howe, P. R.: Rate of dentine formation in incisor teeth of guinea pigs on normal and on ascorbic acid-deficient diets. Arch. Path., *30:*90, 1940.
6. Boyle, P. E., Bessey, O. A., and Wolbach, S. B.: Experimental production of diffuse alveolar bone atrophy type of periodontal disease by diets deficient in ascorbic acid. J.A.D.A., *24:*1768, 1937.
7. Burrill, D. Y.: Oral conditions in experimental vitamin C and B deficiency. J.A.D.A., *33:*594, 1946.
8. Crandon, J. H., Lund, C. C., and Dill, D. B.: Experimental human scurvy. N. E. J. Med., *223:*353, 1940.
9. Glickman, I.: Acute vitamin C deficiency and periodontal disease, periodontal tissue of guinea pig in acute vitamin C deficiency. J. D. Res., *27:*9, 1948.
10. Glickman, I.: Acute vitamin C deficiency and periodontal tissues; effect

of acute vitamin C deficiency upon response of periodontal tissues of guinea pig to artificially induced inflammation. J. D. Res., *27:*201, 1948.
11. Hanke, M. T.: Diet as a factor in the control of gingivitis and diet as a factor in the control of dental caries: a report on nutritional studies at Moosehart, Ill. J. D. Res., *12:*518, 1932.
12. Hunt, A. H.: The role of vitamin C in wound healing. Brit. J. Surg., *28:*436, 1941.
13. Kruse, H. D.: Gingival manifestation of avitaminosis C. Milbank Mem. Fund Quart., *20:*290, 1942.
14. Lind, J.: A treatise on the scurvy. Edinburgh, 1753.
15. Marshall-Day, C. D.: The effect of antiscorbutic deficiency on the pregnant organism and dental tissues. J.A.D.A., *20:*1745, 1933.
16. McBeath, E. C.: Experiments on the dietary control of dental caries in children. J. D. Res., *12:*723, 1932.
17. Meyer, E., and Meyer, M. B.: The pathology of staphylococcus abscesses in vitamin C deficient guinea pigs. Bull. Johns Hopkins Hosp., *74:*98, 1944.
18. Radusch, D. F.: Vitamin C therapy in periodontal disease. J.A.D.A., *29:*1652, 1942.
19. Restarski, J. S., and Pijoan, M.: Gingivitis and vitamin C. J.A.D.A., *31:*1323, 1944.
20. Stuhl, F.: Vitamin C subnutrition in gingivo-stomatitis. Lancet *1:*640, 1943.
21. Waerhaug, J.: Effect of C avitaminosis on the supporting structure of the teeth. J. Perio., *29:*87, 1958.
22. Wolbach, S. B., and Howe, P. R.: Intercellular substance in experimental scorbutus. Arch. Path. and Lab. Med., *1:*1, 1926.

The B Complex Vitamins

The first of the B complex vitamins, the beriberi factor, was discovered at the end of the nineteenth century as a result of original work by Takaki,[4] Eijkman and others.[2] McCollum and Davis[3] in 1915 called this factor "water-soluble B." Ordinary yeast was known to be an excellent source of this antineuritic vitamin, but when heated it lost its ability to cure beriberi. Goldberger[1] in 1926 discovered that even after this treatment a heat stable nutrient that could cure pellagra remained in the yeast. Vitamin B_1 was designated as that fraction that was heat labile and absorbable on Fuller's earth; the term vitamin B_2 was applied to the other fraction that was heat stable and not absorbed on Fuller's earth. Soon after, the heat stable fraction of the B complex was found to contain other vitamins which were chemically different but functionally similar.

All B complex vitamins are (1) natural constituents of yeast and liver, (2) water soluble and (3) growth promoting for microorganisms. In the body they function primarily as energy-releasing and hematopoietic factors. Thiamine, niacin, riboflavin, pantothenic acid and biotin belong primarily to the enzyme activator (energy-releasing group), while folic acid and vitamin B_{12} belong to the group that deals with the formation of red blood cells. Vitamin B_6 (pyridoxine) functions both as a coenzyme and as an antianemic factor. Other fractions of this B complex group, like para-aminobenzoic acid, choline and inositol (the classification of these last two as vitamins is doubtful), have functions that are more specific for species lower than man.

REFERENCES

1. Goldberger, J., and Lillie, R. D.: Experimental pellagra-like condition in the albino rat. Pub. Health Rep., *41:*1025, 1926.
2. Jansen, B. C. P.: Early nutritional researches on beriberi leading to the discovery of vitamin B_1. Nut. Abs. & Rev., *26:*1, 1956.
3. McCollum, E. V., and Davis, M.: The nature of dietary deficiencies of rice. J. Biol. Chem., *23:*181, 1915.
4. Takaki, K.: Health of the Japanese Navy. Lancet, *2:*86, 1887.

THIAMINE

The story of thiamine, a deficiency of which causes beriberi, has already been mentioned several times in the text because its discovery represented one of the milestones in the development of our knowledge about vitamins. Thiamine also has been called vitamin B_1, antineuritic or antiberiberi vitamin and "aneurin." The latter name was suggested by two Dutch workers, Jansen and Donath,[3] who isolated the natural substance in 1926 as a pure crystalline material. Ten years later, Cline et al.[2] identified this vitamin as a sulfur-containing compound which they later synthesized and named thiamine hydrochloride.

Chemistry

Thiamine hydrochloride is a colorless crystalline compound with a faint yeastlike odor. It dissolves easily in water, alcohol and most acid solutions but not in fat solvents. It is more stable to heat than vitamin C but, if heated above the boiling point of water for any extended period, it is destroyed, especially in the presence of alkali. However, destruction is retarded in acid media.

Thiamine contains a pyrimidine and a thiazole component connected by a methylene bridge. Its structural formula is:

```
                                  CH3
                                   |
      N=C—NH2HCl                   C=C—CH2CH2OH
      |   |                       /   |
      |   |                    + /    |
H3C—C   C——CH2——N                 |
    ||  ||                -Cl  \\     |
    ||  ||                      \\    |
      N—CH                         C—S
                                   |
                                   H
```

Thiamine hydrochloride

Thiamine occurs naturally in yeast, liver, beef, pork, legumes and nuts. During the refinement of flour and sugar, this vitamin is partially destroyed. Because of this, most of the milled flour and most flour products manufactured in the United States today are enriched with this vitamin. Since thiamine is heat labile above 100°C., and since it is leached out from meat and vegetables during the cooking process, nutritionists recommend that the water in which these foods are cooked be used as soups, gravies or sauce garnishings and not be discarded.

Thiamine occurs in the body as the free form or as a coenzyme, cocarboxylase, also known as diphosphothiamine (DPT) or a thiamine pyrophosphate (TDP).

Physiology

Like all water-soluble vitamins, thiamine is readily absorbed from the upper intestinal tract into the blood stream. In the body it is phosphorylated and then functions as cocarboxylase. Conditioning factors, such as excessive vomiting, diarrhea or any other prolonged gastrointestinal disturbance, can interfere with the retention of this nutrient and can produce a deficiency. Although the storage of this vitamin is neither very great nor long lasting, it does appear in the muscles, liver, heart, kidneys and brain.

Thiamine functions in the body primarily as a coenzyme required for the intermediary metabolism of carbohydrates. As cocarboxylase, its participates actively in the removal of CO_2 from keto acids as pyruvate. In the absence of thiamine, pyruvic acid accumulates in the blood. Vitamin B_1 is also required for other reactions in the body, such as oxidation, dismutation and condensation.

Requirements

The requirement for thiamine is influenced by age, level of activity and diet. Greater thiamine intakes are indicated when the caloric intake is increased as a result of the greater metabolic requirements of spurt growth, pregnancy or lactation. Diets high in carbohydrate content require more thiamine than normal for complete metabolism. The recommended daily allowance varies with age from 0.3 mg. for the infants to 1.9 mg. for the adolescent. The average adult should ingest approximately 1.5 mg. of thiamine per day, or 0.5 mg. for every 1,000 calories.

General Systemic Pathology of Thiamine Deficiency

Most thiamine deficiencies have their origin in faulty diets. This deficiency is most prevalent in areas where polished rice or refined, unenriched flour products are widely used. Food faddists, chronic alcoholics and very low income groups are most likely to suffer from inadequate intake. Ulcer patients, diabetics and others who have to be on special diets may also suffer from a low thiamine intake unless precautions are taken. In gastrointestinal or hepatic diseases thiamine is not absorbed very efficiently. Increased caloric needs such as are required in febrile conditions, hyperthyroidism, vigorous muscular activity, pregnancy and lactation should be accompanied by a proportionately increased thiamine intake.

In man, thiamine deficiency produces the beriberi syndrome, which affects the heart and the nervous system. Dry beriberi is characterized by neuromuscular effects without edema; wet beriberi, by neuromuscular effects with edema; and cardiac beriberi, by cardiac decompensation.

The initial symptoms of this deficiency are loss of appetite, fatigue, burning numbness in the lower extremities and cramps in the calf muscles indicative of a peripheral neuritis. The pain and tenderness ultimately affect the extensors of the foot, the muscles of the calf and the extensors and flexors of the thigh. There is toe and foot drop. The muscles supplied by the affected nerves may degenerate and atrophy. These are some of the clinical signs of dry beriberi.

In contrast, cardiac beriberi, in addition to the neuritic signs of dry beriberi, is characterized by precordial pain, dyspnea, edema, slightly elevated venous pressure, tachycardia, cardiac murmurs and thready pulse. Edema, resulting from inadequate protein intake and cardiac decompensation, usually begins in the feet and legs and extends to the rest of the body. Heart failure due to vitamin B_1 deficiency differs from that caused by other forms of heart disease in that a decreased circulation time is superimposed upon a failing circulatory system.[5]

A syndrome described by Wernicke in 1881, which is produced by a thiamine deficiency, occurs most often in association with chronic alcoholism and is characterized by clouding of consciousness, ataxia and ophthalmoplegia. Autopsies revealed that there were symmetrical lesions in the gray matter of the brain which were prominent in the region of the third ventricle and corpora quadrigemina.

Oral Pathology of Thiamine Deficiency

The oral tissues like other tissues of the body are markedly sensitive to thiamine deficiency. Weisberger[6] noted the presence of herpes-like lesions in the oral mucosa of patients who were thiamine deficient. Except for hyperesthesia of the oral mucosa, pain in the tongue, teeth and jaws, and hypersensitive dentin, there are no lingual or labial lesions that are characteristic of a thiamine deficiency. Some patients with trigeminal neuralgia have been reportedly helped by the administration of massive doses of this vitamin.[1]

Because dental caries is a bacterial disease and because thiamine, like other members of the B complex group, is so important in bacterial growth, a deficiency in the B complex group may effect a lower dental caries experience. In underfed and malnourished population groups Mann et al.[4] noted an unusually low incidence of dental decay.

Toxicity

Thiamine is ordinarily nontoxic even when large amounts are taken. However, some transient allergic manifestations may arise if doses above 500 mg. are given over extended periods.

REFERENCES

1. Borsook, H., Kremers, M. Y., and Wiggins, C. G.: The relief of symptoms of major trigeminal neuralgia following use of vitamin B_1 and concentrated liver extract. J.A.M.A., *114:*1421, 1940.

2. Cline, J. K., Williams, P. R., and Finkelstein, J.: Studies of crystalline vitamin B_1. XVII. Synthesis of vitamin B_1. J. Am. Chem. Soc., *59*:1052, 1937.
3. Jansen, B. C. P.: Early nutritional researches on beriberi leading to the discovery of vitamin B_1. Nut. Abstr. & Rev., *26*:1, 1956.
4. Mann, A. W., Dreizen, S., Spies, T. D., and Hunt, F. M.: A comparison of dental caries activity in malnourished and wellnourished patients. J.A.D.A., *34*:244, 1947.
5. Robbins, S.: Textbook of Pathology. Philadelphia, W. B. Saunders Co., 1957.
6. Weisberger, D.: Lesions of oral mucosa treated with special vitamins. Am. J. Orth. and Oral Surg., *27*:125, 1941.

RIBOFLAVIN

Riboflavin has been called vitamin B_2, vitamin G and lactoflavin. In 1879 an English food chemist, Winter-Blyth,[3] observed in the whey of milk some pale yellow-colored material which he called lactoflavin. In 1933 Kuhn[1] isolated crystals of lactoflavin and two years later synthesized the vitamin.

Chemistry

Riboflavin is an orange-yellow crystalline compound, practically odorless but bitter in taste. It is heat stable and water soluble. In water it produces a yellowish-green fluorescence. When exposed to light, it breaks down into lumiflavin, which also exhibits a greenish fluorescence. It is stable in acid solutions, but very labile in alkaline solutions.

Riboflavin contains a molecule of D-ribose and the flavinoid molecule, dimethyl isoalloxazine. The empiric formula is $C_{17}H_{20}N_4O_6$. The structural formula is:

```
                 H   H      H      H
                 |   |      |      |
              H—C—C——C——C—CH2OH ← D-Ribityl group
                 |   |      |      |
                 |   OH     OH     OH
       H         |
       C         N         N
     //  \     /   \     //  \
H3C—C      C         C         C=O
    |      ||        |         |          ← Dimethyl isoalloxazine
H3C—C      C         C         N—H
     \\  /   \     //  \     /
       C         N         C
       H                   ||
                           O
```

Milk is the best natural source of riboflavin. Other animal foods, such as liver, kidney, fish and eggs, and many leafy vegetables are also excellent sources. In the body riboflavin is phosphorylated to riboflavin mononucleotide (riboflavin-5-phosphate) or converted to the more complex flavin adenine dinucleotide. These combine with specific apoenzymes (proteins) to form such enzymes as "Warburg's yellow enzyme," cytochrome-c-reductase, D-amino acid oxidase, and many others.

Physiology

Riboflavin is rapidly absorbed from the upper intestinal tract and passes into the circulation in the phosphorylated form.

Its primary function as the mono- or di-nucleotide is as a co-enzyme for the flavoprotein group of oxidative enzymes. As such, it participates in the exchange of oxygen and hydrogen between plasma and tissue cells. It also plays a role in the conversion of the amino acid, tryptophan, to niacin and in the intermediary metabolism of fat and carbohydrates. Because of its interrelationship with other vitamins of the B complex group, such as thiamine and niacin, a riboflavin deficiency may often induce a deficiency of the other B vitamins as well.

Requirements

There appears to be no direct relationship between riboflavin requirements and caloric needs, such as increased muscular activity, as was observed with thiamine. However, there is positive relationship between body weight, growth, pregnancy and lactation and the daily intake of riboflavin necessary for optimum health. Skin lesions and angular stomatitis may become apparent when the daily intake is below 0.75 mg. The recommended daily allowance is between 1.5 and 2.5 mg.

General Systemic Pathology of Riboflavin Deficiency

An inadequate dietary intake is usually the basis for a riboflavin deficiency. As in the case of avitaminosis B_1, the riboflavin deficiency may be found in areas like the Orient where refined, unenriched cereal products are used. Alcoholics and people in low income groups usually do not ingest foods that are rich in this vitamin. There is no clinical picture that is exclusively that of ariboflavinosis because it is usually accompanied by other B complex deficiencies. The usual clinical symptoms are weakness, anorexia, nervousness and confusion. Skin, eye, mouth and lip changes are usually associated with this deficiency.

A dermatitis develops in the skin around the nasolabial folds, which is characterized by a greasy and scaly erythematous lesion and which may extend in a butterfly pattern to the cheeks. There are also seborrheic lesions about the chin and, sometimes, at the canthi of the eyes and the lobes of the ears. In addition, there may be scrotal skin lesions.

The principal eye lesion is a superficial vascularizing keratitis with circumcorneal injection. There is an increase in the number of capillary vessels in the cornea, which may be an attempt to increase the oxygen supply to the tissues through hemoglobin, thus overcoming the consequences of an inefficient group of respiratory enzymes. The symptoms accompanying this vascularization are burning and itching of the eyes, mild photophobia, lacrimation and visual fatigue.

Oral Pathology of Riboflavin Deficiency

Cheilosis and glossitis are the two clinical lesions that are seen in and around the mouth in a riboflavin deficiency. The lips develop vertical fissuring or rhagades and a redness along the line of closure due to superficial denudation. The lesions at the angles of the mouth start as areas of pallor and then, as a result of secondary infection, become macerated and radiate yellow encrusted fissures (Fig. 64).

In the tongue a distinctive type of glossitis sometimes develops which is characterized by a purplish red or magenta color due to the engorgement of the fungiform papillae. The dorsum of the tongue may be shiny, smooth and atrophic with flattened and mushroom-shaped papillae, thus giving the tongue a pebbly texture. In severe deficiencies the entire dorsum is flat and has a deeply fissured surface. Irregular areas of denudation with fissuring and indentations of the lateral borders from the teeth may also be possible.

The symptoms associated with these clinical signs are the following: soreness of lips and tongue, persistent burning, paresthesia, pain on opening of the mouth due to stretching of the

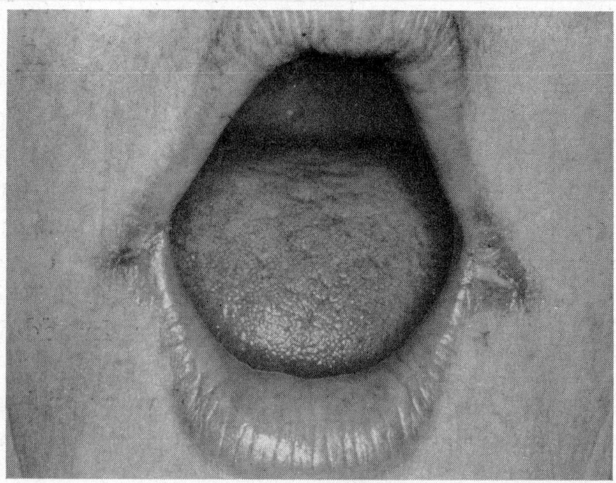

FIGURE 64. Angular cheilosis. (Courtesy Dr. G. Shklar.)

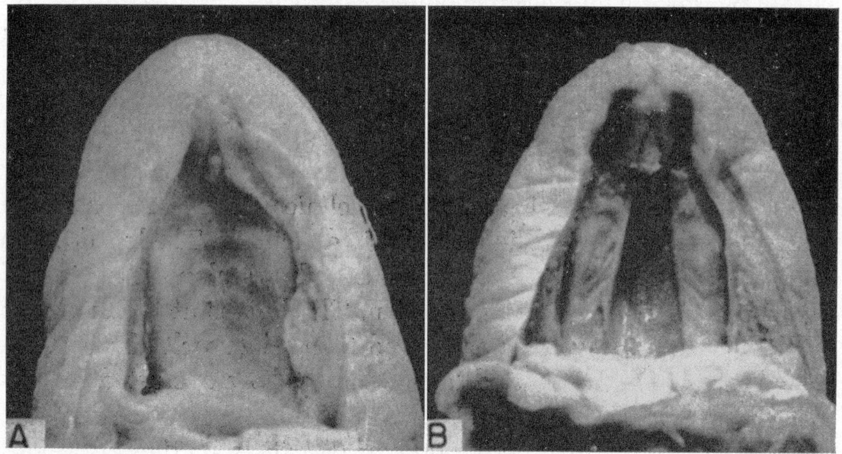

FIGURE 65. Riboflavin deficiency. Congenital malformations. A. normal palate of newborn rat in contrast to B, cleft palate of animal born to riboflavin-deficient mother. There is a communication between the nasal cavity, nasopharyngeal ducts and mouth. (Courtesy of Dr. Joseph Warkany and The Milbank Memorial Fund Quarterly.) (Follis, R. H., Jr.: Deficiency Disease. Charles C Thomas, 1958.)

commissural fissures, and dysphagia due to tenderness of the tongue.

Besides these human clinical manifestations of riboflavin deficiency, congenital malformations of the jaws of young experimental rats have resulted from a riboflavin deficiency in the mother.[4] (See Fig. 65.) Growth of mandibular condyles in mice has been retarded as a result of riboflavin deficiency.[2]

Toxicity

There is no evidence that large doses of riboflavin produce any signs of toxicity.

REFERENCES

1. Follis, R. H., Jr.: Deficiency Disease. Springfield, Ill., Charles C Thomas, 1958.
2. Levy, B. M.: The effect of riboflavin deficiency on the growth of the mandibular condyle of mice. Oral Surg., Oral Med. and Oral Path., *2:*89, 1949.
3. McCollum, E. V.: History of Nutrition. Boston, Houghton Mifflin Co., 1957.
4. Warkany, J., and Schraffenberger, E.: Congenital malformations induced in rats by maternal nutritional deficiency. VI. Preventive factor. J. Nut., *27:*477, 1944.

NIACIN (NICOTINIC ACID)

In the 1920's pellagra was endemic amongst the "poor whites" of the South. At that time many believed that this disease was the result of bacterial infection. The results of a controlled clinical study of twelve convicts in a prison farm showed that pellagra was a deficiency, and not an infectious, disease.[7] Goldberger and his associates selected a control and an experimental group from among volunteer prisoners. Both groups were housed in the same type of wards, which were meticulously clean and identical in all respects except for the diets that were served. The experimental group was fed the diet typical of the pellagrin, consisting of cornmeal, cornstarch, sweet potatoes, rice, syrup and pork fat. This ration was known as the "3M" ration—maize, molasses, and meat (pork fat). The control group was fed the regular prison fare. After six months on their respective diets, the experimental group succumbed to pellagra, whereas the control group did not. As a more convincing proof that pellagra was indeed a dietary deficiency, it was possible to cure the sick of their illness by simply improving their diet with meat, eggs, vegetables and fruits. Attempts to transmit the disease from a pellagrin to a healthy person by inoculation failed; this was added proof that pellagra did not result from a bacterial infection.[6]

Goldberger speculated that the active nutrient, which he called the pellagra-preventive (P-P) factor, was an amino acid.[10] We know now that there was some validity to his theory, for tryptophan has been shown to be interrelated with niacin in the cure of pellagra.

In 1928[3,9] it was reported that experimental black tongue in dogs was similar to pellagra in human beings. In 1937 Elvehjem and his group[5] demonstrated that they could cure black tongue with nicotinic acid and nicotinic acid amide. Further experimentation showed that nicotinic acid was the factor that cured both black tongue and pellagra. Therefore, the P-P factor which, in 1926, Goldberger[11] obtained from the heat-stable portion of yeast was identical with nicotinic acid.

Chemistry

To prevent any unfounded fears in the minds of the lay person who might think that nicotinic acid was a type of acid and, therefore, injurious, the name niacin was recommended in the place of nicotinic acid.

Properties. Niacin is a white, odorless, needlelike, crystalline solid. It is stable in the dry state and soluble in boiling water; it is not destroyed at ordinary cooking temperatures.

Source. The most abundant sources of niacin are yeast, lean meats and liver. In addition, milk, tomatoes, canned salmon and several of the leafy green vegetables are good sources of this vitamin. Because of the compulsory enrichment program, bread and flour contribute about 40 per cent of the daily niacin requirement of the average adult.

A small amount of niacin is synthesized by body tissue and by intestinal bacteria.

The structural formulae of these pellagra preventive factors are:

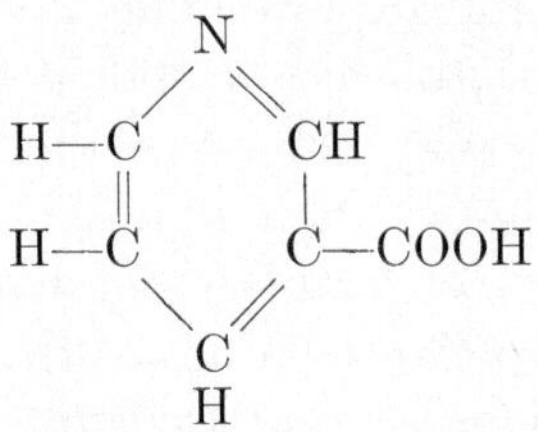

```
          N                              N
        /   \\                         /   \\
   H—C         CH                H—C         CH
     ||         |                  ||         |
   H—C         C—COOH            H—C         C—CONH2
        \\    //                      \\    //
          C                              C
          H                              H
    Nicotinic acid                  Nicotinamide
```

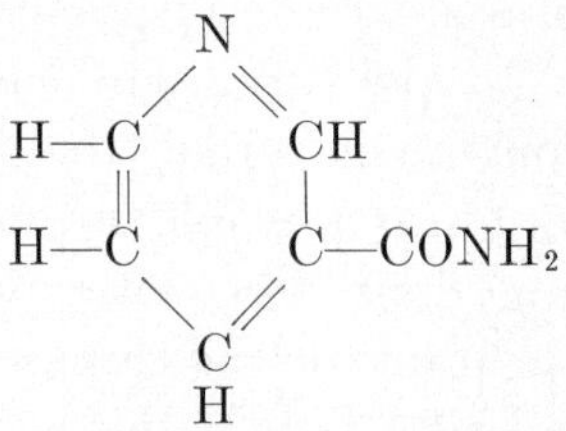

Physiology

Niacin is absorbed from the upper portion of the small intestine and, after being converted to the amide, is transformed primarily to nucleotide structures, which function as coenzymes. These coenzymes are codehydrogenase I or coenzyme I (DPN—diphosphopyridine nucleotide) and codehydrogenase II or coenzyme II (TPN—triphosphopyridine nucleotide). They act as catalysts in cellular respiration by accepting and releasing hydrogen. They are of prime importance in the aerobic catabolism of carbohydrates.

Requirements

Since tryptophan is closely related metabolically to niacin, the recommended daily allowance for niacin must be considered in relation to the amount of tryptophan normally consumed. The minimal amount of niacin required to prevent pellagra in adults is about 9 mg. per day.

The daily recommended niacin allowance was formerly calculated to be ten times that of thiamine, or 10 to 16 mg. However, this was shown to be too generous because it did not consider the niacin precursor, tryptophan. Now the term "niacin equivalent" is used, which includes both the preformed vitamin and the vitamin formed from tryptophan. The average American diet contains approximately 500 mg. of tryptophan or, on the basis that 60 mg. of tryptophan are equivalent to 1 mg. of niacin, about 8 mg. of derived niacin. The recommended daily allowance is based on body weight and calorie intake and is expressed in niacin mg. equivalents. For children the recommended daily allowance is from 8 to 17 niacin mg. equivalents and for adults, 17 to 21 niacin mg. equivalents. Periods of spurt growth such as in adolescence, pregnancy and lactation increase the requirement.

General Systemic Pathology of Niacin Deficiency

Niacin deficiency may be caused by an inadequate intake of the vitamin. Other factors that may induce a deficiency are the following: poor gastrointestinal absorption due to diarrhea, vomiting, or conditions in which demand for this vitamin is greater than the amount that may be normally consumed, e.g., alcoholism, pregnancy and lactation.

Pellagra is a niacin deficiency disease; its name is derived from "pelle" meaning skin and "agra" meaning rough, the pathognomonic lesion of this disease. The typical dermal lesions are symmetrical rough areas which are usually found over sites of irritation and in areas that are exposed to sunlight, such as the dorsum of the hands, wrists, elbows, face, neck and knees.

Before the dermal lesions appear, other clinical signs of the deficiency become manifest; these are lassitude, irritability, general nervousness and alimentary tract disturbances. These are not pathognomonic of the disease but may be considered indicative of a state of anxiety, or neurasthenia.

However, when dermatitis, diarrhea and dementia—the three D's of the disease—appear, a diagnosis of pellagra is justified.

The symmetrical dermatitis is a well demarcated lesion. In the early stages the areas of the skin are red and swollen; vesicles may develop later. These rupture, and the epidermis desquamates. As the disease becomes more chronic, the lesions turn brown and scaly and the skin becomes thickened. Diarrhea is due to an inflammation of the mucosal lining of the intestine. Dementia is due to a degeneration of the ganglion cells of the brain and the tracts of the spinal cord.

Oral Pathology of Niacin Deficiency

Dental Caries. Becks and Morgan found no dental or osseous changes in dogs who were niacin deficient. Several studies from the nutrition clinic in Birmingham, Alabama,[4,13,14] indicated that the incidence of dental caries was lower in the malnourished pellagrin than in normal individuals.

Glossitis. The tongue is one of the first tissues that manifests clinical signs of niacin deficiency. During acute stages, the fungiform, and then the filiform, papillae undergo vascular hyperemia and become edematous. The tip, the lateral borders and the anterior half of the dorsum of the tongue become swollen and red in appearance (Fig. 66). The pressure of the swollen tongue against the teeth may create indentation along the lateral borders. With time the papillae begin to atrophy, thus imparting to the tongue a smooth, dry, glazed appearance. Isolated patches of vesicles and ulcers may form in parts of the dorsum. Fissures and crevices may form, leaving a thin tongue with marginal serrations. The appearance of "black tongue" in dogs as a result of the niacin deficiency was the first step in a chain of events that helped Goldberger,[8] in 1920, identify niacin as the pellagra-preventive factor.

Oral Mucous Membrane. The epithelial lining of the buccal mucosa may degenerate, thus permitting the development of a grayish-white necrotic membrane as a result of secondary bacterial invasion. Excessive salivation or ptyalism accompanies the fiery-red swollen mucosa.

Gingiva. Classical work on the relationship between nicotinic acid and acute necrotizing gingivitis was conducted by King,[12] who

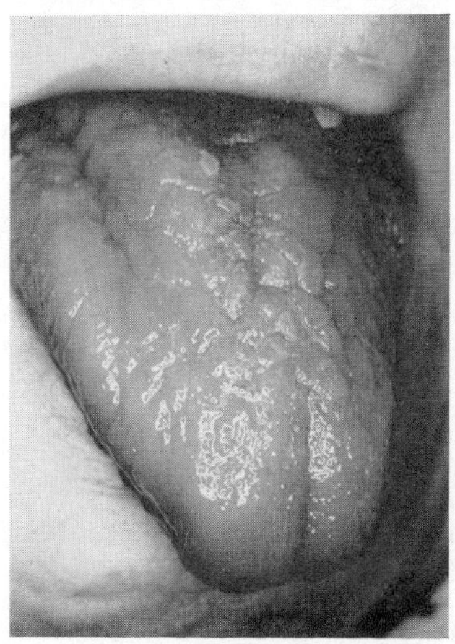

FIGURE 66. Acute glossitis in patient with cirrhosis of liver.

reported the results in several communications. Two hundred and seventy-six patients, all of whom were diagnosed as having "trench mouth," were divided into four groups and given the following treatments: (1) nicotinic acid therapy, (2) local scaling and currettage, (3) combination of nicotinic acid with local therapy, and (4) ascorbic acid and hydrogen peroxide treatment. He found that patients in group (3) i.e., receiving local therapy and nicotinic acid supplements, were relieved of the acute symptoms in 4 days, whereas the patients receiving only local therapy required 10 to 15 days for the same degree of cure. The nicotinic acid therapy group took 5 to 10 days to clear up. No satisfactory response was obtained from ascorbic acid and hydrogen peroxide.

He also showed that the fusiform bacilli and spirochetes, found in the ulcerated dental papillae with grayish pseudomembrane exudate, were secondary invaders. The gingival tissues were predisposed to the infection because of such conditioning factors as local traumatic irritants and systemic nutritional inadequacy.

Spies[16] found that Vincent's infection was very common in pellagrins and that the administration of nicotinic acid did alleviate this condition. However, a preliminary report by Miller et al.[15] failed to show the beneficial effect of the use of large doses of nicotinic acid in ten cases of acute Vincent's infection.

In monkeys[17,18] and dogs,[1,2] a niacin deficiency produced gingival disturbances similar to those in the pellagrin.

Toxicity

Large doses of nicotinic acid will cause flushing, nausea and abdominal pain. Since the amide of nicotinic acid releases nicotinic acid more slowly, thus preventing these undesirable side effects, it is the vitamin of choice. Even in large doses, it has been shown to be nontoxic.

REFERENCES

1. Becks, H., and Morgan, A. F.: Effect of deficiencies of the filtrate fraction of vitamin B complex and of nicotinic acid on teeth and oral structures. J. Perio., *13:*18, 1942.
2. Becks, H., Wainwright, W. W., and Morgan, A. F.: Comparative study of oral changes in dogs due to deficiencies of pantothenic acid, nicotinic acid and unknowns of B vitamin complex. Am. J. Ortho. and Oral Surg., *29:*183, 1943.
3. Denton, J.: A study of tissue changes in experimental black tongue of dogs compared with similar changes in pellagra. Am. J. Path., *4:*341, 1928.
4. Dreizen, S., Mann, A. W., Spies, T. D., and Skinner, T. A.: Prevalence of dental caries in malnourished children: a clinical study. Am. J. Disease Child., *74:*265, 1947.
5. Elvehjem, C. A., Madden, R. J., Strong, F. M., and Woolley, F. W.: Relation of nicotinic acid and nicotinic acid amide to canine black tongue. J. Am. Chem. Soc., *59:*1767, 1937.
6. Goldberger, J.: The transmission of pellagra: experimental attempts at transmission to the human subject. Pub. Health Rep., *31:*3159, 1916.
7. Goldberger, J., Waring, C. H., and Willets, D. G.: The prevention of pellagra: a test diet among institutional inmates. Pub. Health Rep., *30:*3117, 1915.
8. Goldberger, J., and Wheeler, G. A.: Experimental black tongue of dog compared with similar changes in pellagra. Pub. Health Rep., *43:*172, 1920.
9. Goldberger, J., and Wheeler, G. A.: Experimental black tongue of dogs and its relation to pellagra. Pub. Health Rep., *43:*172, 1928.

10. Goldberger, J., and Wheeler, G. A.: Experimental pellagra in the human subject brought about by a restricted diet. Pub. Health Rep., *30:*3336, 1915.
11. Goldberger, J., Wheeler, G. A., Lillie, R. D., and Rogers, L. M.: Further study of butter, fresh beef and yeast as pellagra preventives with consideration of factor P-P of pellagra and black tongue of dogs to vitamin B_1. Pub. Health Rep., *41:*297, 1926.
12. King, J. D.: Nutritional and other factors in "trench mouth" with special reference to the nicotinic acid component of vitamin B_2 complex. Brit. D. J., *74:*113, 141, 169, 1943.
13. Kniesner, A. H., Mann, A. W., and Spies, T. D.: Relationship of dental caries to deficiencies of vitamin B group. J. D. Res., *21:*259, 1942.
14. Mann, A. W., Dreizen, S., Spies, T. D., and Hunt, I. M.: A comparison of dental caries activity in malnourished and well nourished patients. J.A.D.A., *34:*244, 1947.
15. Miller, S. C., Greenhut, W. M., and Roth, H.: Nicotinic acid and Vincent's infection (a preliminary report). N. Y. J. Dent., *10:*424, 1940.
16. Spies, T. D., Vilter, R. W., and Ashe, W. F.: Pellagra, beriberi and riboflavin deficiency in human beings; diagnosis and treatment. J.A.M.A., *113:*931, 1939.
17. Tomlinson, T. H., Jr.: Oral pathology in monkeys in various experimental dietary deficiencies. Pub. Health Rep., *54:*431, 1939.
18. Topping, N. H., and Fraser, H. F.: Mouth lesions associated with dietary deficiencies in monkeys. Pub. Health Rep., *54:*416, 1939.

PANTOTHENIC ACID

Pantothenic acid has been called the liver filtrate factor, the chick antidermatitis factor, the chick antipellagra factor and the antichromotrichia factor (antigray-hair factor). In 1933 R. J. Williams and his co-workers[4] recognized its existence in "bios," a yeast growth factor. Because it was ubiquitous, the word "pan" derived from the Greek meaning "from everywhere" was made part of its name, pantothenic acid. In 1940 Williams and Major[5] determined the structure of pantothenic acid and then synthesized it.

Chemistry

Pantothenic acid occurs in nature probably as the free acid, but it is marketed as the calcium salt. The free acid is a yellow viscous oil, soluble in water and glacial acetic acid, only slightly soluble in ether, and insoluble in benzene and chloroform. It is unstable in the presence of hot acid, hot base and dry heat. Calcium pantothenate is a white crystalline powder, odorless, with a slightly bitter taste. It is soluble in water and is more stable to heat than the naturally occurring pantothenic acid. However, it is insoluble in acid and is precipitated out of solution by alkali, ferric salt and calcium precipitants.

Sources. Pantothenic acid occurs in all tissues of plants and animals. Some of the best food sources are liver, kidney, eggs, lean beef, skim milk, buttermilk, crude molasses, bran and whole grain cereals, peas, cabbage, cauliflower, peanuts, broccoli, sweet potatoes, kale and yeast. The structural formula is:

$$
\begin{array}{ccccccccccccccccc}
 & & OH & & CH_3 & & OH & & O & & H & & H & & H & & O \\
 & & | & & | & & | & & \| & & | & & | & & | & \diagup\!\!\diagup & \\
H & - & C & - & C & - & C & - & C & - & N & - & C & - & C & - & C \\
 & & | & & | & & | & & & & & & | & & | & & \diagdown \\
 & & H & & CH_3 & & H & & & & & & H & & H & & OH
\end{array}
$$

Physiology

Pantothenic acid is required by the lower and higher forms of life. It is necessary for the growth of chicks, rats and microorganisms. It is a component of coenzyme A, which is concerned with acetylation and the metabolism of fat and carbohydrate. It releases energy from carbohydrate and is necessary for the degradation and synthesis of fatty acids, sterols and steroid hormones. As part of coenzyme A, it plays a role in the metabolism of choline, sulfa drugs and para-aminobenzoic acid. Pantothenic acid is intimately related with the functioning of the adrenal glands; both influence skin and hair pigmentation (the vitamin prevents achromotrichia, or graying of the hair).

Requirements

The results of the experimentally induced pantothenic acid deficiency studies in human volunteers indicate that this vitamin is essential for human beings. The amount of pantothenic acid found in the average diet is about 8.7 mg.

General Systemic Pathology of Pantothenic Acid Deficiency

In black rats, a deficiency of pantothenic acid causes graying of the hair. In white rats, the nose and the hair around the nose become covered with red pigment, presenting typical "blood-caked whiskers." As in a biotin deficiency, there may be a loss of hair around the eye, thus giving the spectacle eye appearance. There is atrophy of the adrenal glands with necrosis and hemorrhage. Peripheral nerves undergo degeneration.

Because this vitamin is so widespread in the daily dietary, a pantothenic acid deficiency in the human is almost impossible. However, experimental deficiency was produced in four human beings by feeding them the pantothenic acid antagonist, omega-methylpantothenic acid. Within a few weeks they developed fatigue and cardiovascular and gastrointestinal disturbances. Neurologic symptoms, such as numbness and tingling of the extremities, abnormal gait, hyperactive reflexes and muscular weakness, were also noted. Pantothenic acid was administered, but it did not completely cure the condition because of an adrenal insufficiency. It was necessary to withdraw the antagonist and inject cortisone in order to effect a restoration to normal.

Oral Pathology of Pantothenic Acid Deficiency

In pantothenic acid-deficient rats, ulceration and hyperkeratosis of the oral mucous membrane and marked gingival and periodontal necrosis were evident.[3]

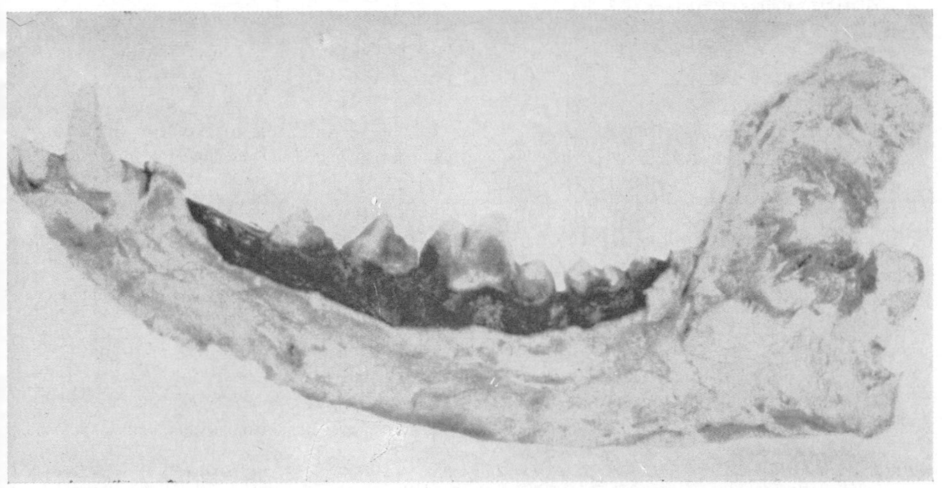

FIGURE 67. Left lower jaw of dog 11 after a period of 343 days on a diet deficient in filtrate fraction and nicotinic acid. Severe gingival and paradental infections are accompanied by marked marginal atrophy. The bifurcations of most molars and premolars are involved. (Becks, H., and Morgan, A. F., in Journal of Periodontology, Vol. 13, No. 1, 1942.)

Becks[1] fed dogs a diet which was deficient not only in pantothenic acid but in other factors as well, because the addition of crystalline pantothenic acid did not cure the oral pathology that had developed. Dental and oral pathology seen in the deficient dogs included rampant decay, root deformities, as well as resorption and osteoporosis of the supporting bone (Fig. 67). This was accompanied by gingival inflammation, necrosis and degeneration of the epithelium. The clinical and histological appearance was similar to that seen in man. However, since this study was done with only two animals, confirmation of the results would be most desirable.

Levy[2] studied the effect of a pantothenic acid-deficient diet upon the growth and development of the mandibles of mice and upon their periodontal structure. He found hypertrophic cartilage in the mandibular condyle and an inhibition of the proliferation process, resulting in a retarded growth of the mandible. The alveolar bone showed evidence of continued resorption, the periodontal membrane was wider than normal, and there was a downward proliferation of the epithelium along the roots of the teeth.

When a pantothenic acid-deficient diet supplemented with zinc carbonate was fed to rats, hyperkeratosis and ulceration of the mucosa of the mouth and tongue and fissuring at the angles of the mouth were apparent.[6]

REFERENCES

1. Becks, H., and Morgan, A. F.: The effect of deficiencies of the filtrate fraction of vitamin B complex and nicotinic acid on teeth and oral structures. J. Perio., *13*:18, 1942.
2. Levy, B.: Effects of pantothenic acid deficiency on the mandibular joints and periodontal structure of mice. J.A.D.A., *38*:215, 1949.
3. Wainright, W. W., and Nelson, M. M.: Changes in the oral mucosa accompanying acute pantothenic acid deficiency in young rats. Am. J. Ortho. and Oral Surg., *31*:406, 1945.
4. Williams, R. J., Lyman, C. M., Goodyear, G. H., Truesdail, J. H., and Holiday, D.: "Pantothenic acid" a growth determinant of universal biological occurrence. J. Am. Chem. Soc., *55*:2912, 1933.
5. Williams, R. J., and Major, R. T.: The structure of pantothenic acid. Science, *91*:246, 1940.
6. Ziskin, D. E., Stein, G., Gross, P., and Runne, E.: Mouth conditions in rats under low pantothenic diet with addition of zinc carbonate. J. D. Res., *23*:152, 1944.

BIOTIN

In 1916 Bateman[1] observed that the feeding of large amounts of egg whites to rats produced toxic effects. Boas,[3] in 1927, reported that a similar diet produced dermatitis, loss of hair, and muscular incoordination in rats, symptoms which could subsequently be cured by the administration of yeast and liver. In 1936 Kögl and

Tönnis[6] isolated a substance from dried egg yolk that promoted growth of yeasts; it was called biotin. Allison et al.[2] obtained from Rhizobium a substance of identical chemical structure which was called "coenzyme R." György[5] had earlier called this substance vitamin H. In 1940 vitamin H, coenzyme R and biotin were declared to be one and the same substance. Du Vigneaud and his coworkers[4] determined the empirical and structural formulae for biotin in 1942.

Chemistry

Biotin is an organic acid which is sparingly soluble in water and alcohol and insoluble in fat solvents. It is stable to heat, light and most reducing agents but is inactivated by strong acids, alkalis and oxidizing agents. Its structural formula is:

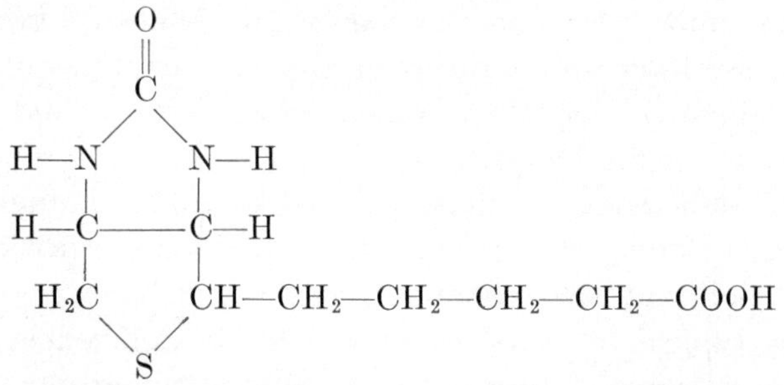

```
            O
            ‖
            C
          /   \
     H—N       N—H
       |       |
     H—C———————C—H
       |       |
      H2C      CH—CH2—CH2—CH2—CH2—COOH
         \    /
           S
```

Source. Biotin is widely distributed in foods, especially in beef liver. Common dietary sources containing biotin in fair quantities are meat, most vegetables, milk, molasses, chocolate and peanuts. Biotin can also be synthesized by intestinal bacteria.

Physiology

Biotin, like all other water-soluble vitamins, is absorbed readily from the upper part of the small intestine. However, avidin, a protein which is found in raw egg whites, can combine with biotin and make it unavailable.

Biotin functions in many enzyme systems found in animals, human beings or bacteria. As a coenzyme in carbon dioxide fixation reactions, it plays an important role in the synthesis of aspartic acid from pyruvate. The vitamin also participates in many decarboxylation reactions. Biotin influences the synthesis of acetoacetic acid, citrulline and oleic acid.

Requirements

The amount of biotin synthesized by intestinal bacteria is sufficiently high to supply its need by most animals. However, excessive use of antibiotics or sulfa drugs will decrease this amount. The average daily American diet provides 150 to 300 micrograms of biotin, an amount which is adequate for the average human being.

General Systemic Pathology of Biotin Deficiency

The spontaneous deficiency of this vitamin is unlikely to occur in man because of its wide distribution in food and its synthesis by intestinal bacteria. However, experimental biotin deficiency has been repeatedly produced in rats by feeding them large amounts of raw egg white containing avidin. The syndrome of the so-called "egg white injury" is characterized by an extensive brown scaly dermatitis, swelling and redness of the lips, circumocular loss of hair to produce the so-called "spectacle eye" effect, and spasticity or paralysis of the hind legs.

A biotin deficiency has been induced in human beings by feeding diets rich in egg whites. They developed a nonpruritic dermatitis, grayish pallor of skin and mucosa and muscle pains.

Lesions typical of many other B vitamin deficiencies, such as anemia, neurological symptoms and electrocardiographic changes, were also noted. The administration of biotin effected a prompt relief from these symptoms. This induced deficiency indicates that biotin is an essential nutrient for man.

REFERENCES

1. Anon: Nutritional Data. Pittsburgh, H. J. Heinz Co., 1956.
2. Allison, F. E., Hoover, S. R., and Burk, D.: A respiration coenzyme. Science, *78:*217, 1933.
3. Boas, M. A.: An observation on the value of egg white as the sole source of nitrogen for young growing rats: the effect of desiccation upon the nutritive properties of egg white. Biochem. J., *21:*712, 1927.
4. Du Vigneaud, V.: A Trail of Research in Sulfur Chemistry and Metabolism and Related Fields. Ithaca, Cornell University Press, 1952.
5. György, P.: The curative factor (vitamin H) for egg white injury, with particular reference to its presence in different foodstuffs and in yeast. J. Biol. Chem., *131:*733, 1939.
6. Kögl, F., and Tönnis, B.: Uber das Bios-Problem: Darstellung von krystallisierten Biotin aus Eigelb. Ztsch. Physiol. Chem., *242:*43, 1936.

VITAMIN B_6 GROUP

Vitamin B_6 was recognized as a vitamin in 1934 by György, who demonstrated that there was another factor besides riboflavin in the heat-stable fraction of B complex that could cure a scaly dermatitis in rats; he called this vitamin the "anti-acrodynia factor." The following investigators played important roles in the isolation, identification and synthesis of this vitamin: Kuhn, Lepkovsky, György, Ichiba, Folkers, Snell and many others.[3]

György chose the name pyridoxine for this vitamin because, chemically, it was a pyridine derivative containing several oxy (methoxy) groups.

Chemistry

Pyridoxine hydrochloride forms white crystals or platelets, is soluble in water, insoluble in ether. It is stable to heat, strong acids and alkalis but is destroyed by light.

Pyridoxine can be converted to the amine form, which is called pyridoxamine or to the aldehyde form, which is called pyridoxal. Both forms are found in nature. Pyridoxamine and pyridoxal are biologically active like pyridoxine, but they are more labile compounds; they are rapidly destroyed when exposed to air, ultraviolet light or heat.

Source. The members of the B_6 group are found in many plant and animal foods. Wheat germ, milk, yeast, legumes, liver, kidney and certain fruits and vegetables are excellent sources. Whole grain cereals contain good quantities of this vitamin but, as is the case with all B complex vitamins, 80 to 90 per cent is lost in the milling or refining process. Pyridoxal appears to be the predominant form in animal products, whereas pyridoxamine is the predominant form in plants. Vitamin B_6 may also be synthesized by microorganisms in the intestinal tract.

The structural formulae of each of the three compounds of the B_6 group are:

CH_2OH	CHO	CH_2NH_2
HO, CH_2OH, H_3C, N	HO, CH_2OH, H_3C, N	HO, CH_2OH, H_3C, N
Pyridoxine	Pyridoxal	Pyridoxamine

Physiology

After members of the B_6 group are ingested and absorbed from the upper intestinal tract, they are converted primarily to pyridoxal-5-phosphate, in which form this group of vitamins exerts its biological activity.

Vitamin B_6 plays an important role in the metabolism of protein and fat.

In a B_6 deficiency an abnormal end product of tryptophan metabolism, xanthurenic acid, appears in the urine. B_6 functions as a coenzyme in the decarboxylation of amino acids and in the transamination reactions between amino acids and keto acids; it also participates in the dehydration of hydroxyamino acids and in the desulfhydration of sulfur amino acids.

Vitamin B_6 has been shown to be essential for the conversion of limited amounts of dietary fatty acids to the essential fatty acid, arachidonic acid. Because essential unsaturated fatty acids are active in reducing cholesterol accumulation, a necessary step in the control of atherosclerosis, the presence of adequate dietary B_6 becomes an important consideration in the prevention of coronary heart disease.

Requirements

The ratios of fat, carbohydrate and protein in the diet govern the amount of vitamin B_6 required. When large amounts of protein and carbohydrate are given, requirements are increased. On the other hand, if the diet is rich in fat, the requirement is decreased. It has been estimated that the daily human requirement for B_6 is 1 to 2 mg.

General Systemic Pathology of Vitamin B_6 Deficiency

A frank vitamin B_6 deficiency in man is rare because of its widespread distribution in natural foodstuffs and its intestinal synthesis. An experimental deficiency was produced in humans by feeding a vitamin B_6-low diet together with a vitamin antagonist, desoxypyridoxine. Experimental subjects developed clinical signs and symptoms of burning and itching seborrheic dermatitis with erythema in the nasolabial folds, around the eyes and at the angles of the mouth (Fig. 68). Subjective symptoms were anorexia, nausea and drowsiness.

Severe sensory neuritis, numbness and tingling in the hands and feet, and hyperesthesia are other sensory symptoms that may arise. Vitamin B_6 deficiency produces a degeneration of the myelin sheath of the nerves.

A microcytic hypochromic anemia accompanied by a lymphocytopenia may develop in this deficiency.

In 1954 a very interesting episode occurred which conclusively demonstrated that the pyridoxine was essential for man.[3,4] A group

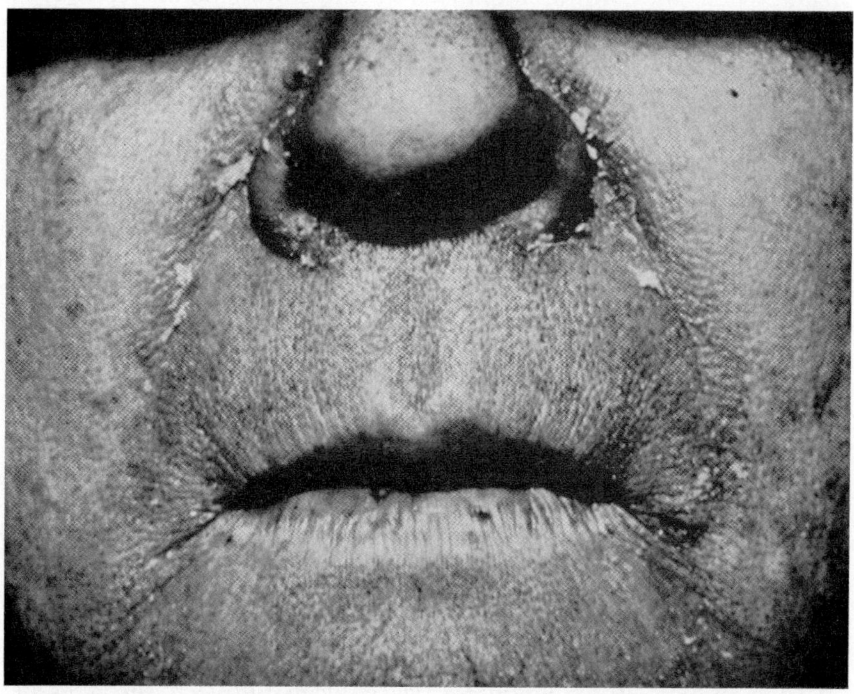

FIGURE 68. Pyridoxine deficiency. Seborrheic dermatitis about the nose from individual experimentally depleted of pyridoxine. (Courtesy of Dr. R. W. Vilter.) (Follis, R. H., Jr.: Deficiency Disease. Charles C Thomas, 1958.)

of infants, aged 6 weeks to 6 months, who were being fed the same type of liquid canned milk formula developed severe convulsions. Alert pediatricians recognized that this syndrome resembled that seen in vitamin B_6 deficiency. Within minutes after an injection of this vitamin, the convulsive seizures ceased and electroencephalographic tracings returned to normal. The reason for the apparent B_6 deficiency was traced to a low vitamin B_6 content of the formula which resulted from changes in the formulation and processing techniques. As a result of this unfortunate accident, many infant foods are now enriched with B_6.

In rats a vitamin B_6 deficiency produces acrodynia in the paws, tips of the ears, tail and nose. The animals develop fatty livers, microcytic hypochromic anemia, and brain and nerve damage.

Oral Pathology of Vitamin B_6 Deficiency

Tongue and Oral Mucous Membrane Changes. Vilter and his associates[9] observed clinical signs of a B_6 deficiency in thirty patients when they were administered the antimetabolite, desoxypyridoxine. Changes in the tongue and mucous membrane, resembling those in a niacin deficiency, were noted. The tongue was so red that it looked as if it had been scalded.

Dental Caries. Rhinehart[5] noted that pyridoxine deficiency produced an increased incidence of dental caries in rhesus monkeys. However, little or no effect was noted in the teeth of the animals on short-term experiments. Only animals which had been on experimental diet for two years or longer showed this difference in the incidence of caries. In the animals receiving 1 mg. of pyridoxine a day, there was 7 per cent less caries than the B_6-deficient group. It appears that the slow, chronic, degenerative change is a local oral environmental one.

Strean[8] observed that 5 hamsters that had received twenty times more vitamin B_6 in their cariogenic diet than the controls had only one-sixth the caries score of the control group. In a subsequent paper he suggested that vitamin B_6 exerted its cariostatic effect by acting preferentially on the oral flora.[6] The mode of action of B_6 appeared to be local in nature, because mandibular teeth were more affected than the maxillary.

In a human study involving 28 children between the ages of 10 and 15 years, those who took pyridoxine lozenges (3 mg.) for a period of one year showed less dental caries than a similar group of children who received placebo lozenges.[7] Others[1] have also reported on the ability of pyridoxine lozenges to suppress dental caries.

Toxicity

Vitamin B_6 is practically nontoxic; the amount of vitamin necessary to produce adverse effects is many times greater than the therapeutic dose of 5 mg./kg.

REFERENCES

1. Cohen, A., and Rubin, C.: Pyridoxine supplementation in the suppression of dental caries. Bulletin, Philadelphia County Dent. Soc., *22:*84, 1958.
2. Coursin, D. B.: Convulsive seizures in infants with pyridoxine deficient diet. J.A.M.A., *154:*406, 1954.
3. György, P.: Symposium on rule of some of newer vitamins in human metabolism and nutrition; the history of vitamin B_6. Am. J. Clin. Nut., *4:*313, 1956.
4. Maloney, C. J., and Parmelee, A. H.: Convulsions in young infants as a result of pyriodoxine (vitamin B_6) deficiency. J.A.M.A., *154:*405, 1954.
5. Rinehart, J. F., and Greenberg, L. D.: Symposium on role of some of newer vitamins in human metabolism and nutrition; vitamin B_6 deficiency in rhesus monkey. Am. J. Clin. Nut., *4:*318, 1956.
6. Strean, L. P.: The importance of pyridoxine in effecting a change in the microflora of the mouth and intestines. N. Y. State D. J., *23:*85, 1957.
7. Strean, L. P., Bell, F. T., Gilfillan, E. W., Emerson, G. A., and Howe, E. E.: The importance of pyridoxine in the suppression of dental caries in school children and hamsters. N. Y. State D. J., *24:*133, 1958.
8. Strean, L. P., Gilfillan, E. W., and Emerson, G. A.: Suppressive effect of pyridoxine as dietary supplement on dental caries in Syrian hamsters. N. Y. State D. J., *22:*325, 1956.
9. Vilter, R. W., Mueller, J. F., Glazer, H. S., Jarred, T., Abraham, J., Thompson, C., and Hawkins, V. R.: The effect of vitamin B_6 deficiency induced by desoxypyridoxine in human beings. J. Lab. and Clin. Med., *42:*335, 1953.

FOLIC ACID

The name folic acid, or folacin, was suggested for this group of B vitamins because the active principle was first obtained in concentrated form from deep green leaves. Since then it has been found in yeast, nuts, cereals and animal tissues, especially in liver. This compound is sometimes called pteroylglutamic acid (PGA). It is the *Lactobacillus casei* factor found in liver.

Other names conferred on this vitamin by different investigators are: vitamin B_c, vitamin M, factor U, SRL factor and norite eluate factor.[1]

Chemistry

Folic acid occurs as bright yellow, spear-shaped leaflets, is slightly soluble in water but insoluble in fat solvents. It is readily destroyed by heat and acid and is labile when exposed to sunlight. Chemically, it is composed of para-aminobenzoic acid, glutamic acid and pteridine, which confers the yellow color to the molecule.

Structurally, it may be written as:

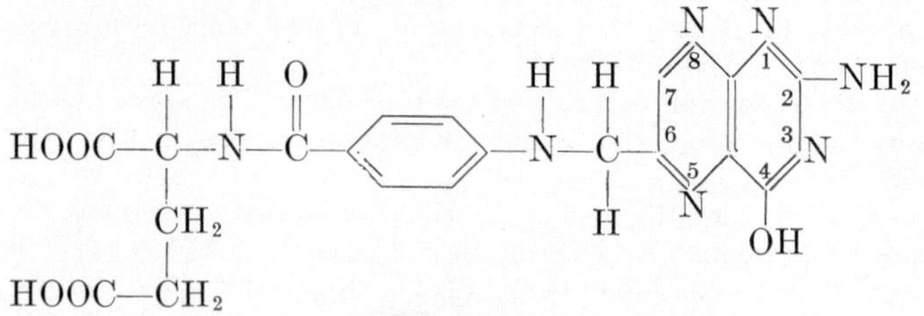

```
                                                       N   N
         H  H  O                      H  H            //8\ /1\
         |  |  ||                     |  |          |7  ||   2|—NH2
HOOC—C—N—C—<benzene ring>—N—C—|6  ||   3|N
         |                               |           \\5/ \4//
         CH2                             H            N     |
         |                                                  OH
HOOC—CH2
```

Folic Acid
(Pteroylglutamic acid)

Folic acid can be converted into the biologically active form, known as folinic acid or citrovorum (CF) factor. The latter is concerned with the formation of normal red blood cells.

Physiology

Folic acid is required for the normal functioning of the hematopoietic system. It has been used in the treatment of sprue and macrocytic anemia. It has a therapeutic value in the treatment of anemias characterized by megaloblastic maturation arrest in the bone marrow.

Folic acid plays an important role in the metabolism of one-carbon compounds such as formate. It participates actively in the synthesis and transfer of methyl groups and in the oxidation of tyrosine.

Requirements

The human requirement for folic acid is not known. The daily dosage used in the treatment of macrocytic anemia is 200 mg. orally or 10 to 30 mg. intravenously.

General Systemic Pathology of Folic Acid Deficiency

A dietary source of the vitamin is required by all types of vertebrates with the possible exception of ruminants. A deficiency will interfere with the growth of chicks, guinea pigs and monkeys.

In man, a deficiency will cause anemia. Sprue, which is common in some tropical areas, is a disease that is related to a deficiency of this compound. Fat utilization is impaired and severe diarrhea may result which will produce a general vitamin deficiency if it is allowed to continue for any length of time. A megaloblastic bone marrow is also the result of a deficiency.

A folic acid deficiency adversely affects the furry coat of rats and feather formation in chicks. It also produces in chicks and turkeys a crippling disease called perosis, or slipped tendon disease.

Toxicity

Large doses of folic acid have not been shown to produce toxic effects in animals or man.

REFERENCE

1. Anon.: Present knowledge of folacin, in Stares, F. J., ed.: Present Knowledge in Nutrition. New York, The Nutrition Foundation, Inc., 1956.

VITAMIN B_{12} (CYANOCOBALAMIN)

Vitamin B_{12} is the anti-pernicious anemia factor which is identical with Castle's extrinsic factor. It was discovered and isolated from liver after more than two decades of research. In 1926 Minot and Murphy[3] used whole liver in the diet to treat pernicious anemia, a disease which had previously been invariably fatal. In 1948 several papers[4,5,6,8] were published which announced the isolation of pure, crystalline vitamin B_{12} from liver and described its microbial and clinical activity.

Chemistry

Chemically, vitamin B_{12} is a complex coordination compound containing trivalent cobalt. Several active forms of B_{12} have been found in addition to cyanocobalamin, such as hydroxocobalamin, and nitritocobalamin. The empiric formula for cobalamine is $C_{63}H_{90}H_{14}O_{14}PCo$.

Vitamin B_{12} is a red crystalline compound, stable at normal temperatures but slowly decomposed by ultraviolet or strong visible light; it also can be inactivated by treatment with dilute acid or alkali. Crystalline vitamin B_{12} is soluble in water, alcohol and phenol but insoluble in acetone, chloroform and ether.

Sources. Liver is the richest source of vitamin B_{12}. Foods of animal origin such as meats, eggs, milk, cheese and fish are also very good sources of this vitamin. Many bacteria require vitamin B_{12} for growth, while others can synthesize it.

Physiology

Human beings do not appear able to absorb vitamin B_{12} from foods unless the intrinsic factor is present in the gastric juice at the same time. The intrinsic factor facilitates the passage of the extrinsic factor across the intestinal mucous membrane. Orally administered crystalline B_{12} is also poorly absorbed unless the intrinsic factor is present. However, when very large amounts of B_{12} are administered, some absorption of the vitamin may occur without the mediation of the intrinsic factor.

Vitamin B_{12} promotes the maturation of erythrocytes. In its absence, red cell maturation is arrested in the megaloblastic stage of development. The vitamin is also concerned with normal neuronal function and the maintenance of nerve cells. Young animals require the vitamin for normal growth.

Biochemically, vitamin B_{12} plays an important role in the synthesis and metabolism of labile methyl groups.

Requirements

The minimum daily human requirement for vitmain B_{12} has not been established but it is considered essential.

General Systemic Pathology of Vitamin B_{12} Deficiency

A vitamin B_{12} deficiency causes certain anemias to develop as a result of a disturbance in the hemapoietic function of bone marrow.

Addisonian pernicious anemia is characterized by a reduced red blood cell count and a low hemoglobin value. The number of enlarged erythrocytes, macrocytes, megaloblasts and reticulocytes is increased. The bone marrow is megaloblastic and hyperplastic. Other characteristic clinical signs of the deficiency are a pallor or yellowish tint to skin, papillary atrophy of the tongue (Fig. 69), and lesions in the gastric mucosa, accompanied by achlorhydria. Changes in the bone marrow, peripheral blood and nervous system may occur. Other clinical symptoms of the disease are weakness, anorexia, sore tongue, paresthesia, incoordination and mental disturbances.

The nutritional macrocytic anemia that is found in malnourished people who eat little protein is similar to pernicious anemia with respect to hematologic findings and mucous membrane changes. However, there are no neurologic or gastric disturbances in the

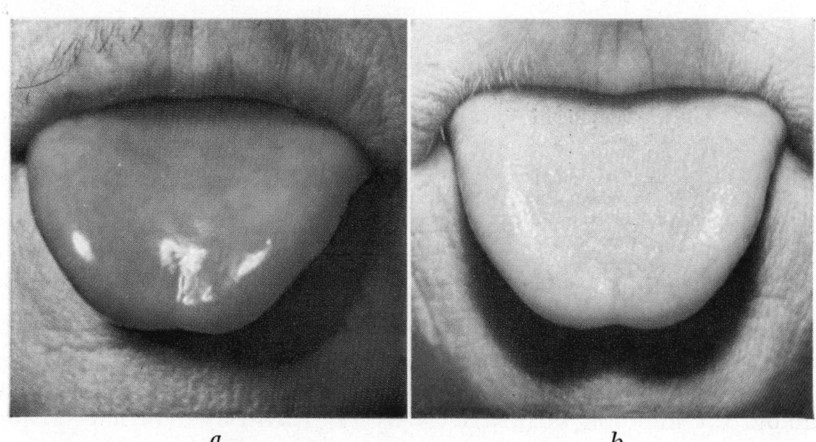

FIGURE 69 *a.* Slick, denuded tongue of a patient with pernicious anemia in relapse, showing striking atrophy of the lingual papillae and discoloration of the tongue. *b.* Same patient after two weeks' treatment with vitamin B_{12}, now shows regrowth of lingual papillae and disappearance of the abnormal color of the tongue. (Dreizen, S., Stone, R. E., and Spies, T., in Dental Clinics of North America, July, 1958.)

former. Both folic acid and vitamin B_{12} are necessary to treat this disease successfully.

Oral Pathology of Vitamin B_{12} Deficiency

The parenteral administration of large doses of vitamin B_{12} has relieved some cases of trigeminal neuralgia.[2,7]

Toxicity

Doses as large as 1,000 micrograms or more have been administered parenterally without local irritation or side effects. Single oral doses as large as 10,000 micrograms have produced no toxic effects.

REFERENCES

1. Castle, W. B.: Medical progress; development of knowledge concerning the gastric intrinsic factor and its relation to pernicious anemia. N. E. J. Med., *249:*603, 1953.
2. Fields, W. S., and Hoff, H. E.: Relief of pain in trigeminal neuralgia by crystalline vitamin B_{12}. Neurology, *2:*131, 1952.
3. Minot, G. R., and Murphy, W. P.: Treatment of pernicious anemia by a special diet. J.A.M.A., *87:*470, 1926.
4. Rickes, E. L., Brink, N. G., Koniuszy, F. R., Wood, T. R., and Folkers, K: Crystalline vitamin B_{12}. Science, *107:*396, 1948.
5. Shorb, M. S.: Activity of vitamin B_{12} for the growth of *Lactobacillus lactis*. Science, *107:*397, 1948.
6. Smith, E. L.: Purification of anti-pernicious anemia factors from liver. Nature, *161:*638, 1948.
7. Surtees, S. J., and Hughes, R. R.: Treatment of trigeminal neuralgia with vitamin B_{12}. Lancet, *1:*439, 1954.
8. West, R.: Activity of vitamin B_{12} in addisonian pernicious anemia. Science, *107:*398, 1948.

PARA-AMINOBENZOIC ACID

P-aminobenzoic acid (PABA) is one of the so-called growth factors for microorganisms. It is widely distributed in nature and is especially abundant in yeast, liver and whole wheat. P-aminobenzoic acid and sulfanilamide resemble each other chemically. Because of this, they participate in a bio-chemical concept known as "competitive inhibition." Sulfanilamide is bacteriostatic because it prevents microorganisms from receiving PABA.

CHOLINE

Choline is required in gram rather than microgram quantities. Some, therefore, do not consider it a vitamin; they state that it acts as a structural component of the body rather than as a biocatalyst. With betaine and methionine, choline constitutes a group of organic compounds that participate actively in transmethylation reactions.

It occurs in nature as a component of certain phospholipids, such as lecithin and sphingomyelin, or as acetylcholine.

Acetylcholine performs an important function in the animal body as a transmitter of nerve impulses across the synapse. Choline furnishes free methyl groups for transmethylation. Methionine, which is an amino acid, also serves as a source of labile methyl groups. These three compounds, choline, methionine and betaine, prevent the accumulation of fat in the liver; therefore, they are called lipotropic factors.

Choline prevents renal hemorrhagic degeneration in rodents and perosis, or slipped tendon disease, in chicks. Further investigation is needed to establish more fully the relationship between choline and methionine and their ability to prevent or cure liver pathology that is seen in liver cirrhosis and kwashiorkor.

INOSITOL

Inositol has not been shown to be necessary for human beings. It is required in such small amounts that sufficient quantities are present even in a poor diet to prevent the development of a deficiency in man. However, in rats and mice a deficiency produces alopecia. Inositol can prevent the accumulation of fat and cholesterol in the liver under certain conditions. It does, therefore, have lipotropic properties.

BIOFLAVONOIDS

Szent-György, in 1936,[1] reported the existence in lemon peel of citrin, a mixture of flavonoids. The active principals in citrin are hesperidin and eriodictin. Its principal function is to maintain normal capillary permeability and fragility.

LIPOIC ACID

This is a new factor which is necessary for the oxidation of pyruvic acid.

REFERENCE

1. Kleiner, I. S., and Orten, J. M.: Human Biochemistry. 5th ed. St. Louis, The C. V. Mosby Co., 1958.

Chapter X

Dietary Interrelationships and Antimetabolites

BY SANFORD MILLER, PH.D.

INTRODUCTION

Life is a series of dynamic, interrelated systems in which the whole is greater than the sum of its parts. To enable this ultimate synthesis of life to take place, all of the constituent systems must be balanced in the quantity and the quality of their components. The body can be compared to an extremely precise machine in which all the parts must be balanced against one another for maximum efficiency of operation. Since the diet serves as a source of raw materials for these systems, it must comply with the basic rules of balance in the universe. It is obvious that, as with all other aspects of life, the diet-metabolism relationship is a two-way street. A good diet should attempt to fulfill the needs of metabolism; conversly, metabolic activity is an expression of diet.

The diet itself, therefore, must in all areas reflect the vagaries and interrelationships of metabolism. The concept of a diet balanced in amounts as well as types of nutrients is a relatively new idea. For example, the quantity of calcium and phosphorus in a diet may seem adequate when each is considered separately. If, however, the ratio of calcium to phosphorus is not optimal, the body will not be able to utilize these nutrients fully. The result may then be a deficiency syndrome, such as rickets in children. For the first time dietetic treatments of deficiency syndromes are available that are based on fundamental metabolic knowledge in a more precise manner than had heretofore been possible.

In recent years it has become increasingly evident that many deficiency syndromes cannot be explained on the basis of an insufficient dietary supply but rather must be based on antimetabolic activity.

An antimetabolite is a substance that is structurally related to an essential nutrient. On this basis it can interfere with the metabolism or function of the essential nutrient. In other words, it is a sterile or nonfunctioning imitation. If the concept of antimetabolite activity was of use in the laboratory alone, it would be of theoretical value only. Today, however, it has been extended beyond the laboratory and is applicable to practical dietary problems.

In this chapter we shall attempt to consider briefly the principles of interrelationships of dietary components and the influence of antimetabolites in nutritive function. While there is no attempt to consider these subjects exhaustively, it is hoped that some appreciation of the areas can be developed.

The history of dietary interrelationships probably began with research into the cause of pellagra. During the course of these investigations, it was observed that the relationship between an amino acid and a vitamin was an important aspect of the etiology of this disease. This was, of course, the niacin-tryptophan interrelationship. The concepts developed in this work have been extended into all other areas of nutrition. For example, interrelationships have been found among the vitamins themselves as well as among vitamins and many other nutrients. Similar interrelationships have been discovered among nearly all of the known nutrients. Since these interplays can influence the utilization of the dietary components, they are of major importance to the clinical nutritionist.

We shall first consider a number of specific nutrient relationships that the dentist should be aware of when reviewing the diet of his patients. For example, the dentist is interested in bone growth and factors affecting it. He is, therefore, concerned with calcium and phosphorus and their interrelationships. Since tissue growth is also part of his area of interest, vitamins A and C and their interrelationship concern him. The amino acids interrelationships involved in tissue growth will be discussed in a later section.

In addition, an appreciation of the interrelationship of folic acid and vitamin B_{12} and that of copper and iron is necessary for an understanding of hematopoiesis, a vital clinical consideration in dentistry.

Secondly, our discussion will turn to the broad classes of nutrient interplay. In this way we shall attempt to indicate the complexities of the problem. In addition, we shall attempt to show that the concept of a single nutrient influencing a particular tissue may not be completely acceptable. For example, an angular cheilosis may not necessarily be the result of a simple riboflavin deficiency but rather may be the end result of a series of interrelated activities among several vitamins.

As indicated in Table 12, these interplays are broad and varied. All of the known seventy or more nutrient materials are involved in one or more relationships, so that to discuss all of the possible combinations is clearly beyond the scope of this chapter. Within each category, examples will be given with the understanding that these by no means exhaust the known interrelationships.

SOME SPECIFIC DIETARY INTERRELATIONSHIPS THAT HAVE DENTAL APPLICATIONS

Calcium—Phosphorus Interrelationships

Of all the nutrients, calcium and phosphorus exert the most direct control over bone structure and formation. Since bone consists essentially of an organic matrix upon which mineral matter is deposited, the relationships of the components of the mineral phase, mostly calcium and phosphorus, are of vital importance to proper bone growth. In fact, there is some evidence that both minerals must be present in the proper proportions at the active sites for deposition of bone apatite to take place. From what has been discussed earlier, it would seem likely that the ratio of dietary calcium and phosphorus should reflect the optimum metabolic proportions.

The dietary calcium-phosphorus ratio is of little significance in an adequate, well-balanced ration. Under conditions of inadequate dietaries, however, this ratio does assume some importance. Since calcium phosphate is not very soluble at the *p*H of the intestine, exaggerated amounts of calcium can decrease phosphate absorption. The reverse is also true. Estimates for the optimum calcium-phos-

TABLE 12. SOME DEMONSTRATED INTERRELATIONSHIPS AMONG THE VARIOUS NUTRIENTS

	Minerals	*Vitamins*	*Proteins (Amino Acids)*	*Fats*	*Carbohydrates*
Minerals	1. Ca-P 2. Ca-Mg 3. Fe & Mn-P 4. Cu-Fe 5. Cu-Mo 6. Fe-Pb 7. Na-K	1. Ca-Vitamin D 2. Fe-Choline 3. Cu-Pantothenate 4. Thiamine-*p*H of dietary salts	1. Ca & Mg-dietary level of Protein 2. K-dietary level of Protein 3. P-dietary level of Protein	High fat increases need for certain minerals, particularly K	1. Ca-lactate (*p*H effect) 2. High carbohydrate increases Ca requirements 3. High carbohydrate decreases K requirements
Vitamins	See listing under Vitamins above	1. B_1-B_2 2. B_1-B_6 3. B_2-Pantothenic acid 4. B_2-B_6 5. B_6-Niacin 6. C-A, B_1, B_6, Biotin, Pantothenic acid 7. B_{12}-Folic acid	1. Choline-Methionine 2. Vitamin D-Protein 3. Niacin-Tryptophan 4. Protein-B_1, B_2, B_6, E, C, Pantothenic acid	1. High fat increases need for B_1, B_2 2. Unsaturated fatty acids destroy Vitamin E	1. Increased carbohydrate increases need for B_1, B_6, Pantothenic acid 2. Dextrin increases absorption of Pantothenic acid
Proteins (Amino Acids)	See listing under Proteins above	See listing under Proteins above	1. Tyrosine-Alanine 2. Arginine-Proline-Glutamic acid 3. Tryptophan-Threonine 4. Methionine-Cystine 5. Tryptophan-Phenylalanine 6. Casein-Threonine	Dietary fat level can decrease requirement for Protein	Dietary glucose can decrease requirement for Protein
Fats	See listing under Fats above	See listing under Fats above	See listing under Fats above	1. Cholesterol and type of fatty acid 2. Saturated fatty acids—Unsaturated fatty acids	1. Carbohydrate-fat ratio to prevent ketosis 2. Fat-Galactose
Carbohydrates	See listing under Carbohydrates above	See listing under Carbohydrates above	See listing under Carbohydrates above	See listing under Carbohydrates above	Dextrin increases the absorption of sucrose

phorus ratio for various ages range from 1.5:1 to 2:1 for infants, to about 1:1 in adults.[46] A calcium-phosphorus ratio of 2:1 represents the proportion of these minerals in mother's milk.

Vitamin D is, of course, known to exert a powerful regulatory effect on calcium and phosphorus utilization. Much experimental work has indicated that vitamin D increases the absorption of calcium from the intestine. While phosphorus is not affected directly by vitamin D, its intimate association with calcium increases its absorption with the use of vitamin D.[18] It is interesting to note that the most rapid absorption of calcium, and thus phosphorus as well, takes place within 2 to 4 hours after their ingestion. This phase is *not* affected by vitamin D. After this period, absorption takes place *only* in animals receiving this vitamin.[22] Apparently, vitamin D extends the conditions optimum for calcium absorption to the lower intestines, allowing a longer period for absorption to take place.[47] The manner in which vitamin D exerts this action is obscure.

Under conditions of abnormal fat absorption (e.g., sprue), excessive amounts of calcium are lost in the feces as calcium soaps. A certain amount of vitamin D is also lost in the feces. On the other hand, fat ingestion under normal conditions actually favors calcium absorption. This would obviously be an important consideration in formulating diets for pathological conditions.[1]

Similar results are seen when protein intakes are examined. Both whole protein and peptones have been found to exert a beneficial effect upon calcium absorption and retention. This is presumably due to the formation of soluble calcium—amino acid compounds upon digestion of the protein.[19] It would seem likely that rickets or rachitic-like changes may be associated with conditions of protein malnutrition.

Although oxalic acid is not generally considered to be a normal nutrient, its effect on calcium absorption is of interest. The formation of the insoluble calcium oxalate is the cause of the loss of calcium in high oxalic acid diets. The most notable example is that of spinach, which contains sufficient oxalic acid to prevent the absorption of all of its own calcium as well as that of the rest of the diet. Spinach, however, does not usually comprise a sufficiently large proportion of the diet to be a serious nutritional problem.

Vitamin C — Unsaturated Fatty Acids Interrelationship

The exact role of vitamin C in metabolic events is difficult to define. This nutrient is involved in so many reactions that relationships with it could fill a book. There are a few interrelationships, however, which can characterize the place of vitamin C in metabolism.

There is today a great interest among cardiac research workers in the factors influencing fatty acid metabolism. It has been known for some time that vitamin C was a necessary cofactor in fatty acid metabolism, in fact, that high fat diets seem to increase the organism's requirement for ascorbic acid.[2,38] If the hypothesis concerning the role of unsaturated fatty acids in atherosclerosis proves correct, the position of vitamin C and its relationship with unsaturated fatty acid metabolism will have to be carefully reevaluated.

Vitamin C — Vitamin A Interrelationship

The fact that vitamin C is concerned with tissue growth makes it likely that this vitamin is related to other tissue growth factors, such as vitamin A. There is some evidence to indicate that this is true. Acute scorbutic symptoms have been found in vitamin A-deficient animals. These symptoms were, in fact, alleviated by the administration of large amounts of vitamin C.[3,31]

The evidence presented thus far can serve to illustrate the fact that deficiencies in one nutrient can often influence the requirements for other nutrients. The dietary concentration of a particular nutrient is no sure way of evaluating its effect on the condition of the patient. More important, perhaps, are the relationships among the various dietary components. The vitamin C picture clearly demonstrates this. Any careful evaluation of the adequacy of a diet must include careful consideration of possible imbalances. As we have shown, this is particularly true of vitamin C.

Vitamin A — Fat Interrelationships

Since vitamin A is intimately concerned with synthesis of epithelial tissue, its importance in dental disease is obvious. In addition to its relationships with vitamin C, vitamin A utilization is influenced by a number of other nutrients.

Much evidence has been collected to show that vitamin A is quickly destroyed by rancid fats.[37] In fact, fats that have been previously used in cooking may be rancid enough to cause measurable destruction. There is no question that the manner of preparation of food can determine, in part, the extent of destruction of a vitamin. In the evaluation of a ration, the preparation of foods should not be overlooked.

Vitamin A — Vitamin D Interrelationship

Since both vitamin A and vitamin D are concerned with dental problems, it should be interesting to note that a relationship between them has been reported. Hypervitaminosis D has been alleviated by the simultaneous feeding of vitamin A.[35] In fact, some evidence of hypervitaminosis D has been found in vitamin A-deficient animals fed "normal" levels of vitamin D in the diet. Again, the requirement for one vitamin is influenced by the availability of another.

Vitamin A — Vitamin E Interrelationship

There is also some evidence that the requirement for vitamin A increases with vitamin E deficiency.[34] In fact, prolonged vitamin E deficiency may lead to a secondary vitamin A deficiency. Although the role of vitamin E in human nutrition has not been fully established, its influence on other, more directly involved nutrients must be considered. This kind of effect may very well be significant in a number of instances where diagnoses are obscure. Consideration of the influence of little understood nutrients on other better defined ones may offer a solution.

Some Interrelationships Affecting Hematopoiesis

The function of vitamin C in hematopoiesis requires careful evaluation. Evidence has been collected which demonstrates clear relationships among folic acid, vitamin B_{12} and vitamin C. For example, folic acid utilization is apparently decreased considerably in the scorbutic human.[17] On the other hand, vitamin C synthesis is disturbed in folic acid-deficient animals.[53] As far as vitamin B_{12} is concerned, there is some indication that vitamin C can restore growth in animals deficient in B_{12}.[50] Other data[24,39] also support these contentions.

Copper and iron are also necessary for optimum hemoglobin synthesis. Apparently copper is necessary for oxidation of inorganic iron. When the proper balance of these minerals is not maintained, anemia is found even in diets high in iron.[12]

There is no question that proper hematopoietic function requires the presence, at least, of all five of these nutrients in the proper amounts and proportions. It is wise for the practitioner who is confronted with possible faulty hematopoietic activity to consider these nutrients carefully and to keep their relationships in mind when evaluating the diet.

GENERAL DIETARY INTERRELATIONSHIPS

Vitamin — Vitamin Interrelationships

As might be anticipated from their key role as coenzymes in metabolism, the interplay among the various vitamins was one of the earliest areas of this field to be studied.

Thiamine has been found to be involved with the activities of a number of vitamins. Deficiencies of this vitamin have caused extensive losses of riboflavin in the urine, decreased niacin storage, and a loss of ascorbic acid from the liver, kidney, lung and other tissues.[49] On the other hand, excesses of thiamine have induced pyridoxine deficiencies,[40] showing that an excess can be as damaging as a deficiency.

A number of other known relationships deserve mention. Among these are folic acid—vitamin B_{12},[3] biotin, pantothenic acid and folic acid,[55] and folic acid—vitamin E.[7] Others are given in Table 12.

Vitamin — Protein Interrelationships

The influence of the vitamins on the metabolism of proteins and protein-containing substances is easily apparent. Protein-vitamin combinations form many enzyme systems in the body. Some of these enzymes, in turn, are involved in the metabolism of the amino acids.[51] Immunological responses can be altered by some of the vitamins.[33] Many other examples could be given to demonstrate these general responses.

Specifically, the requirement for thiamine is thought to be directly related to protein need.[10] Similar data have been collected for riboflavin,[43] pyridoxine,[5] pantothenic acid,[36] ascorbic acid[6] and the tocopherols.[23] In all cases, increasing protein needs increase the organism's need for these vitamins. In all probability these vitamins are directly involved in protein anabolism. There is no doubt that the relationship can work the other way, i.e., a deficiency of the vitamin decreases protein utilization.

Much evidence has also been collected to indicate that even the relationships between specific amino acids and vitamins must be considered in an optimum diet. The nicotinic acid-tryptophan interplay[45] has already been discussed. Work has also been reported to indicate that ascorbic acid is involved in tyrosine and phenylalanine metabolism.[27] Folic acid and ascorbic acid are known to be necessary for the proper utilization of tyrosine.[54] Methionine requires folic acid or vitamin B_{12}[52] and pyridoxine[8] to fulfill its metabolic functions. The effect of choline on sulfur amino acid requirements is well known.[9] Table 12 summarizes much of this data.

Vitamin — Fat Interrelationships

The effect of fat on vitamin requirements and of vitamins on fat utilization stems not only from a metabolic interrelationship but also from the physical characteristics of the fats themselves. A great deal of evidence has been collected to demonstrate the destruction of vitamin E by certain fats and oils. Cod liver oil,[13] lard and oleic acid have all been implicated in this phenomenon. The importance of this activity in the consideration of prepared foods is evident.

Not only can the physical characteristics of the individual fats affect the utilization of vitamins, but the level of dietary fats can also influence vitamin requirements. This effect is variable, however. Thiamine requirements have been found to decrease with high fat diets.[14] Similarly, unsaturated fats in the diet appear to spare pyridoxine so that suboptimal amounts of pyridoxine become optimal when included in a diet containing linoleic acid.[44] On the other hand, thiamine has been reported to be a limiting factor in fat synthesis. To complicate matters even more, high fat diets have been shown to increase the need of the body for riboflavin.[29] It is obvious from these few examples that the optimum dietary level for any of these nutrients cannot be determined by the application of any simple formula. The decision can only be based on a careful evaluation of the entire diet and its function.

Vitamin — Carbohydrate Interrelationships

The relationship between carbohydrate and thiamine was one of the earliest interrelationships investigated. As early as 1914 it was demonstrated that diets high in carbohydrate hastened the outbreak of beriberi.[16] More recent studies have indicated that the role of thiamine as a coenzyme in carbohydrate metabolism may help explain this dietary relationship.

The type of carbohydrates in the diet may also influence vitamin requirements. Dietary riboflavin requirements appear to decrease when dextrin or cornstarch, instead of sucrose or lactose, is used in the ration.[30] Dextrin improves the growth of rats on pantothenic acid-deficient diets. This vitamin-sparing action of dextrin has also been demonstrated for biotin and pyridoxine.[42] On the other hand, deficiencies in thiamine, riboflavin, pyridoxine and pantothenic acid are known to produce lower liver glycogen values, indicating an unbalanced metabolism.[48] If only one of these factors was missing, liver glycogen rose upon administration of the vitamin. Apparently all of these vitamins had to be present in the proper proportions for the efficient utilization of the ration.

Vitamin — Mineral Interrelationships

An interesting interrelationship between vitamins and minerals is represented by the observation that certain vitamins are destroyed when mixed with various salt mixtures. Apparently this response is dependent on the *p*H of the water solution of the salt mix.[41] Thiamine was found to be the most sensitive and riboflavin the most resistent to this *p*H effect. It is possible that the appearance of deficiency syndromes in animals fed supposedly adequate rations might be explained on this basis. The importance of these phenomena in human nutrition is not well documented. However, the *p*H of the ration should be a consideration in the formulation of any diet.

Mineral — Mineral Interrelationships

Much work has been done in recent years in investigations of the trace elements. While most of these nutrients have been found to have specific functions, the efficient utilization of each is in some way dependent upon other minerals. In contrast to the work on the vitamins previously discussed, research in mineral metabolism is not well advanced. The relationship between minerals and protein or fat is not well understood. For example, it is known that high protein diets facilitate the efficient absorption of calcium and magnesium.[32] The reason for this is not known. Moreover, much of this work has been confined to animal studies. The influence of these relationships in human nutrition is little understood. For these reasons, this section will be confined primarily to a consideration of balance among the minerals themselves.

In the feeding of farm animals, the relationship between copper and molybdenum has become important. Animals fed on pastures high in molybdenum content died rapidly; this became a severe economic problem in some parts of Florida.

In potassium deficiency, sodium becomes toxic in some respects. It has been shown that myocardial lesions result when high sodium diets are fed to potassium-depleted animals.[4] This may be the result of the reciprocal intracellular relationship between sodium and potassium, which may produce an accumulation of sodium in cells depleted of potassium and, in this way, possibly injure enzyme activities in these cells.

These few examples serve, it is hoped, to illustrate the dangers of "shot gun" therapy. Destruction of sensitive balances by the overfeeding of specific nutrients is sometimes potentially more dangerous than the initial deficiency itself. "Moderation in all things" applies particularly well in nutrition.

Protein, Fat and Carbohydrate Interrelationships

The relationships of fat, carbohydrate and protein have been discussed in earlier chapters and, to some extent, in previous sections of this chapter. These relationships are generally based on the metabolic conversions of fats and amino acids to carbohydrate and vice versa. There is one area, however, that deserves more extended comment. This is the fairly new field of amino acid imbalance.

Amino Acid Interrelationships

One of the most interesting aspects of nutritional imbalance is of more recent origin. Until 1946 it had been thought that an essential amino acid deficiency in a protein could be corrected by supplying either the amino acid itself or a protein containing the amino acid. No consideration was given to amounts; in fact, excess supplementation was the general practice. In 1946 Elvehjem and his associates[26] published a paper which demonstrated the relationship between tryptophan and several other amino acids, including threonine and cystine.[20] Increases in the dietary levels of these amino acids produced growth inhibitions which were alleviated by the feeding of tryptophan.

Another well known balance is that between leucine and isoleucine. Leucine to isoleucine ratios which vary much from a basic 2:1 produced severe growth depressions.[21] This work led to additional discoveries of relationships between phenylalanine and isoleucine, valine and isoleucine, and phenylalanine and valine.[11]

While it is apparent that nearly all of the amino acids are involved in some type of relationship, the mechanism of these events is not amenable to explanation. Some thought has been given to an antimetabolite-like action and suitable enzyme system. This, however, does not explain the relationships of dissimilar amino acids, such as phenylalanine and valine. Much work remains to be done in this field, an important one in view of the sensitivity of many of these ratios. The severity of protein deficiency disease in many parts of the world adds a note of urgency to this type of research which is not present in other areas of nutrition.

ANTIMETABOLITES

It is perhaps fitting that the discussion of antimetabolites should be contained in a chapter with dietary interrelationships. More often than not, an antimetabolite of a specific nutrient can cause a multiple deficiency simply by reducing available amounts or utilization of other interrelated nutrients.

In general, the action of an antimetabolite is dependent on its structural relationship to a required nutrient. The closer the resemblance, the more potent the antimetabolite. The body uses these analogues as part of enzyme systems, or in any activity in which the nutrient itself is involved. Since the analogue is similar only in structure and not in function, these systems become inactivated and a deficiency syndrome results. Obviously, all other systems that are related to the affected one will also respond, thus leading to apparent deficiencies in those areas as well.

Antimetabolites have been found, or prepared, for nearly all of the known nutrients. In addition to increasing the knowledge of deficiency diseases, antimetabolites have been a potential tool in investigating the function and specific activities of many nutrients. The use of pyrithiamine and oxythiamine in studies of thiamine metabolism and aminopterin in folic acid investigation has been of immeasurable value. Furthermore, the use of antimetabolites as a clinical weapon, e.g., sulfanilamides as antimetabolites of para-aminobenzoic acid, is well known.

Antimetabolites as a practical problem in foods and animal feeds are being investigated with much care today. This is due to the current interest in new methods of processing, such as the use of ionizing radiations and the development of chemical food additives. For example, it has been shown that the treatment of wheat protein with nitrogen trichloride in order to bleach flour results in the formation of methionine sulfoxime. This is a potent antagonist of methionine and is known to cause neurological disorders in dogs. Although this bleaching agent had been used for years, the milling industry has now changed to a less potentially dangerous material.

Another example is dicoumarin, which is found in spoiled sweet clover. This is a vitamin K antagonist and it has been known to cause a hemorrhagic disease in domestic animals given feeds containing spoiled sweet clover. Addition of vitamin K to these rations will alleviate the disease.

The antagonism of acetylsalicylic acid (aspirin) to vitamin K is of more immediate interest to the dentist. It has been demonstrated that regular ingestion of large amounts of aspirin can produce a hemorrhagic syndrome similar to that of vitamin K deficiency. This syndrome can be cleared by treatment with vitamin K. In 1943 Link and his associates demonstrated the induction of hypoprothrombinemia in rats fed salicylic acid. This pathology was alleviated by increasing the vitamin K in the ration.[28] Later these workers demonstrated that acetylsalicylic acid (aspirin) induced the most severe hypoprothrombinemia of all of the salicylates tested.[15] More recently, Kelchner has demonstrated this syndrome in the human and has also indicated the value of vitamin K therapy in its alleviation.[25] The importance of this to the dentist is clear. It is possible for patients who have regularly consumed large quantities of aspirin to develop uncontrolled bleeding after extraction of teeth. Vitamin K or menadione therapy may be indicated in such patients prior to surgery. It seems appropriate for the dentist to determine the need for such treatment before extraction.

REFERENCES

1. Bassett, S. H., Keutman, E. H., Hyde, H. V., and Van Alstine, H. E.: Metabolism of idiopathic steatorrhea. J. Clin. Invest., *18*:121, 1939.
2. Bernheim, F., Wilbur, K. M., and Fitzgerald, D. B.: Studies on a new

metabolite and its oxidation in presence of ascorbic acid. J. Gen. Physiol., *31:*195, 1947.

3. Boyer, P. D., Phillips, P. H., Pounder, W. D., Jensen, C. W., Rupel, W., and Nesbit, M. E.: Certain relations of avitaminosis A to vitamin C in the young bovine. J. Nutr., *23:*525, 1942.
4. Cannon, P. R., Frazier, L. E., and Hughes, R. H.: Sodium as a toxic ion in potassium deficiency. Metabolism, *2:*297, 1953.
5. Cerecedo, L. R., and Foy, J. R.: Protein intake and pyridoxine deficiency in rat. Arch. Biochem., *5:*207, 1944.
6. Dann, M.: Influence of diet on ascorbic acid requirement of premature infants. J. Clin. Invest., *21:*139, 1942.
7. Darby, W. J., Cherrington, M. E., and Ruffin, J. M.: Plasma tocopherol levels in sprue. Proc. Soc. Exp. Biol. & Med., *63:*310, 1946.
8. DeBey, H. J., Snell, E. E., and Baumann, C.: Studies on the interrelationship between methionine and vitamin B_6. J. Nutr., *46:*203, 1952.
9. DuVigneaud, V., Chandler, J. P., Moyer, A. W., and Keppel, D. M.: Effect of choline on the ability of homocystine to replace methionine in the diet. J. Biol. Chem., *131:*57, 1939.
10. Elsom, K. O., and Machella, T. E.: Vitamins in the human subject. Am. J. Med. Sci. *202:*502, 1941.
11. Elvehjem, C. A., and Krehl, W. A.: Dietary interrelationships and imbalance in nutrition, in Borden's Review of Nut. Res., *16:*80, 1955.
12. Elvehjem, C. A., and Sherman, W. C.: Action of Cu in Fe metabolism. J. Biol. Chem., *98:*309. 1932.
13. Evans, H. M., and Burr, G. O.: Vitamin E—Ineffectiveness of curative dosage when mixed with diets containing fats. J.A.M.A., *88:*1462, 1927.
14. Evans, H. M., and Lepkovsky, S.: Sparing action of fat on vitamin B. J. Biol. Chem., *108:*439, 1935.
15. Field, J. B., Spero, L., and Link, K. P.: Hypoprothrombinemia induced in the dog by salicylic acid. Am. J. Physiol., *159:*40, 1949.
16. Funk, C.: Studien uber beriberi XI mitteilung. Die rolle der vitamine beim kohlenhydrat-stoffwechsel. Hoppe-Seyler's Zeitsch. fur Physiol. Chem., *89:*378, 1914.
17. Gabuzda, G. J., Phillips, G. B., Schilling, R. F., and Davidson, C. S.: Metabolism of pteroylglutamic acid and the citrovorum factor in patients with scurvy. J. Clin. Invest., *31:*756, 1952.
18. Greenberg, D. M.: Mineral metabolism. J. Biol. Chem., *157:*99, 1945.
19. Hall, T. C., and Lehmann, H.: Experiments on practicability of increasing calcium absorption with protein derivatives. Biochem. J., *38:*117, 1944.
20. Hankes, L. V., Henderson, L. M., and Elvehjem, C. A.: Liberation of amino acids from raw and heated casein by acid and enzyme hydrolysis. J. Biol. Chem., *180:*1027, 1949.
21. Harper, A. E., Benton, D. A., Winje, M. E., and Elvehjem, C. A.: Antilipotropic effect of methionine in rats fed threonine-deficient diets containing choline. Arch. Biochem. and Biophys., *51:*523, 1954.
22. Harrison, H. E., and Harrison, H. C.: Studies with radiocalcium: The intestinal absorption of calcium. J. Biol. Chem., *188:*83, 1951.
23. Hove, E. L.: Interrelation between alpha-tocopherol and protein metabolism: body weight and tooth pigmentation of rats. Proc. Soc. Exp. Biol. & Med., *63:*508, 1946.
24. Johnson, B. C., and Dana, A. S.: Choline deficiency in the baby pig. Science, *108:*210, 1948.

25. Kelchner, C. H.: Acetylsalicylic acid and vitamin K. Acta Med. Scand., *154* (Supp. 312):471, 1956.
26. Krehl, W. A., Henderson, L. M., de la Huerga, J., and Elvehjem, C. A.: Relation of amino acid imbalance to niacin-tryptophan deficiency in growing rats. J. Biol. Chem., *166:*531, 1946.
27. Levine, S. Z., Marples, E., and Gordon, H. H.: Defects in the metabolism of aromatic amino acids in premature infants. J. Clin. Invest., *20:*199, 1941.
28. Link, K. P., Overman, R. S., Sullivan, W. R., Huebner, C. F., and Scheel, L. D.: Studies on the hemorrhagic sweet clover disease: XI. Hypoprothrombinemia in the rat induced by salicylic acid. J. Biol. Chem., *147:*463, 1943.
29. Mannering, G. J., Lipton, D., and Elvehjem, C. A.: Relation of dietary fat to riboflavin requirements of growing rats. Proc. Soc. Exp. Biol. & Med., *46:*100, 1941.
30. Mannering, G. J., Orsini, D., and Elvehjem, C. A.: Effect of the composition of the diet on the riboflavin requirement of the rat. J. Nutr., *28:* 141, 1944.
31. Mayer, J., and Krehl, W. A.: Scorbutic symptoms in vitamin A deficient rats. J. Nutr., *35:*523, 1948.
32. McCance, R. A., Widdowson, E. M., and Lehman, H.: Effect of protein intake on the absorption of calcium and magnesium. Biochem. J., *36:*686, 1942.
33. Mitchell, H. H.: Chemical and physiological relationship between vitamins and amino acids. Vitamins and Hormones, *1:*186, 1943.
34. Moore, T.: The effect of vitamin E deficiency on the vitamin A reserves of the rat. Biochem. J., *34:*1321, 1940.
35. Morgan, A. F., Kimmel, L., and Hawkins, N. C.: A comparison of the hypervitaminosis induced by irradiated ergosterol and fish liver oil concentrates. J. Biol. Chem., *120:*85, 1937.
36. Nelson, M. M., and Evans, H. M.: Sparing action of protein on the pantothenic acid requirement of the fat. Proc. Soc. Exp. Biol. & Med., *60:*319, 1945.
37. Nelson, E. L., and Lowe, R. A.: Effects of preparation on vitamin destruction. Iowa Agr. Exp. Sta. Report, page 81, 1934.
38. Page, E., and Babineau, L. M.: Effect of cold environment on the hybernating gland of the rat. Can. J. Res., *28:*196, 1950.
39. Proehl, E. C., and May, C. D.: Experimental nutritional megaloblastic anemia and scurvy in the monkey; protoporphyrin, cuproporphyrin, urobilinogen, and iron in blood and excreta. Blood, *7:*671, 1952.
40. Richards, M. B.: Imbalance of vitamin B factors, pyridoxine deficiency caused by additives of aneurin and chalk. B. Med. J., *1:*433, 1945.
41. Rombouts, J. E.: Destruction of B vitamins by certain salt mixtures in purified rations. J. Nutr., *50:*255, 1953.
42. Sarma, P. S., Snell, E. E., and Elvehjem, C. A.: The vitamin B_6 group: VIII. Biological assay of pyridoxal, pyridoxamine and pyridoxine. J. Biol. Chem., *165:*55, 1946.
43. Sarett, H. P., Klein, J. R., and Perlzweig, W. A.: The effect of the level of protein intake upon the urinary excretion of riboflavin and nicotinic acid in dogs and rats. J. Nutr., *24:*295, 1942.
44. Sherman, H.: Pyridoxine and fat metabolism. Vitamins and Hormones, *8:*55, 1951.
45. Singal, S. A., Briggs, A. P., Sydenstricker, V. P., and Littlejohn, J. M.: Ef-

fect of tryptophane on the urinary excretion of nicotinic acid in rats. J. Biol. Chem., *166:*573, 1946.

46. Stearns, G.: Preparation of fecal digests for use in nitrogen and mineral analysis. Am. J. Dis. Child., *42:*749, 1931.
47. Steenbock, H., Bellin, S. A., and Wiest, W. G.: Vitamin D and urinary *p*H. J. Biol. Chem., *193:*843, 1951.
48. Supplee, G. C., Bender, R. C., and Hanford, Z. M.: Interrelated vitamin requirements. J. Am. Pharm. A., *31N:*7, 1942.
49. Supplee, G. C., Jensen, O. G., Bender R. C., and Kahlenberg, O. J.: Factors affecting the riboflavin content of the liver. J. Biol. Chem., *144:*79, 1942.
50. Tappan, D. U., Lewis, U. J., Register, V. D., and Elvehjem, C. A.: Effect of carbohydrate on growth response to vitamin B_{12} in the hyperthyroid gland. Arch. Biochem., *29:*408, 1950.
51. Thompson, R. C., Bakins, R. E., and Williams, R. S.: The extraction of biotin from tissues. Science, *94:*589, 1941.
52. Verly, W. G., Kinney, J. M., and du Vigneaud, V.: Effect of folic acid and leucovorin on synthesis of the labile methyl group from methanol in the rat. J. Biol. Chem., *196:*19, 1952.
53. Williams, J. N., Jr.: Effects of folic acid and aminopterin on enzyme systems. Proc. Soc. Exp. Biol. & Med., *77(2):*315, 1951.
54. Woodruff, C. W., and Darby, W. J.: Effect of pteroylglutamic acid on tyrosine metabolism in the scorbutic guinea pig. J. Biol. Chem., *172:*851, 1948.
55. Wright, L. D., and Welch, A. G.: Folic acid and biotin in the utilization of pantothenic acid by the rat. Science, *97:*426, 1943.

Section II

Applied Nutrition in Dental Practice

Chapter XI

Interpreting Nutritional Needs

BY ISABEL PATTERSON, M.S., M.P.H.

Nutritional standards, whether expressed in recommended amounts of nutrients or of foods, are guides to the practical application of nutrition knowledge to everyday living.

Although several guides or yardsticks relating to nutrition have been formulated during the past 150 years, it was only in the 1930's that sufficient scientific knowledge of nutrition was available to set up a standard based on specific nutrients. It is interesting to note that the first nutritional standard on record related to the compulsory inclusion of "lime" juice (really lemon) in the ration of the Royal British Navy to prevent scurvy.[11] This was in 1796, well over 100 years before vitamin C was isolated and identified. Prior to the 1930's, food standards were usually drawn up at times of emergencies such as wars, famines or industrial depressions to prescribe the amounts of foods or nutrients which would prevent starvation.

As knowledge of the science of nutrition increased, more attention was focused on the relation of nutrition to health. During the decade of the 1930's both the U.S. Department of Agriculture and the League of Nations formulated dietary standards in terms of nutrients with the goal of promoting optimum health.

RECOMMENDED DIETARY ALLOWANCES

In 1940, when we were facing the crisis of World War II, the National Research Council of the National Academy of Sciences established a Food and Nutrition Board. The purpose of this Board was to advise on matters relating to foods and nutrition. One of the first tasks undertaken was the formulation of dietary standards to guide the nation in planning food supplies that would protect the health of our human resources, both military and civilian.

The first set of standards was published in 1943 and was entitled Daily Recommended Dietary Allowances. These allowances are not minimum requirements; they allow a margin of safety sufficient to cover the dietary needs of all healthy people in the United States. However, they are not intended to cover people who are ill or have special dietary problems. Since they allow a margin of safety, an individual who eats less than is recommended is not necessarily malnourished. "The margin of sufficiency above minimal requirements varies widely among single nutrients. This occurs because of the relative differences in storage capacity in the body, in the range of requirements among individuals, in the difficulty of assessing precise requirements, and in possible hazards of excessive intake of some nutrients."[4]

The Recommended Allowances have been revised four times since they were first published in 1943. Revisions appeared in 1945, 1948, 1953 and 1958. Although each revision has had some changes, it is remarkable that so many figures in the 1958 revision are similar to those of the first edition. The allowances are based on the combined judgment of the outstanding nutrition authorities in this country and are not the opinion of a single individual. The fact that they have been revised so frequently since their inception indicates that these allowances are modified as scientific knowledge in nutrition advances.

The 1958 revision of the Recommended Daily Allowances may be seen in Table 13. The allowances are expressed in amounts of specific nutrients. Only those nutrients are included in the table which have been most extensively studied and for which sufficient knowledge is available to indicate a suggested amount. The omission of other nutrients does not mean that they are not essential to human well-being, but if the recommended allowances are met by a mixed diet, other essential nutrients are likely to be provided in adequate amounts. A full explanation of the nutrients not included in Table 13 but believed essential to human health is given in the Report of the Food and Nutrition Board.[5]

Calorie Allowances

Calorie allowances have undergone greater changes in the last two revisions of the recommended allowances than have any of the other nutritional factors. In both the 1953 and the 1958 revisions, a reference man and woman have been used in estimating calorie allowances. In the 1958 revision the reference man is one who weighs 70 kg. (154 lbs.) and is 175 cm. (69 inches) tall; the reference woman weighs 58 kg. (128 lbs.) and is 163 cm. (64 inches) tall. Both are 25 years of age, live in a temperate climate with an average mean temperature of 20°C., and are physically active.

Calorie allowances vary for body size. Table 2, p. 16, gives the suggested calorie allowances for men and women who are smaller or larger than the reference standard. These allowances are based on desirable weights which may be seen in Table 1, p. 16.

Adjustments for calorie needs as a person grows older are also given in Table 2. A 3 per cent reduction is suggested for each decade between 30 and 50 years, a 7.5 per cent decrease from 50 to 70 years, and a 10 per cent decrease between 70 and 80 years. Accordingly, calorie allowances for 45 years are 6 per cent lower than for age 25, and 21 per cent lower for age 65.

Calorie allowances are also affected by climate. Where the average mean temperature is 30°C., a 5 per cent reduction in calories is suggested. For those living in a colder climate, with an average mean temperature of 10°C., a 5 per cent increase is allowed. For each additional 10°C. decrease, a 3 per cent increase in calories is allowed because people living in such areas protect themselves with heavier clothing and indoor heating.

The calorie allowances, as previously mentioned, are given for physically active people. Today, with easy means of transportation and an abundance of labor-saving devices, many people in the United States live sedentary lives. For these people calorie allowances will be less than those shown in Table 13. On the other hand, the person who is very active physically will need more calories. The best criterion for calorie needs is weight. If a person maintains a desirable weight, his calorie intake is probably correct for him. The following statement by Shank is pertinent: "Perhaps a later revision of the Recommended Dietary Allowances will be able to

TABLE 13. FOOD AND NUTRITION BOARD, NATIONAL RESEARCH COUNCIL, RECOMMENDED DAILY DIETARY ALLOWANCES,[1] REVISED 1958

DESIGNED FOR THE MAINTENANCE OF GOOD NUTRITION OF HEALTHY PERSONS IN THE U.S.A.

(Allowances are intended for persons normally active in a temperate climate)

	AGE YEARS	WEIGHT KG. (LB.)	HEIGHT CM. (IN.)	CALORIES	PROTEIN GM.	CALCIUM GM.	IRON MG.	VITAMIN A I.U.	THIAM. MG.	RIBO. MG.	NIACIN[2] MG. EQUIV.	ASC. ACID MG.	VITAMIN D I.U.
Men	25	70 (154)	175 (69)	3200[3]	70	0.8	10	5000	1.6	1.8	21	75	
	45	70 (154)	175 (69)	3000	70	0.8	10	5000	1.5	1.8	20	75	
	65	70 (154)	175 (69)	2550	70	0.8	10	5000	1.3	1.8	18	75	
Women	25	58 (128)	163 (64)	2300	58	0.8	12	5000	1.2	1.5	17	70	
	45	58 (128)	163 (64)	2200	58	0.8	12	5000	1.1	1.5	17	70	
	65	58 (128)	163 (64)	1800	58	0.8	12	5000	1.0	1.5	17	70	
	Pregnant (second half)			+300	+20	1.5	15	6000	1.3	2.0	+3	100	400
	Lactating (850 ml. daily)			+1000	+40	2.0	15	8000	1.7	2.5	+2	150	400
Infants[4]	0–1/12[4]				See								
	2/12–6/12	6 (13)	60 (24)	kg. × 120	Footnote	0.6	5	1500	0.4	0.5	6	30	400
	7/12–12/12	9 (20)	70 (28)	kg. × 100	4	0.8	7	1500	0.5	0.8	7	30	400
Children	1–3	12 (27)	87 (34)	1300	40	1.0	7	2000	0.7	1.0	8	35	400
	4–6	18 (40)	109 (43)	1700	50	1.0	8	2500	0.9	1.3	11	50	400
	7–9	27 (60)	129 (51)	2100	60	1.0	10	3500	1.1	1.5	14	60	400
	10–12	36 (79)	144 (57)	2500	70	1.2	12	4500	1.3	1.8	17	75	400
Boys	13–15	49 (108)	163 (64)	3100	85	1.4	15	5000	1.6	2.1	21	90	400
	16–19	63 (139)	175 (69)	3600	100	1.4	15	5000	1.8	2.5	25	100	400
Girls	13–15	49 (108)	160 (63)	2600	80	1.3	15	5000	1.3	2.0	17	80	400
	16–19	54 (120)	162 (64)	2400	75	1.3	15	5000	1.2	1.9	16	80	400

[1] The allowance levels are intended to cover individual variations among most normal persons as they live in the United States under usual environmental stresses. The recommended allowances can be attained with a variety of common foods, providing other nutrients for which human requirements have been less well defined.

[2] Niacin equivalents include dietary sources of the preformed vitamin and the precursor, tryptophan. 60 milligrams tryptophan equals 1 milligram niacin.

[3] Calorie allowances apply to individuals usually engaged in moderate physical activity. For office workers or others in sedentary occupations they are excessive. Adjustments must be made for variations in body size, age, physical activity, and environmental temperature.

[4] The Board recognizes that human milk is the natural food for infants and feels that breast feeding is the best and desired procedure for meeting nutrient requirements in the first months of life. No allowances are stated for the first month of life. Breast feeding is particularly indicated during the first month when infants show handicaps in homeostasis due to different rates of maturation of digestive, excretory and endocrine functions. Recommendations as listed pertain to nutrient intake as afforded by cows' milk formulas and supplementary foods given the infant when breast feeding is terminated. Allowances are not given for protein during infancy.

offer somewhat more satisfactory procedures for modification of calorie allowances for variations in physical activities."[13]

Nutrient Allowances

Careful scrutiny of Table 13 will show that the nutrients for which specific amounts have been recommended include protein; the minerals, calcium and iron; and six vitamins, namely vitamin A, thiamine, riboflavin, niacin (expressed as equivalents and related to tryptophan, i.e., see footnote which accompanies Table 13), ascorbic acid and vitamin D.

With each of the nutrients except vitamin D the highest recommendations for any age group are for adolescents and for pregnant and lactating women. To provide for growth, the ratio of each of the nutrients to calories is greater for children than for adults.

In regard to vitamin D, 400 units are suggested for infants, children, adolescents and pregnant and nursing women. The following quotation about vitamin D merits special attention:

> "The need for supplemental vitamin D by vigorous adults leading a normal life seems to be minimal. For persons working at night and for nuns and others whose habits shield them from the sunlight, as well as for elderly persons, the ingestion of small amounts of vitamin D is desirable."[5]

Since vitamin D does not occur naturally in many foods, a special preparation is often used to supply it. Recent research indicates that toxic symptoms may result from an overdosage of vitamin D.[6] Caution should be used not to exceed the recommended amount. With vitamin D, as well as with other fat-soluble vitamins, a little (the recommended amount) is good, but a lot is *not* better.

Special mention should be made of iodine, one of the nutrients not included in Table 13. For people living away from the coastal areas, especially those living in the goiter belt of the Midwest, food sources of iodine are apt to be limited. The use of iodized salt needs continuous emphasis. Again a quote from the text of the 1958 revision of the Recommended Dietary Allowances is pertinent:

> "Reliable measurements of iodine . . . indicate that intake averages about 150 micrograms per day. The need for

iodine is increased in adolescence and pregnancy. If iodine intake is reduced so that losses are in excess of intake for a prolonged period of time, thyroid hypertrophy will occur. Ingestion of iodized salt will provide an adequate iodine intake. Unfortunately, less than half of the table salt sold in the United States is iodized."[5]

The recommended allowances are the basis of much of our nutrition teaching. Some people consider them too high, some too low but, over-all, they provide a standard which has wide acceptance. We do not know all we need to know about nutritional needs. Research is continuously revealing new knowledge. As stated previously, we now have a fourth revision of the Recommended Allowances in less than 20 years, which means that the allowances are not static. Hegsted's statement in regard to dietary standards summarizes the need to keep an open mind in regard to their use and interpretation: "Experience has demonstrated that nutritional standards, even when they are based on inadequate information that turns out to be wrong, are necessary and useful. Only when data from various sources are compared to standards is it possible to evaluate standards and, if possible, revise them. The danger lies in the universal acceptance without realization of their limitations. Widespread use and custom may often lead to unjustified assumptions as to the accuracy of facts, making revision of established customs extremely difficult."[9]

U. S. FOOD AND DRUG ADMINISTRATION—MINIMUM DAILY REQUIREMENTS

Although the National Research Council's Recommended Dietary Allowances are the basis of most of our nutrition teaching, mention should be made of another set of nutrient standards in use in the United States. These are the Minimum Daily Requirements of Specific Nutrients prepared by the U. S. Food and Drug Administration and shown in Table 14. These figures are minimum and "the levels chosen were such that amounts less than these would produce demonstrable deficiency signs." They are used primarily in labeling foods or preparations for "special dietary uses." The reader should be aware that if the label on a drug or food package indicates that it contains 25 per cent of the *minimum daily requirement*, this amount of nutrient may be quite different from 25 per

TABLE 14. (FEDERAL SECURITY AGENCY, FOOD AND DRUG ADMINISTRATION, AS ISSUED IN THE REGULATIONS UNDER SECTION 403 [j] AS AMENDED IN THE FEDERAL REGISTER, JUNE 1, 1951.)

MINIMUM DAILY REQUIREMENTS OF SPECIFIC NUTRIENTS

U. S. Food and Drug Administration

	INFANTS	CHILDREN 1-5 YRS. INCLUSIVE	CHILDREN 6 YRS. AND OVER	ADULTS	PREGNANCY OR LACTATION
A—*U.S.P.* units	1500	3000	3000	4000	-------
B_1—*mg.*	.25	.50	.75	1.00	-------
B_2—*mg.*	.60	.90	.90	1.20	-------
Niacin—*mg.*	-------	5	7.5	10	-------
C—*mg.*	10	20	20	30	-------
D*—*U.S.P. units*	400	400	400	400	-------
Calcium—*g.*	-------	.75	.75	.75	1.50
Phosphorus—*g.*	-------	.75	.75	.75	1.50
Iron—*mg.*	-------	7.5	10.0	10.0	15.0
Iodine—*mg.*	-------	0.1	0.1	0.1	0.1

*Cow's milk containing 135 units of vitamin D per quart, and evaporated milk containing 7.5 U.S.P. units per avoirdupois ounce, usually will prevent clinical rickets when fed to normal infants in customary quantities.

cent of the recommended dietary allowance. The differences in the two standards may be seen by comparing the figures in Tables 13 and 14.

FOOD GUIDES

Since the majority of people eat and think in terms of foods rather than nutrients, food guides are practical tools for interpreting the Recommended Dietary Allowances. For several years "The Basic 7 Food Groups," formulated by the United States Department of Agriculture, was the most popular and generally used food guide in the United States. It suggested, "Eat this way every day."

1. Leafy green and yellow vegetables—1 serving or more
2. Citrus fruit, tomatoes, raw cabbage—1 serving or more
3. Potatoes and other fruits and vegetables—2 servings or more
4. Milk, cheese, ice cream—children—3 to 4 cups milk
adults—2 or more cups milk
5. Meat, poultry, fish, eggs, dried peas and beans—1 or 2 servings

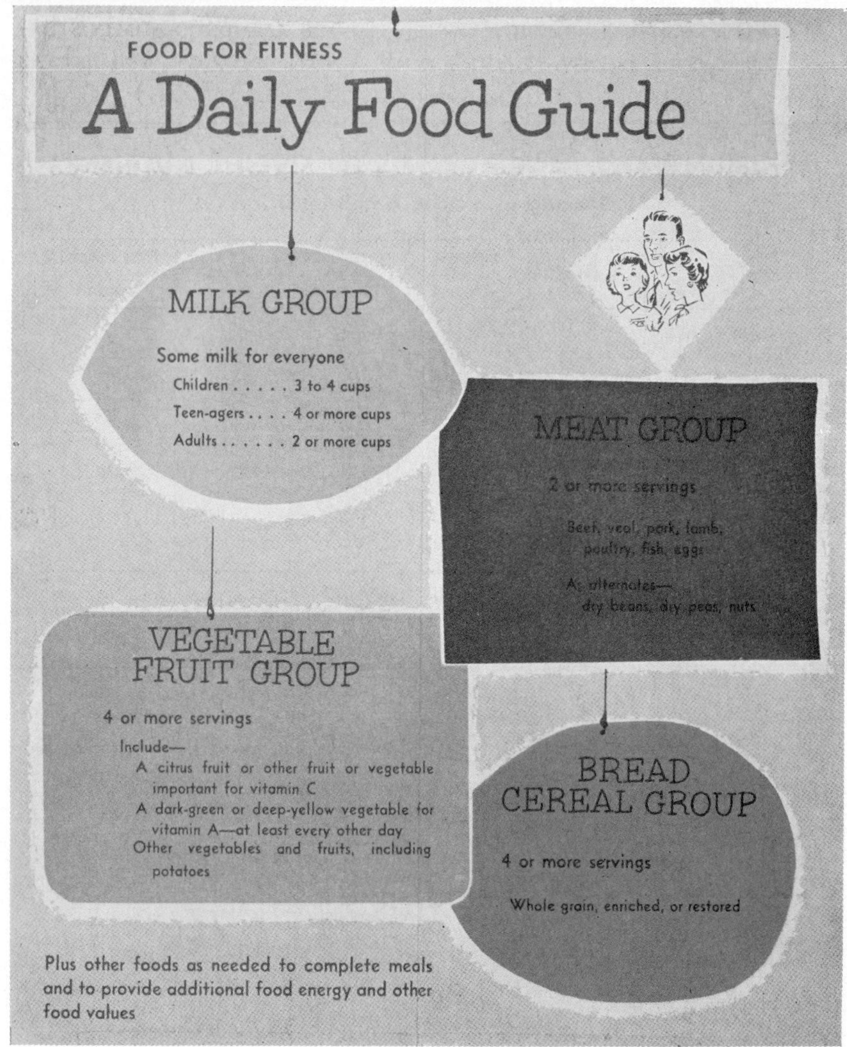

FOOD FOR FITNESS
A Daily Food Guide
MILK GROUP
Some milk for everyone
Children . . . . . 3 to 4 cups
Teen-agers . . . . 4 or more cups
Adults . . . . . . 2 or more cups
MEAT GROUP
2 or more servings
Beef, veal, pork, lamb, poultry, fish, eggs
As alternates— dry beans, dry peas, nuts
VEGETABLE FRUIT GROUP
4 or more servings
Include—
A citrus fruit or other fruit or vegetable important for vitamin C
A dark-green or deep-yellow vegetable for vitamin A—at least every other day
Other vegetables and fruits, including potatoes
BREAD CEREAL GROUP
4 or more servings
Whole grain, enriched, or restored
Plus other foods as needed to complete meals and to provide additional food energy and other food values

FIGURE 70. U. S. Department of Agriculture, Leaflet No. 424, 1958.

6. Bread, flour, cereal (enriched or whole grain)—Some every day
7. Butter and fortified margarine—Some daily

In 1958 the United States Department of Agriculture published a somewhat simpler guide based on "4 Food Groups."[1] (See Fig. 70.) In essence, the guide is similar to the Basic 7 except that butter and fortified margarine are not given group status and fruits and vegetables are grouped together. The 4 Food Groups suggested on this daily food guide are:

1. Milk—children, 3 to 4 cups
   teenagers, 4 or more cups
   adults, 2 or more cups
2. Meat—2 or more servings of beef, veal, lamb, poultry, fish, eggs, dried beans or peas and nuts
3. Vegetable-fruit group—4 or more servings to include a citrus fruit or vegetable important for vitamin C and a dark-green leafy or deep-yellow vegetable for vitamin A
4. Bread-cereal group—4 or more servings of whole grain, enriched, or restored

No one of the above food groups provides all the recommended nutrients but when the food groups, in the amounts recommended, are included in the daily diet, a person may be reasonably assured of meeting the National Research Council's Recommended Dietary Allowances. The milk group will provide most of the calcium, along with high quality protein, riboflavin, vitamin A and other nutrients. The meat group will supply protein, iron and the B vitamins. The vegetable-fruit group will contribute most of the vitamin C and about half of the vitamin A, as well as other minerals and vitamins. The bread-cereal group will furnish the B vitamins, iron, protein and food energy. Other foods such as butter, margarine and other fats and oils, as well as sugars and refined cereal products, may be used to round out the meals and provide food energy. Of course, additional servings from the 4 Food Groups may also be eaten to meet energy needs.

MEAL PLANNING WITH THE 4 FOOD GROUPS

The 4 Food Groups provide a guide to good eating which allows for adjustments in meal planning to fit various cultural patterns, economic levels and individual likes and dislikes. A knowledge of food values in no way detracts from the joy of eating nor from an interest in recipes and meals. In fact, a knowledge of basic nutrition allows a person to choose many different kinds of food, to plan meals with greater variety, and to have confidence that he is eating what he needs to nourish his body adequately. Although a well-adjusted person usually enjoys most foods, everyone is entitled to some likes and dislikes. Nutritionally speaking, there is no single food for which some substitute cannot be found. A look at each of the 4 Food Groups will show the wide variety of choices within each group which may be made to fit individual needs.

Milk Group

Milk may be taken either as whole fresh milk, evaporated milk, buttermilk, yoghurt, dry milk or cheese. Milk may be used in desserts, soups, creamed dishes or on cereals. Milk in an oyster stew has as much value as milk which is drunk from a glass. A generous slice of cheese used in a cheeseburger is equal to a glass of milk.

For the family that lives on a limited food budget, nonfat dry milk is a valuable penny saver. A quart of milk made from nonfat milk solids costs less than half as much as a quart of fresh milk. Nonfat milk is lacking in fat and vitamin A, but the inclusion of a dark green or deep-yellow vegetable in the diet several times a week will provide an adequate supply of this vitamin. Both fat and vitamin A may be obtained economically by using fortified margarine.

Evaporated milk is also an economical food in the milk group. It may be used in cooking or in coffee or tea; not only is it less expensive than cream, it contains more calcium and protein.

Those who prefer fermented milks such as buttermilk or yoghurt may choose these foods from the milk group. Buttermilk is equal to skim milk in food value; yoghurt is equal to whole milk. Despite recent propaganda, yoghurt has no special health values over whole fresh milk. Yoghurt costs more than regular milk and, unless one especially enjoys its flavor and can afford its extra cost, there is no special reason for using it. Buttermilk, on the other hand, usually costs less than regular milk. For those who enjoy it, it may well be used in place of some or all of the regular milk.

Whole milk cheeses such as cheddar cheese are equal to milk in food value. One ounce of cheddar cheese may be used as equivalent to one cup of milk. Unripened cheeses such as cottage cheese have less calcium than whole milk but are richer in protein.

In choosing foods from the milk group, due consideration may be given to various cultural and religious patterns. For example, we are aware that "plain milk is difficult for most Italian-American patients to accept."[7] However, it is often accepted in coffee or in cocoa. For this nationality cheeses are usually well liked and may be used in liberal amounts as foods from the milk group.

For the orthodox Hebrew it is important to remember that milk may be eaten immediately before meat, but not with it. Six hours must elapse after meat has been consumed before milk products may be used.[10] In families who adhere to the Hebrew dietary laws, care needs to be taken to make sure that children receive adequate amounts of foods from the milk group at times when it is permissible.

Meat Group

The choices within the meat group are many: beef, lamb, veal, pork, fish, poultry, eggs, dried beans or peas and nuts.

Foods in this group are usually the most expensive item in the diet. So far as meats are concerned, cost is not related to food value. Cheaper grades and cheaper cuts are just as high in protein and iron as tenderloin. In this group the organ meats (liver, heart and kidneys) deserve special mention for their high nutritional value in relation to cost. If they are disliked and refused, serving them to the garbage can accomplishes nothing. Learning to like these foods is worth the effort.

There is relatively little difference in the protein and iron content of beef, veal, lamb and pork, although pork is richer in thiamine. A family of Southern European extraction will probably choose more veal and lamb, whereas beef and pork will be used more widely by those whose background is Northern European. Fish, poultry and eggs are also complete proteins and may be used as equivalents to meat. Eggs and poultry are well accepted by many cultural groups. Fish, although not universally so well liked as eggs and chicken, is an important and economical member of the "meat" group to many people. For example, Puerto Ricans frequently include salt codfish in their diet.[14] Hebrews often use fish liberally since it is a neutral (parve) food and may be eaten with either dairy or meat meals. Only fish with scales and fins are allowed under the orthodox dietary laws.

Dried beans and peas are also economical foods. Although their protein is not complete, when they are used with milk or cheese or mixed with small amounts of meat, they may well be used to meet the requirements of the meat group. Such dishes as chili con carne, pea soup with ham, or frankfurters and beans, which combine meat and a dried legume, are commendable nutritionally and economically. In the Southwest, among the Spanish Americans, dried pinto beans are often a mainstay of the diet and may be eaten several times each day.[8]

To obtain full advantage from the foods in the meat group, it is recommended that a small amount of food from this group be eaten at each meal rather than a large amount at one meal. To make the most efficient use of protein foods, it is preferable to have an egg for breakfast, a fish, meat or cheese sandwich at noon, and some meat, fish or poultry at night, rather than to have a large serving of meat, fish or poultry at only one meal and no food from this group at the other meals.

Vegetable-Fruit Group

Too frequently the term nutrition has been associated with eating green salads and raw vegetables. Granted these foods are excellent, nevertheless one can be well nourished and never touch a salad or a raw vegetable. Fruits are an excellent substitute for vegetables. They are delicious served with a main course. For example, fried apple slices with pork, baked pears or peaches with chicken, or grilled pineapple with ham may be used in place of a vegetable.

People who claim they do not like vegetables may change their minds when they are served fresh vegetables properly cooked in a small amount of water and delicately seasoned. No wonder some people dislike vegetables when their only conception of a vegetable is a watery mixture of dull green peas and soft carrots which have been soaking on a steam table for several hours.

In considering cultural patterns many adaptations may be made within the vegetable-fruit group. Scandinavians may have some of their servings from this group in the form of delicious fruits soups. Other nationalities may obtain theirs largely from vegetable soups, such as borsch or minestrone. Foods from this group may be used as a first course, as vegetables and salad with the main course or as dessert.

Two groups of fruits and vegetables are singled out for special attention: those rich in vitamin C, and those rich in vitamin A. Within these two groups, choices are wide.

Many of us rely on our daily glass of orange juice for vitamin C. However, for those in areas where the mango or the guava are plentiful, these may well be used. A generous serving of cabbage as a salad at lunch or dinner or a large fresh tomato may be the choice of others to fulfill the recommended serving of foods rich in vitamin C. Nor should the potato be overlooked for its contribution of ascorbic acid, especially when it is cooked in its skin. No doubt the statement that the lowly potato prevents more scurvy than the lordly orange is as true today in some areas as in former years.

When it comes to dark-green or deep-yellow vegetables, our Southern neighbors are more apt to use collards or mustard greens, whereas in the North people will use spinach, kale or winter squash.

From an economical standpoint the use of fresh fruits and vegetables in season is recommended. Fresh tomatoes in season are often an excellent buy, but for much of the rest of the year canned tomatoes are kinder to the food budget. This same principle applies to many other fruits and vegetables. However, there are some, like potatoes, carrots, oranges, squash, cabbage and apples, almost always obtainable. Modern methods of processing, packaging and transportation have greatly increased the variety of fruits and vegetables available for year round use. Today, most of us can enjoy many frozen fruits and vegetables at all times at reasonable prices.

Many young children seem to dislike cooked vegetables but eagerly accept fruits and raw vegetables. From the standpoint of both their nutrition and their happiness, fruits and raw vegetables may well be used to provide the servings of vegetables and fruits recommended. There is no need to force cooked carrots on youngsters who will more readily accept raw ones.

Bread-Cereal Group

Breads and cereals are the most economical source of nutrients in our daily diets. For many people they are truly the staff of life, as they provide well over 50 per cent of the food energy. A wide variety of cereal grains is available, including wheat, rice, corn, rye, oats and barley.

It should be noted that the 4 Food Groups recommends breads and cereals which are *whole* grain or enriched. These are the ones which contain substantial amounts of the B vitamins and iron; the completely refined breads and cereals are much lower in these nutrients (Table 15). The purpose of enrichment is to restore bread and flour to the original nutritive value of whole grain prior to refinement by adding specified amounts of iron, thiamine, riboflavin and niacin.

TABLE 15. COMPARISON OF THREE B VITAMINS AND IRON

(In wheat flour [by the pound][1] and in wheat bread [pound loaves].[2])

	Thiamine mg.	Riboflavin mg.	Niacin mg.	Iron mg.
Wheat Flour				
Unenriched	.28	.21	4.1	3.6
Enriched (all-purpose)	2.–2.5	1.2–1.5	16.–20.	13.–16.5
Whole Wheat	2.49	.54	19.7	15.
Wheat Bread				
Unenriched	.24	.48	4.1	2.7
Enriched*	1.1–1.8	.7–1.6	10.–15.	8.–12.5
Whole Wheat	1.34	.59	13.4	10.

* Enriched bread may also furnish as an optional ingredient added vitamin D in such quantity that each pound of the finished bread will contain not less than 150 U.S.P. units and not more than 750 U.S.P. units of vitamin D. It may also contain as an optional ingredient added harmless calcium salts in such quantity that each pound of the finished bread will contain not less than 300 milligrams and not more than 500 milligrams of calcium.[2]

[1] *Composition of Foods,* U. S. Department of Agriculture, Handbook No. 8, Washington, D.C., 1950.

[2] Bread Standards, Federal Security Agency, Food and Drug Administration, as issued in the Federal Register, May 15, 1952.

In 29 states and Puerto Rico all white flour, bread and rolls are required by law to be enriched. The states in which such enrichment laws exist may be seen in Figure 71. In addition, several Southeastern states where corn is a major item of the diet require the enrichment of degerminated corn meal and grits. In Puerto Rico and South Carolina white rice is required to be enriched. Table 16 summarizes the levels of enrichment in the U. S. of several other food products in addition to those just mentioned.

In those states where no enrichment laws are in effect, care should be taken to read labels carefully. Since over half of the states have enrichment laws, companies which sell bread and flour in interstate commerce are likely to enrich all their products. In this way states in which enrichment is compulsory benefit the others.

The United States Food and Drug Administration has set standards for the amounts of iron, thiamine, riboflavin and niacin which must be present if a product is to be labeled enriched. Some "dark" breads made largely of white flour with only a small amount of whole grain flour added may be of lower nutritional value than the white ones which are enriched. Since there is no legislation controlling the enriching of "dark" bread, careful reading of labels is recommended to determine if the product is enriched or of whole grain.

Cultural patterns affect choices in the bread-cereal group. In the Northern United States, wheat flour and bread are most commonly used. In the South more corn meal, grits and rice are consumed. Those of Italian background may use large amounts of spaghetti, macaroni and other pastas as their choice from the bread-cereal

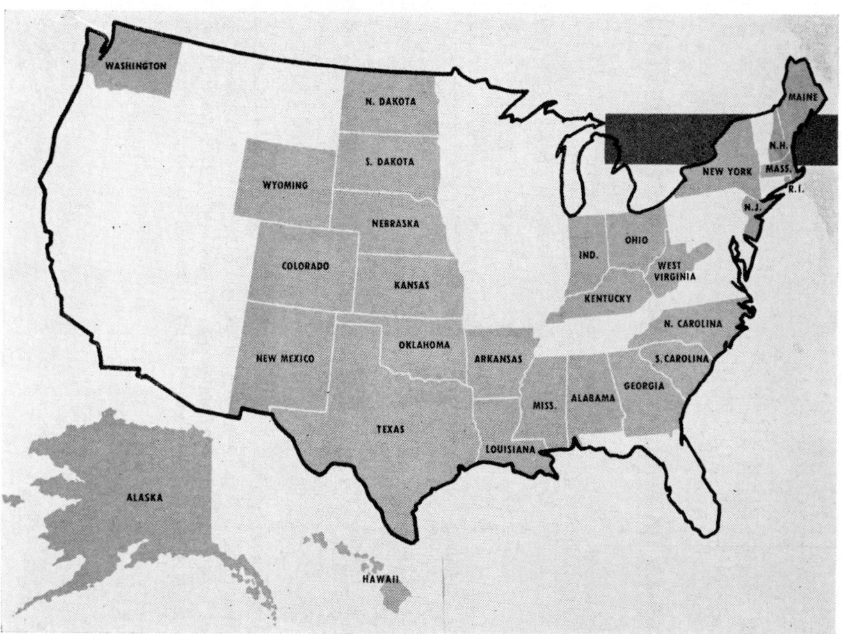

FIGURE 71. The 29 states designated on this map and Puerto Rico passed enrichment laws prior to April, 1959. (Courtesy, American Institute of Baking.)

group; those from the Far East use rice; and those from the Latin American countries are apt to choose more corn meal and use it in tortillas.

Foods from the bread-cereal group are generally well liked; they are bland and used frequently by most people.

From a nutritional standpoint care should be taken not to use cereal foods which are unduly sweetened. Too frequently sweet rolls, doughnuts, cookies and cakes replace the recommended whole grain and enriched breads and cereals. Sweet or refined breads and cereals supply little other than carbohydrates, whereas those recommended supply iron and the B vitamins.

TABLE 16. LEVELS OF ENRICHMENT OF U.S. FOODS (MG./LB.)

Enriched product	Thiamine		Riboflavin		Niacin		Vit. D[a] (U.S.P. units)		Iron		Calcium[a]	
	min.	max.	min.	max.	min.	max.	min.	max.	min.	max.	min.	max.
Bread	1.1	1.8	0.7	1.6	10.0	15.0	150	750	8.0	12.5	300	800
Flour[b]	2.0	2.5	1.2	1.5	16.0	20.0	250	1000	13.0	16.5	500	625
Farina[c]	2.0	2.5	1.2	1.5	16.0	20.0	250	...	13.0	...	500	...
Macaroni[d]	4.0	5.0	1.7	2.2	27.0	34.0	250	1000	13.0	16.5	500	625
Noodles[a]	4.0	5.0	1.7	2.2	27.0	34.0	250	1000	13.0	16.5	500	625
Corn meal	2.0	3.0	1.2	1.8	16.0	24.0	250	1000	13.0	26.0	500	750
Corn grits[e]	2.0	3.0	1.2	1.8	16.0	24.0	250	1000	13.0	26.0	500	750
White rice	2.0	4.0	1.2[a]	2.4[a]	16.0	32.0	250	1000	13.0	26.0	...	...
Whole milk	...	...	...	...	...	...	150	400	...	...	...	...

[a] Enrichment is optional; [b] in enriched self rising flour, Ca 500–1500 mg./lb. required; [c] no maximum for iron; [d] levels allow for 30–50% losses in kitchen procedures; [e] levels must not fall below 85% after washing and rinsing.

(Harris, R. S.: Supplementation of foods with vitamins. Reprinted from Journal of Agricultural and Food Chemistry, Vol. 7, p. 100, February, 1959. Copyright, 1959, by the American Chemical Society and reprinted by permission of the copyright owner.)

Today, with the current emphasis on weight control, bread is unjustly maligned as being fattening. Even for the weight-conscious individual some whole grain or enriched bread or cereals should be included in the daily diet to insure adequate amounts of the B vitamins and iron.

The 4 Food Groups serve as an excellent basis for daily menu planning. In addition to the recommended amounts of the 4 Food Groups, iodized salt should be used regularly; 400 U.S.P. units of vitamin D should be included in the diet of children and pregnant and nursing mothers; and additional foods should be added to meet individual energy needs.

THE 4 FOOD GROUPS—A GUIDE TO TEACHING

The 4 Food Groups provide a comparatively simple guide for the busy dentist, physician or nurse to use in checking on the adequacy of a patient's food intake. It may also be used as a teaching device for effecting improvement in eating habits.

A simple method by which a clinician may use the 4 Food Groups for patient teaching is as follows:

1. Find out what the patient is eating. This may be done by asking him to recall what he has eaten during the past 24 hours. Of course, questions should determine if this 24-hour period is typical of his usual eating pattern.
2. Compare the patient's eating pattern with the 4 Food Groups. Note both the foods which meet those recommended in the guide and those which are lacking.
3. Praise the foods in his diet which are commendable. Since choice of food is a very personal matter, as much comment should be made about what is "good" as about what needs to be changed.
4. If changes are indicated, make one or two suggestions. If more extensive changes are indicated, make note to discuss these at a later date. If the diet is good, do not hesitate to tell the patient so.

A more detailed method of patient teaching, using the 4 Food Groups, will be explained in the chapters which apply this nutritional knowledge to the clinical dental problem.

REFERENCES

1. Anon.: Food for Fitness—A Daily Food Guide. U. S. Department of Agriculture, Leaflet No. 424, 1958.
2. Anon.: Minimum Daily Requirements. U. S. Drug and Food Administra-

tion, Federal Food, Drug and Cosmetic Act, Section 403, Federal Register, Washington, D.C., June 1, 1951.
3. Anon.: National Food Guide. Institute of Home Economics, U. S. Department of Agriculture, Leaflet No. 288, August, 1946.
4. Anon.: Recommended Dietary Allowances. National Research Council Reprint and Circular Series No. 115, 1943.
5. Anon.: Recommended Dietary Allowances, Rev. 1958. Pub. No. 589. Washington, National Academy of Sciences-National Research Council, 1958.
6. Anon.: Vitamin preparations as dietary supplements and as therapeutic agents. J.A.M.A., *169:*41, 1959.
7. Cantoni, M.: Adapting therapeutic diets to the eating patterns of Italian-Americans. Am. J. Clin. Nut., *6:*548, 1958.
8. Hacker, D. B., and Miller, E. S.: Food patterns of the Southwest. Am. J. Clin. Nut., *7:*224, 1959.
9. Hegsted, D.: Establishment of nutritional requirements in man, in Borden's Review of Nut. Res., *20:*13, 1957.
10. Kaufman, M.: Adapting therapeutic diets to Jewish food customs. Am. J. Clin. Nut., *5:*676, 1957.
11. Leitch, I.: The evaluation of dietary standards. Nut. Abst. and Rev., *11:*509, 1941–1942.
12. Roberts, J. L.: Beginnings of the Recommended Dietary Allowances. J. Am. Diet. A., *34:*903, 1958.
13. Shank, R. E.: The 1958 revision of Recommended Dietary Allowances. J. Am. Public Health Asso., *49:*1001, 1959.
14. Torres, R. M.: Dietary patterns of Puerto Rican people. Am. J. Clin. Nut., *7:*349, 1959.

Chapter XII

Applying Nutrition Knowledge

BY ISABEL PATTERSON, M.S., M.P.H.,
AND A. E. NIZEL, D.M.D., M.S.D.

The preceding chapter has dealt with the primary dietary factors —foods and the nutrients of which they are composed. The physiological and environmental factors which influence the selection of the food as well as the systemic conditioning factors are of equal importance in nutrition. Conditioning factors will be discussed in Chapter XIII. We shall consider here: (1) some of the factors that influence food selection; (2) normal diets for the different age groups in the life cycle, because only through an understanding of the normal can we intelligently apply nutritional knowledge to therapeutic diets; (3) special dietary considerations and some brief points on quantitative calculation of diets; and (4) food fads and misconceptions.

FACTORS IN FOOD SELECTION

Physiological and Psychological Influences

Hunger, appetite and satiety regulate food intake. It would be difficult for the dentist to understand the motivation for his patient's food cravings and aversions without having some fundamental concept of some of the theories involved in the mechanisms of hunger and appetite.

Hunger. Several theories have been advanced over the years on the mechanism of hunger. One of the first was probably that of Cannon and Washburn,[14] in 1911, who related hunger sensations to the peristaltic contractions of the gastric wall. Two other theories have been advanced in the last few years, namely the "thermostatic" theory of Brobeck[12] and the "glucostatic" theory of Mayer[17] According to the thermostatic theory "animals eat to keep warm and stop eating to prevent hyperthermia." The glucostatic theory of hunger is based on the utilization of glucose by the tissue cells. There are glucoreceptor cells in the hypothalamus which are stimulated by the differences in blood sugar level between the arterial and venous blood. Blood taken from the capillary bed in the finger and venous blood drawn simultaneously from the cubital fossa of the arm will give different blood sugar levels. The arterial blood is from 10 to 30 mg. per cent higher. If a meal is eaten and blood samples are drawn about an hour later, the arterial blood may be 120 to 130 mg. per cent glucose and that of the venous blood 100 to 105 mg. per cent. This difference in blood glucose level between the finger tip and the arm is the amount of glucose that the tissues in this area of the forearm are using for cell metabolism. When the A-V glucose difference is found to be more than 10 to 15 mg. per cent, the subject is not hungry. On the other hand, if there is a low glucose utilization by the tissues and the A-V glucose difference is below 10, the sensation of hunger will be felt. But even this latter theory has its dissidents.[10] At the moment a completely acceptable explanation of the mechanism of hunger is not yet available.

Appetite. Appetite is an acquired rather than inborn sensation like hunger. It is dependent upon previous experience; in short, there is a psychic element present. In addition to the mental attitude, there is a gastric element in the production of appetite. For example, alcohol warms the gastric mucosa and this effect may arouse appetite. Gastric tone also influences appetite. Suggestions of pleasant things will stimulate gastric tone whereas anxieties, worry and fear will depress gastric tone. Attractive, well-balanced meals may be left untouched on the table if one is emotionally upset; worry, anger or fear can remove all desire for food. Emotions also can cause a person to overeat. Some people nibble continuously when "nervous" or upset, often on easily available foods such as candy or sweets.

Environmental Influences

Food selection is primarily influenced by many environmental factors, some of which are culture, religion, geography, economics and education.

Cultural. From a cultural standpoint we know that, despite hunger, people will often refuse foods with which they are unfamiliar. Many of us would go hungry rather than eat insects or grasshoppers, which are relished by people in other parts of the world. People accustomed to eating large quantities of rice daily as their staple food would probably find great difficulty in substituting potatoes or corn meal. Culturally, people vary in the amount of prestige they attach to food. For some a "good table" well laden with home-cooked foods is of prime importance in their daily living. Others give little thought to meals and are satisfied with simple fare.

Religious. Religion also influences food choices. Some people eat fish on Fridays and fast during Lent and on Holy Days; others forego pork. Still others eliminate all animal flesh from their meals.

Geographic. Geographic availability of food will affect its choice. Wheat, for example, is used in the United States and Canada as the cereal food, whereas rice is the grain of choice in Far Eastern countries.

Economic and Educational. The practical item of money cannot be ignored in considering nutrition; an adequate diet cannot be purchased without adequate funds. For people on limited incomes, a knowledge of food values is of the utmost importance if they are to secure the foods they need to be well nourished. Facetiously, it may be said that a college education in foods and nutrition is needed to eat adequately on a welfare budget. Knowledge and appreciation of the value of a good diet favorably affect food choices. In a study of pregnant women in Iowa it was found that the wives of college students living on a meager income ate a better diet than the wives of laborers receiving about the same amount of money.[16]

NORMAL DIETS

If a person is to realize his potential of health, physically, emotionally and intellectually, he must receive the nutrients he needs at each period in the life cycle.

Early Life

During infancy, a baby's nutritional needs are high. This is obvious when we realize that in 5 to 6 months an infant usually doubles his birth weight and before his first birthday triples it. At no other time in the life cycle is growth so rapid, unless it is during the preceding 9 months of intra-uterine life.

Milk is the principal item of the infant's diet and provides the protein and calcium he needs for growing muscles and bones, plus some of the other essential nutrients. Most authorities agree that either breast milk or a carefully prepared formula will nourish an infant adequately if he is given the necessary cuddling along with the breast or bottle. No mother who wants to breast feed her baby should be denied the opportunity to do so. In addition to milk, a baby needs vitamin D and vitamin C daily. These are usually started during the first month of life. Some pediatricians give diluted, strained orange juice to provide the vitamin C, others prefer a preparation containing vitamin D as well as C.

There is considerable controversy over the best time for a baby to start solid foods. Some pediatricians feel solids should be delayed until the baby is about 3 months of age to allow his swallowing and digestive structures to mature sufficiently. Again, doctors vary as to which is the best "first food" to use. Strained fruit, such as apple sauce or prunes, may be the first solid food because the flavor is generally liked. Some babies may receive cereal as their first solid food. Whatever food is used, the infant may not accept it well because of its newness and strange "feel." If a food is refused, it should not be forced on the baby; it is better to try again in a few days. Fruits and cereals have usually been included in the daily diet by the time the child is 3 to 4 months of age. Egg yolk and strained meats are frequently started about this same period. Vegetables are added sometime during the first 6 months of life. As a baby's teeth appear, he is given dried bread to chew on. Babies vary in regard to the exact time they are ready to start the various foods. Infant Care[6] gives an excellent discussion of the many factors involved in feeding a baby during the first year.

By the end of the first year some foods from each of the 4 Food Groups have become part of the infant's diet. Happy feeding experiences during the first year help to establish good food habits for all the years ahead.

Preschool Years

Throughout the preschool years a child's diet includes the same basic foods he received during the first year. A greater variety of foods from each of the 4 Food Groups will be used and they will be served in forms which require more chewing. For example, strained foods will give way to chopped and, eventually, to "whole" foods. During these early years the use of a minimum of refined sugars will promote good physical and dental health.

Often between 18 and 24 months of age there is a diminution in appetite. A little anticipatory guidance in regard to this lessened interest in food may help parents not to become unduly concerned when their 2 year old eats less than he did at 12 months. When the appetite slows down, it is advisable that the foods available be of the highest quality, nutritionally speaking. Foods from 4 Food Groups will better meet the preschooler's physical and dental needs than those foods which contain a great many calories.

Developing good food habits during the preschool years is a continuous process. Unlike other health measures such as immunizations, which once accomplished last for years, the formation of good food habits takes time, patience and understanding.

School Years

During the school years youngsters are away from home more during the day. This often means that more food is eaten outside of home than during the earlier years. Some children may already have had group experience in eating at nursery school, but for many eating lunch at school is the first regular outside eating experience. Fortunate, indeed, are those children who attend a school where they may partake of lunch, classed as Type A, which meets the nutritional standards set by the U. S. Department of Agriculture. A Type A lunch provides a complete meal composed of ½ pt. milk as a beverage, 2 oz. of a protein food, ¾ cup of fruit or vegetable and a serving of whole grain or enriched bread with margarine or butter. Schools serving lunches which meet the above specifications receive a government subsidy and operate on a nonprofit basis so that the cost to the students is lower than would otherwise be possible.

Children may also carry an adequate lunch from home or go

home to an adequate meal. But too frequently school lunch money is spent at a nearby drugstore or snack shop for sweet foods, soft drinks or other foods of low nutritional value. Today, with many mothers employed outside of the home, care and planning is needed to make sure the noon lunch is an adequate one.

During the school years, breakfast is often a problem. In many cases it is the lack of adequate time which causes the trouble. Rectifying the "time" problem may require an earlier bedtime. A child needs to arise early enough to have sufficient time to dress and eat without worry over missing the school bus or being late for school. Such worry affects the appetite. A little planning the night before can facilitate the serving of breakfast. The table may be set, the fruit juices prepared and refrigerated and the nonperishable foods assembled for easy serving.

Growth continues throughout the school years. Attention to nutrition, both in regard to providing good food and to including instruction in nutrition as a part of health education at home and in school, will aid children in attaining and retaining their best health during these important years.

Adolescence

Of the "growing" years, with the exception of infancy, adolescence is the period of most rapid growth and development. Nutritional needs are consequently among the highest in the life cycle. (See Table 13, p. 246). Adolescence is also a period involving emotional upsets. A desire for independence is often accompanied by a desire for dependence, either simultaneously or alternately. These feelings affect appetite and, thus, nutrition. Telling an adolescent what to eat because it is good for him accomplishes little. However, both adolescent boys and girls are interested in their personal appearance, and if they are helped to understand that wise food choices will improve their appearance, they will accept advice more readily. Clear skin, good figures, pep and energy are desired by adolescents, and adequate nutrition helps to bring these about. Fad diets or drastic weight control measures which may be indulged in, especially by girls, are dangerous because they can impair the health, sometimes permanently.

Today many young girls are marrying and having babies before they are 20 years old. Pregnancy superimposed on a period of rapid growth will tax a girl's strength to the utmost. Adequate nutrition during the adolescent years cannot be too strongly stressed. Since parents' admonitions and suggestions during this period are often not too well received, counsel from the family dentist, physician or other professional person will often be more readily accepted and followed.

Pregnancy

A relationship between good nutrition during pregnancy and the health of both the mother and her infant has been proved in controlled scientific studies.[13,18] During pregnancy the need for protein, minerals, especially calcium, and the vitamins is increased. Caloric needs may be slightly higher than for the nonpregnant woman, but any increased need for calories is usually offset by a decrease in activity. In order to obtain the increased nutrients recommended during pregnancy without increasing caloric intake, foods need to be chosen carefully. When we stop to consider that in nine months a fetus grows from a pair of invisible cells to a fully formed baby weighing about 7 pounds, we realize the importance of his receiving all the nutrients he needs to build various tissues of the body—muscles, bones, blood, teeth, and so forth. If the mother's diet is inadequate, both she and the baby suffer. The diet during pregnancy is a special one in that it is increased in quality to a much greater degree than in quantity.

Teaching good nutrition to pregnant mothers is a rewarding experience. Their interest is high because of their desire to bear a healthy baby. However, care must always be taken not to emphasize nutrition as the only important factor of prenatal health. There are many factors which contribute to a successful pregnancy, and nutrition is only one.

Lactation

The recommended dietary allowances during lactation are about the highest of any time in adult life. Wishik's statement helps us to understand why. He states, "During the period of lactation, however, the amount of output of milk in a single month is greater than the increased mass of the whole nine months of pregnancy."[20] A nursing mother who produces 850 cc. of milk a day requires about 1000 additional calories to produce this milk. She also needs extra protein, minerals and vitamins. The contention that breast feeding is cheaper than formula feeding is a poor one to use in advocating breast feeding. The extra foods a mother needs for lactation are about equal in cost to the baby's formula. For a nursing mother, 1½ quarts of milk, plus generous amounts of fruits and vegetables as well as other foods are recommended to meet dietary allowances for lactation. After the baby has been weaned, a mother who has breast fed her baby may need to reduce her food intake to avoid excessive weight gain.

Adulthood

To maintain and to repair tissues requires a constant supply of all nutrients even when physical growth is complete. As age increases, calorie needs decrease (providing activity is the same), but the need for protein, minerals and vitamins does not. This means that food should be chosen carefully on the basis of its nutritional content if all nutrients are to be included without an excess of calories. Since obesity is a health hazard which predisposes to many of the chronic diseases which appear in the middle years, emphasis needs to be put on the fact that energy needs decrease with age. This means that, if a person is not to gain weight as he grows older, either calories must be reduced or energy expenditure must be increased through more exercise or activity. This latter does not usually happen. Instead of increasing activity, people are apt to participate in fewer sports, to ride more and to walk less.

Programs and methods for losing weight have not been very successful. Therefore, increased attention must be directed toward preventing weight gain through reduction in calorie intake. The old adage that an ounce of prevention is worth a pound of cure certainly holds in regard to the prevention of obesity in the adult years.

Although more publicity has been directed toward the hazards of obesity than toward extreme thinness, the markedly underweight adult should not be ignored nutritionally. Fatigue, proneness to infections, anemia and lack of pep and vigor may be found in the person who is undernourished or eats too little.

Although a desirable weight is not the only criterion for good nutrition, it is one of the most tangible and easily determined measures. Even though our knowledge is far from complete in regard to the best weight for any individual, the range of weights given in Table 2, p. 16, is an excellent guide. The mirror will also help to determine if weight needs to be lost or gained.

Old Age

The general food needs of the older person do not differ greatly from those in the middle years. He needs ample amounts of protein, minerals and vitamins for maintenance and repair of his tissues; his caloric needs are lower because of a slowing down of metabolism and a decrease in physical activity.

The nutritional status of the older person is affected by the many things that have happened to him through the years. Some of the physiological factors will include a decreased ability to absorb nutrients, impaired circulation, difficulty in eating due to poor teeth or dentures, and a diminution of digestive juices, which may cause discomfort and indigestion. Other factors which also influence eating habits of older people are loneliness, reduced income, loss of family and friends, inadequate cooking facilities, diminished interest in foods and lack of appreciation of the need for adequate nutrition.

Often concern on the part of a professional person will stimulate an older person to take more interest in eating. Since protein foods are apt to be eaten in too small amounts, suggestions as to how to use more eggs, milk, meat, fish or poultry may be helpful. Nonfat milk solids (dry skim milk) are an economical food, rich in both protein and calcium. Their use in cooking or as a beverage is highly recommended and often accepted by the older person. Other protein foods are too often neglected because of the bother of cooking them. Encouragement may well be given for use of those which are easily available, such as hamburger or canned meat, chicken or fish. Since a low protein intake may be the cause of habitual fatigue, an improvement in protein intake may help the person to take a greater interest in eating better and in life in general.

In addition to protein foods from the milk and meat group, care also needs to be taken to include fruits and vegetables and whole grain or enriched breads and cereals. Frozen or canned fruits or vegetables require little effort to prepare. Since these are equal in food value to the fresh, their use may appeal to the older person who has less energy to put into food preparation. Vitamin C foods often need special attention since the foods rich in this vitamin are not too numerous and are found almost entirely in the vegetable-fruit group. Although citrus fruits are one of the best sources of ascorbic acid, sometimes tomato juice or some of the other less acid-tasting juices are more readily accepted by the older person.

Today many of these, including apple, pineapple and cranberry, may be fortified with vitamin C. Labels will indicate whether vitamin C has been added. Potatoes cooked in their skins are often well accepted by older people and their use should be encouraged. Even though they are less rich in ascorbic acid, their daily use provides a considerable amount of this vitamin. Breads and cereals are also generally well liked by older people. Cooked cereals such as oatmeal and other whole grain or enriched cereals served with milk not only provide B vitamins and other nutrients but are easily digested, economical and easy to eat. The use of bread stuffs such as doughnuts, sweet rolls and cakes which contain much sugar and refined flour needs to be discouraged, since these may either replace the nourishing whole grain or enriched breads and cereals or add extra, unnecessary calories.

Since more people today are living longer than ever before, medical science is focusing increased attention on ways of improving health during these added years. Adequate, but not overabundant, nutrition is one of the factors which enables older people to enjoy improved health and well being during the later years. The benefits of good nutrition throughout the early and adult years will be reflected in a healthier, happier old age.

SPECIAL DIETARY CONSIDERATIONS

So far in this chapter we have been discussing the need for a well-balanced diet, sometimes called the "normal" diet, to promote health at all ages and to aid in preventing disease. At times therapeutic or modified diets are used to help in treating certain diseases or conditions and as a part of rehabilitation. In recent years there has been a definite trend toward simplifying therapeutic diets and planning them as modifications of the normal diet. As Dr. Stare states, "Intelligent diet therapy should be molded around a basic food plan selected to provide adequately the essentials of good nutrition but yet designed with consideration to the disease under treatment and the food habits of the individual patient."[19]

In general, dietary modifications may be made (1) in the texture of foods, (2) by increasing or (3) by decreasing one or more of the elements of the regular diet, and (4) by elimination of certain specific foods.

The bland, soft or low-fiber diet used in gastrointestinal disturbances is an example of diets which are modified in texture. Such coarse foods as bran, stringy meats and fruits or vegetables high in cellulose or containing seeds are restricted.

The calorie-restricted diet used in obesity, the restricted carbohydrate diet used in diabetes and the sodium-restricted diet used in certain types of heart disease are examples of diets in which some element of nutrition is decreased.[5]

The high protein diet used in some types of liver disease and during convalescence following surgery or a debilitating illness is an example of increasing the diet with a nutrient.

Food allergies require the elimination of a specific food.

Calculating Diets

Occasionally, a dentist may see a diet prescription in the order sheet for a hospitalized patient. It expresses a diet in the amounts of each of the major nutrients that will be required to meet the patient's needs. For example, a diabetic patient whose requirements are 1800 calories per day might have a diet prescription that reads 180C: 80P: 80F (180 grams of carbohydrate: 80 grams of protein: 80 grams of fat). The physician has based the diet prescription on the caloric requirements of the patient. These are influenced by the patient's desirable weight, activity and body size. To fill this prescription the dietitian may use an exchange list for the following groups of foods: milk, vegetables, fruit, bread, meat and fat. Foods within each grouping may be exchanged for one another. Appendix VIII, p. 422, gives the values used in calculating each food exchange in terms of carbohydrate, protein and fat. Appendix IX, p. 423–426, gives lists of foods in each exchange list, as does a special publication of The American Dietetic Association.[7]

The procedure that is used in calculating a diet consists of providing the patient with limits of his desired amount of milk, vegetable and fruit intake and then determining the number of servings of bread, meat and fat exchanges required to complete the diet prescription. Because in this text the use of 4 Food Groups as a standard for evaluating and prescribing diets is used, techniques for actual calculations such as are used in diabetic diets are not included but can be ascertained in many standard texts[15,19] by the interested reader.

After the total amount of food that should be eaten each day has been determined from the prescription, the food is divided into meals. The meal pattern and menu plan are designed to meet the individual's own tastes and environmental problems. This latter point has been discussed in the early part of this chapter.

Appendix II, Food Composition Table for Short Method of Dietary Analysis, pp. 404–409, gives a more detailed analysis of food groups in terms of nutrients. Mineral and vitamin values for various foods are included as well as caloric, carbohydrate, protein and fat. This table is a valuable reference for the professional person who needs to know the nutrient value of individual foods. The bibliography also includes several references to more detailed tables of food values.[1,11,19]

FOOD FADS AND FALLACIES

In the process of eliciting a dietary history as well as prescribing diets, the dentist may encounter food fads and misconceptions. A food fad may connote that a certain food concentrate or mixture of foods (e.g., seaweed, alfalfa and salt) is essential to one's well-being, and it is represented by the charlatan to be a cure-all for any ailment from toothache to flat feet. These pseudo-scientists associate food with magic and mysticism, just as was done in ancient times when special foods were offered at the altars of gods to drive away evil spirits. In our grandparent's day the peddling of concoctions of herbs and tonics by the medicine man in the horse and buggy was probably a carry-over from these early superstitions. Nowadays we have so-called nature food advocates, a modern version of the ancient medicine man.

The following statement from a recent publication of the Federal Food and Drug Administration emphasizes the importance of the problem of food quackery:

> "Nothwithstanding the abundance and quality of the American food supply, a persistent campaign is being carried on to undermine public confidence in the nutritional value of staple foods. False ideas about food are circulated by food faddists and by fringe promoters of vitamin and mineral products. Such products are sometimes offered as cure-alls for serious disease conditions. This may be dangerous to health, especially if ailing people are led to put off getting proper medical attention.
>
> "Modern as well as ancient myths and superstitions about food are utilized by faddist promoters. Such notions as the old idea that fish and celery are 'brain foods' are harmless, but when garlic pills are promoted for high

blood pressure, or grapes for the treatment of ulcers and cancer, the price of ignorance may come high. There is quackery in the field of nutrition as well as in the field of medicine."[4]

The quacks have a few stock arguments that they present rather glibly and persuasively. But the true scientific facts refute each of their ideas.

The points that the faddist emphasize are: (1) Most of our diseases are diet deficiency diseases. (2) The vitamin and mineral value of most foods is inferior because they are grown in depleted soil or soil that is fertilized with chemical rather than organic fertilizers. (3) Therefore, expensive nature food concoctions need to be eaten every day to counteract the ever-present subclinical vitamin and mineral deficiency.

The true facts are: (1) that deficiency disease in America is practically nonexistent, insofar as it is manifested in gross anatomic change. Furthermore, food alone cannot promote health; factors like rest and proper mental and physical environment are equally important. (2) The composition of the soil is not the vital factor in determining the quality of the food; it is the genetic strain of the seed that is important. For example, the breeding and inbreeding of corn determines its nutritive value. Soil enriched with fertilizer will increase the yield of the corn crop. Chemical fertilizers are as effective in increasing the crop yield as the less available organic fertilizers. (3) A wide variety of foods is preferable to any concentrate in promoting adequate nutrition.

In addition to food fads, food fallacies make up another aspect of nutritional misinformation. Old wives' tales and misconceptions are often handed down to succeeding generations. In addition, a fallacy may be compounded by personal dislikes of the individual. Within each of the 4 Food Groups there are specific foods and food preparations that are condemned or praised without scientific basis. The following are only a few examples of several of the fallacies and the true facts that invalidate them. More information about this subject can be found in the American Dietetic Association's leaflet, Food Facts Talk Back.[3]

Milk Group

Pasteurization of milk is described as being detrimental because it produces "dead" milk and the process removes the cream. The fact is that the fat content of pasteurized milk is the same as that of raw milk. Pasteurization kills the bacteria that can produce undulant fever.

Milk is said to have a constipating effect. The fact is that when people drink milk in large quantities and do not eat other foods high in crude fiber and bulk, they are omitting the type of food that promotes peristalsis. Milk does not cause constipation.

Yoghurt is claimed to be superior to whole milk. The fact is that yoghurt is fermented milk which is thick in consistency. There is no difference in nutritive value between fresh and fermented milk, but the cost of yoghurt is greater.

Meat Group

Brown shell eggs are fallaciously thought to be more nutritious than white shell eggs. There is no difference. The color of the shell is determined by the breed of the hen.

Raw or rare meat is held to be more nourishing. The fact is that cooking does not damage protein. In fact, it has the advantage of making meat more palatable and thorough cooking of pork, for instance, will prevent trichinosis.

Fish is spoken of as brain food. Actually, fish is rich in phosphorus, which is an important element in the brain tissue, but no food has been found to be specific for increasing mental activity or capacity.

Vegetable-Fruit Group

Some say that frozen orange juice is not so nutritious as fresh oranges or their juice. The fact is that the vitamin C content of frozen and fresh orange juice is about the same.

Tomatoes are said to help clear the brain. Tomatoes merely supply nutrients and have no such special properties.

Vegetables are said to be more nutritious if they are drunk as juices. The fact is that whole vegetables have the same amount of vitamins or minerals as their juice and, in addition, have the advantage of supplying bulk to the diet.

Bread-Cereal Group

Toasted bread is thought by some to be less fattening. The fact is that toasting changes some of the starch to dextrin and removes water but does not reduce caloric value.

White bread and white flour are condemned as being nutritionally inferior. When they are enriched with iron, niacin, thiamine and riboflavin, as is required by law in most of the states in this country, they are equally nutritious and more palatable than unmilled flour products.

Sugar

Blackstrap molasses is a thick, dark syrup which is an end product of sugar manufacture and is used as a food for livestock. Some say it is the way sugar should be eaten because it contains vitamins and minerals that will cure "tired blood." These same nutrients can be obtained in larger quantities from other foods at much lower cost.

In conclusion, if the dentist is suspicious of any food fad, suspected fallacy or fraudulent scheme, he can receive authentic information about any food by writing the Federal Food and Drug Administration in Washington. This administration has control over foods, drugs, cosmetics and therapeutic devices shipped in interstate commerce or imported into this country to insure that they are "pure and wholesome," safe to use, prepared under sanitary conditions and truthfully labeled.[9] Many states have laws similar to the federal law (in 1956, 26 states had such laws)[4] to cover foods and drugs sold within the state. In 1958 a milestone was passed when the President signed the Food Additive Law which provides that any chemical used in processing food must be proved safe before use.[2] The American Medical Association's Council on Foods and Nutrition carries on a continuous educational campaign to inform both professional workers and the public about false food schemes and misleading advertising.[8] The American Dietetic Association's leaflet, Food Facts Talk Back,[3] is a valuable leaflet which presents the scientific facts which refute many of the common misconceptions about foods.

The dentist needs to stress the following facts to his patient who might be a food faddist: (1) food faddism can lead to malnutrition; (2) the so-called nature foods are very expensive and supply no more in the way of nutrition than the usual foods; and (3) using food concoctions to cure ailments which need medical attention can lead to serious consequences.

REFERENCES

1. Anon.: Composition of Foods. Washington, U. S. Department of Agriculture, Handbook #8, 1950.

2. Anon.: Food Additives Law of 1958. J. Home Economics, *50:*682, 1958.
3. Anon.: Food Facts Talk Back. Chicago, The Amer. Dietetic Assoc., 1957.
4. Anon.: Food Facts vs. Food Fallacies, Washington, U. S. Food and Drug Administration, 1958.
5. Anon.: Guide to Planning Therapeutic Diets. Boston, The Mass. Dietetic Association, 1959.
6. Anon.: Infant Care. Washington, U. S. Department of Health, Education, and Welfare, Children's Bureau, Pub. #8, 1955.
7. Anon.: Meal Planning with Exchange Lists. Chicago, The Amer. Dietetic Assoc., 1950.
8. Anon.: Statements and Decisions of the Council on Foods and Nutrition of the American Medical Association. Chicago, Am. Med. Assoc., 1957.
9. Anon.: You and Your Foods, Drugs and Cosmetics. Washington, U. S. Department of Health, Education, and Welfare, Food and Drug Administration, 1956.
10. Bernstein, L. M., and Grossman, M. L.: An Experimental Test of the Glucostatic Theory of Regulation of Hunger. Rep. No. 165. Denver, Med. Nutrition Lab., 1955.
11. Bowes, A. deP.: Food Values of Portions Commonly Used. 8th ed. Philadelphia, Fife-Hamill Memorial Health Center, 7th. and Delancey Streets, 1956.
12. Brobeck, J. R.: Food intake as a mechanism of temperature regulation. Yale J. Biol. & Med., *20:*545, 1948.
13. Burke, B. S.: Nutrition during pregnancy: a review. J. Am. Diet. A., *20:*735, 1944.
14. Cannon, W. B., and Washburn, A. L.: An explanation of hunger. Am. J. Physiol., *29:*441, 1911.
15. Cooper, L. F., Barker, E. M., Mitchell, H. S., and Rynberger, H. S.: Nutrition in Health and Disease. Philadelphia, J. B. Lippincott Co., 1958.
16. Jeans, P. C., et al.: Dietary habits of pregnant women of low income in a rural state. J. Am. Diet. A., *28:*27, 1952.
17. Mayer, J.: Genetic, traumatic and environmental factors in the etiology of obesity. Physiol. Rev., *33:*472, 1953.
18. Stearns, G.: Nutritional state of the mother prior to conception. J.A.M.A., *168:*1655, 1958.
19. Turner, D.: Handbook of Diet Therapy. 3rd ed. Chicago, University of Chicago Press, 1959.
20. Wishik, S. Nutrition in pregnancy and lactation. Fed. Proceedings, *18:*4, 1959.

Chapter XIII

Clinical Malnutrition—
Its Pathogenesis and Assessment

The subject of clinical malnutrition will be more clearly understood if the terms nutrition, diet, nutritional status, adequate diet, insufficient diet, undernutrition, malnutrition and deficiency disease are defined and differentiated.

Nutrition and diet have been used carelessly and inaccurately as synonymous terms, but actually they are quite different. According to Kruse,[6] "Nutrition is a bodily process; diet, in contradistinction refers to a regimen of food which supports nutrition." In other words, when one considers a patient's total nutrition, he should include a consideration of nondietary as well as dietary factors.

Nutritional status or "nutriture"[7] is the state of health resulting from food ingestion and utilization.

An adequate diet is one that contains sufficient kinds and amounts of food for normal growth, maturation, maintenance and reproduction of the living organism under the stress of its environment. An insufficient diet contains less food than is needed for these functions. The distinguishing factor between undernutrition and malnutrition is that the latter results from eating a diet that is unbalanced in one or more nutrients, whereas the former is due to a generalized lower intake of all nutrients.

Deficiency disease is the direct result of a severe degree of malnutrition. It is manifested by physiologic and, frequently, also by anatomic defects. The state of impaired health that lies between a good state of nutrition and a deficiency disease is referred to as latent or subclinical malnutrition. This type of malnutrition is probably the most prevalent, and also the most difficult to detect.

NUTRITIONAL DEFICIENCY

A deficiency disease is produced when a cell or tissue lacks one or more of the indispensable nutrients. An indispensable nutrient is one that is necessary for growth, maturation, maintenance or reproduction; a deficiency in it will result in metabolic defects and morphologic changes.[3]

To understand how a deficiency is brought about, the following equation suggested by Kruse helps to explain which factors contribute to nutritional balance in tissues:

$$\frac{\text{Supply to tissue}}{\text{Tissue requirement}} = \text{Nutritional balance}$$

Therefore, for a deficiency state to occur, the need must exceed the supply. It may be equally undesirable for the supply to exceed the requirement. For example, an intake of calories in excess of requirements will produce obesity. In other words, for maintenance of nutritional balance there is an optimum zone for this ratio. For most nutrients the zone of injurious excess is not frequently reached, and the problems in clinical malnutrition are usually concerned with a higher requirement for nutrients than is supplied.

Kruse[6] has classified the conditions which affect nutritional balance as (1) external environment, (2) bodily environment, and (3) genetic pattern. See Table 17. The time factor, which is one of the subheadings in the external and bodily environmental conditions, determines the chronicity of the deficiency state. A factor that is not generally recognized is that the acute state frequently represents an exacerbation of an underlying chronic one. Classifying nutritional diseases into acute and chronic types is useful because the speed of response to treatment can be anticipated. In acute deficiencies where tissues are drastically depleted of their nutrients and where cellular metabolism is altered markedly a rapid dramatic response can be expected when therapy is instituted. On the other hand, the subtle changes that are produced by long-standing, low-nutrient utilization by the tissues and cells will respond slowly to

TABLE 17. CLASSIFICATION OF CONDITIONS

	1. *External Environment*		
a. *Socio-Economic*	b. *Physical and Chemical*	c. *Time*	d. *Dietary*
Living conditions	Radiant energy		1) Form of nutrient
Working conditions	Light infrared		Provitamin: analogue
Available foods	Ultraviolet, x-ray		Potential or intrinsic biological activity
Ability to seek them	Radioactive		2) Level
Income	Temperature		3) Imbalance—Disproportion
Education	Mechanical		4) Interrelations
	Trauma		a. Protein-Carbohydrate-Fat
	Physical movement		b. Vitamin-Vitamin
	Pressure; irritation; friction		c. Vitamin: Protein, Carbohydrate, Fat
	Occlusion		
	Dentures		
	Toxicants		
	2. *Bodily Environment*		
a. *Digestive and Metabolic Channels*	b. *Functions and Reactions*	c. *Time*	5) Inhibitors—Antagonists
Functional form of nutrient	Disease: Degenerative, Neoplastic, Organic, Toxic, Infectious		Anti-vitamins
Appetite			6) Enzymatic destruction
Ingestion			7) Autoxidation-rancidity
Digestion			Oxidants-autoxidants
Absorption			8) Processing of foods
Transport	Chemotherapy		9) Availability of nutrients
Formation of enzyme	Endocrine relationship		Precipitation
Breakdown of enzyme	Nutritional status		Phytic acid—Iron
Elaboration, Utilization: Metabolism	Morphology and physiology of tissue		Oxalic acid—Ca
Storage	Growth		10) Acceptability—Palatability
Metabolic level	Pregnancy		
Excretion	Lactation		
Biosynthesis	Work		
Intestinal synthesis	Psychobiology		
Biodegradation	Food habits		
Intestinal destruction	Psychosomatic reactions		
	3. *Genetic Patterns*		

Classification of conditions affecting the ratio according to their natural location and character. The list is not exhaustive.

therapy. The intensity of the disease, mild or severe, also contributes to the rate of recovery. Severe diseases will obviously take longer to respond to treatment than mild ones.

Jolliffe[5] states that a nutritional deficiency may be caused by a nutritional inadequacy which is produced by a dietary inadequacy (a primary nutritional inadequacy), and may also result from various environmental or bodily states that interfere with ingestion, absorption or utilization of essential nutrients (secondary nutritional inadequacy). In addition, there may be physiological stress factors which cause an increased requirement, destruction or abnormal excretion of these nutrients. The conditioning factors may be described as follows:

(1) Various conditions can interfere with food intake, for example, (a) improper or inadequate natural or artificial teeth to masticate food, (b) loss of appetite due to fever, infection, food allergy or nausea of pregnancy, (c) special diets such as are prescribed for obesity, hypertension, etc.

(2) Requirements for nutrients are increased by stress factors, such as fever, physical exertion, hyperthyroidism, growth, pregnancy and lactation.

(3) Interference with absorption by anatomic, physiologic or chemical changes is manifested by reduced absorbing surfaces, altered secretions and hypermotility of the intestinal tract. For example, diarrhea causes hypermotility of the intestine so that there is a rapid transit of ingested food through the intestinal tract, allowing insufficient time for absorption. Achlorhydria, frequently found in elderly people, interferes with the absorption of ascorbic acid, thiamine, calcium, phosphorus and iron.

When absorption of fat is impaired, as for example in sprue, ulcerative colitis, dysentery and celiac disease, absorption of the fat-soluble vitamins A, D, E and K may be seriously curtailed.

Substances in the diet such as oxalic acid or phytic acid will interfere with the normal absorption of calcium.

(4) Interference with utilization of nutrients may result from liver failure. Alcoholics with cirrhosis of the liver have an inability to convert thiamine to cocarboxylase. Adrenal dysfunction will affect vitamin C utilization. Some thyroid diseases hamper concentration and utilization of iodine.

(5) Increased excretion of urine in uncontrolled diabetes affects water and electrolyte balance. Infections generally result in a greater loss of nitrogen in the urine.

PATHOGENESIS OF NUTRITIONAL DEFICIENCY

The body has some reserves of nutrients such as nitrogen and vitamin A upon which it can draw when either primary or secondary nutritional deficiencies are present. When these reserves are exhausted or when the body has no appreciable reserves, as is the case for the water-soluble vitamins, tissue depletion follows. Then

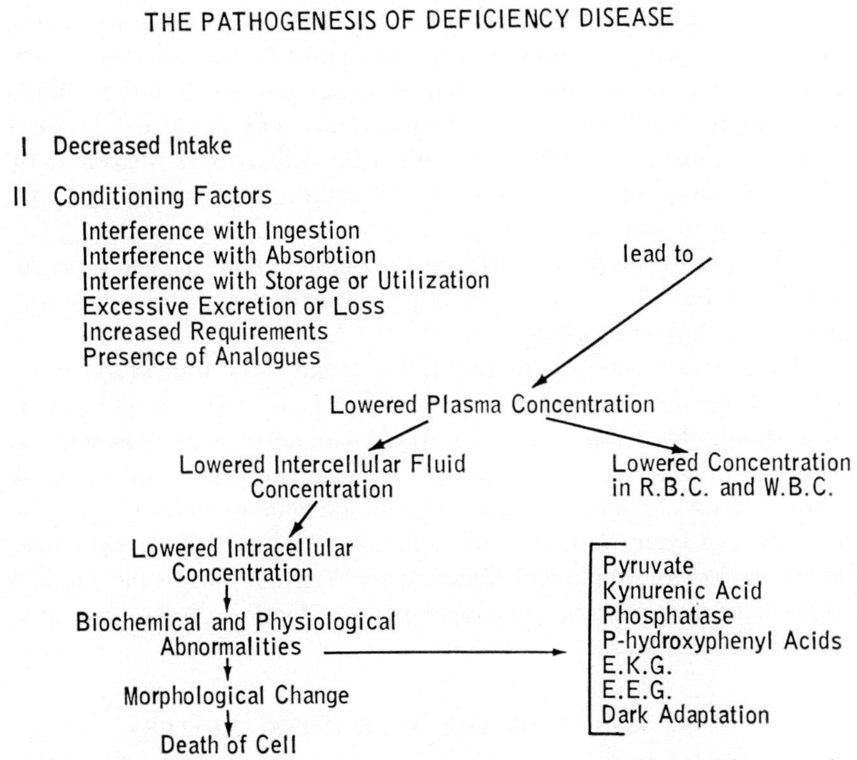

THE PATHOGENESIS OF DEFICIENCY DISEASE

I Decreased Intake

II Conditioning Factors
Interference with Ingestion
Interference with Absorbtion
Interference with Storage or Utilization
Excessive Excretion or Loss
Increased Requirements
Presence of Analogues

lead to

Lowered Plasma Concentration

Lowered Intercellular Fluid Concentration

Lowered Concentration in R.B.C. and W.B.C.

Lowered Intracellular Concentration

Biochemical and Physiological Abnormalities

Pyruvate
Kynurenic Acid
Phosphatase
P-hydroxyphenyl Acids
E.K.G.
E.E.G.
Dark Adaptation

Morphological Change

Death of Cell

FIGURE 72. Schematic representation of factors which contribute to the various stages of deficiency disease. (Follis, R. H.: Deficiency Disease. Charles C Thomas Co., 1958.)

come biochemical, functional, miscroscopic and even gross changes (Fig. 72).

For some nutrients such as vitamin C there is a decreased concentration in the blood and extracellular fluids long before tissue depletion occurs, while for others, such as protein and vitamin A, serum levels are maintained long after considerable loss from the tissues has occurred. Therefore, the value of determining the blood plasma level of a nutrient depends upon which pattern of response it follows. In either case, tissue changes eventually begin to be noted and the deficiency can be considered to enter a second stage, the first stage being a decrease in plasma levels.

In general, the concentration of a nutrient in a tissue is a more reliable laboratory index of nutritional status. Saturation tests and the determination of some nutrient levels in the white cell-platelet layer, as well as in liver and muscle biopsies, are fairly reliable indices of nutritional status.

As a nutritional deficiency progresses to the third stage, there are physiological changes which are manifested as metabolic disease. Abnormal metabolites such as pyruvates are found in blood (in thiamine deficiency) and xanthurenic acid in urine (in pyridoxine deficiency). There may be cardiac changes as measured by electrocardiograph (in potassium and protein deficiencies) or poor adaptation to sudden darkness (in vitamin A deficiency).

The fourth stage of nutritional disease manifests itself microscopically by cellular breakdown and other histologic changes and, grossly, by anatomic changes.

However, it needs to be pointed out that these four stages overlap and are not necessarily clearly defined and separate entities. It also should be made clear that the term nutritional deficiency is also applicable to subclinical as well as clinical conditions. A patient need not show a frank morphologic change before he can be classified as being nutritionally deficient. Biochemical changes may serve to reveal subclinical deficiencies. Vague, nonspecific clinical signs may also precede the development of clinically recognizable nutritional disease.

ASSESSMENT OF THE NUTRITIONAL STATUS

Present knowledge of the procedure for nutritional assessment is based largely on surveys that have been done on population groups.[8] In the past the lack of agreement on standards and the subjective nature of the observations has confused the definition and recognition of clinical signs of malnutrition. Recently, the Interdepartmental Committee on Nutrition for National Defense has published a Manual for Nutrition Surveys[4] which stresses the importance of formulating a mutually agreeable standard for all examiners.

There is still much to be done to clarify what constitutes a "normal" nutriture for an individual, because slight differences in color, texture, dryness, pigmentation, vascularity, etc., are almost impossible to interpret. However, the occurrence of signs commonly found in population groups suffering from specific nutritional deficiencies can be considered suggestive of these deficiencies in an individual.

The nutritional status, or nutriture, of a patient is ascertained by analysis of dietary history, interpretation of symptoms and observation of physical and biochemical signs of disease as well as by the response of the patient to food or specific nutrients which are recommended to correct the disturbance.

HISTORY

Chief complaints frequently associated with nutritional deficiencies are general weakness, loss of appetite, sore mouth and tongue, lassitude, night blindness, muscle tenderness and even numbness of the extremities. Often there is a skin eruption or rash of some type that persists despite any local cleansing or medication.

Inquiries into the *present* and *past illnesses* may elicit information on systemic conditions such as gastrointestinal disease, allergies, gallbladder disease, etc., which interfered with the proper ingestion, absorption and utilization of foods.

The *family history* may reveal a familial tendency toward a disease. Restricted diets may be consumed by the entire family if one member of the family has diabetes or gallbladder disease. The attitude of parents toward food may suggest reasons for the offspring's food habits.

In the *personal history* information on the occupation, food habits, and socio-economic as well as educational status is elicited. It reveals the individual as a whole, his personality and mental make-up as well as the environmental factors that influence his daily activities.

A *dietary history* is obtained through questioning as to usual diet practices by recording total food intake over a week's period. The diet is then evaluated as to adequacy in terms of nutrients or food groups. The recommended allowances of the Food and Nutrition Board of the National Research Council are a guide to the relative adequacy of the diet groups. However, since they are planned to provide a safe margin to cover the needs of almost all individuals, they are considerably in excess of the requirements of many. Only in the case of calories do they offer a precise guide to individual requirements. For dental problems, rampant caries or periodontal disease, comparing the patient's actual intake of the 4 Food Groups with that suggested by the U. S. Department of Agriculture can give qualitative dietary information that is useful for planning and recommending an improved diet.

EXAMINATION

The examination for nutritional deficiencies is largely concerned with exposed parts of the body such as hair, eyes, tongue, lips and skin of the face, neck and arms, and these are the most significant aspects of the examination. In fact, palpation of the spleen and liver and other parts of the examination which are more time-consuming or require the patient to disrobe, are often omitted. Similarly, where thiamine deficiency is known not to be a problem, evaluation of knee and ankle jerks may not be included; and careful examination for beading of the ribs, swelling of the costochondral junctions, etc., will be indicated only in geographical areas and age groups in which rickets or scurvy are known to be occurring.

There are certain systemic conditions or structural changes that are characteristic of a particular age group. For example, edema in a child suggests protein malnutrition, although kidney disease is sometimes responsible; in an adult it is more likely to indicate cardiovascular disease than protein deficiency. Bowing of the legs in a child suggests nutritional deficiency of vitamin D and calcium. In an adult the bowed legs are usually indication of a long past period of malnutrition.

Height, weight and skin-fold thickness are the major physical measurements considered in clinical nutritional evaluation. The skin-fold is measured by picking up a fold of skin over the posterior surface of the upper arm or other specified area and actually measuring it with a caliper. It gives a good indication of the fatness or leanness of a person.

Hair

Even though there is marked genetic and racial variation in color and other characteristics of hair, changes such as discoloration and thinning, particularly in children, may be indications of protein malnutrition. Lusterless, dry, brittle and easily detached hair are other related signs.

ABBREVIATED PHYSICAL EXAMINATION CARD

DATE ______ CARD # ______ (1-5) LOCATION ______ (6) ACTIVITY ______ (7)

NAME ______ SEX ☐ M ☐ F RANK ______ UNIT ______

TIME IN SERVICE ______ ______ (8) AREA OF ORIGIN ______ (9) ☐ RURAL (10) ☐ URBAN

AGE ______ (11-12) YR. HT. ______ (13-14) IN. WT. ______ (15-17) LBS. STD. WT. ______ (18-20) %STD. WT. ______ ______ (21-23)

GLANDS

24 ☐ Thyroid Enlarged

SKIN - FACE & NECK

25 ☐ Nasolabial Seborrhea

EYES

26 ☐ Bitot's Spots

LIPS

27 ☐ Angular Lesions
☐ Angular Scars
☐ Cheilosis, General

TONGUE

28 ☐ Magenta Colored
☐ Filiform Papillary Atrophy
☐ Slight ☐ Moderate ☐ Severe

29 ☐ Glossitis

GUMS

30 ☐ Scorbutic Type

SKIN - GENERAL

31 ☐ Follicular Keratosis
☐ Arms ☐ Back

32 ☐ Scrotal Dermatitis
☐ Pellagrous Lesions

LOWER EXTREMITIES

33 ☐ Bilateral Edema
☐ Loss of Ankle Jerk ☐ R ☐ L

34 ☐ Calf Tenderness
☐ Slight ☐ Moderate ☐ Severe

35 ☐ Studied Further

Special Card No. ______ (36-40)

IBM #	1 - 5	6 - 10	11 - 17	18 - 23	24 - 29	30 - 34	35 - 40
CODE							
ITEM	CARD #	LO ACTS AO RU	AGE HT. WT.	STD.WT. %STD.WT	T NS B MF G LIPS TONGUE	F SP BE-A CT GUMS SKIN L. EXT.	SF CARD NO

ICNND-7

FIGURE 73. From Manual for Nutrition Surveys. 1957 Interdepartmental Committee on Nutrition for National Defense.

Glands

An enlarged thyroid is detected by palpation as well as inspection and is usually due to iodine deficiency. Parotid and submaxillary enlargement may be associated with protein deficiency, as well as with infectious parotitis or mumps.

Skin, Face and Neck

Seborrhea is characterized by greasy, yellowish scaling or filiform excrescences in the nasolabial angles and is sometimes associated with riboflavin deficiency. These smooth, greasy, seborrheic

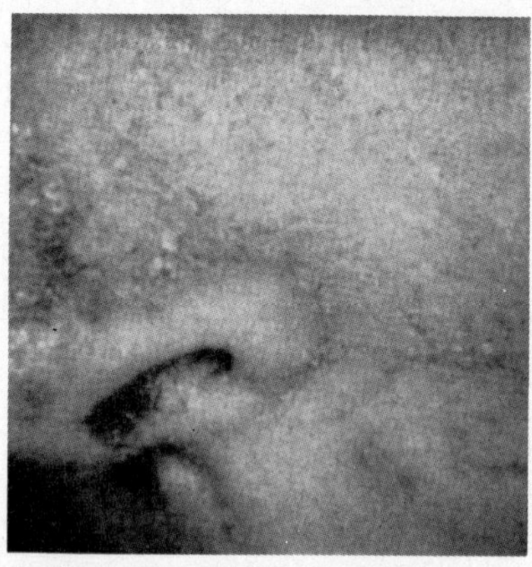

FIGURE 74. Advanced dyssebacea with seborrheic dermatitis. (Jolliffe, N., Tisdall, F. F., and Cannon, P. R.: Clinical Nutrition. Paul B. Hoeber, Inc.)

changes are also noted behind the ears, at the outer canthi of the eyes and on the forehead.

Splotchy erythema of the cheeks over the malar prominences and light brown pigmentation under the eyes and extending down over the malar prominences are commonly seen in undernourished populations. Their significance and their specific nutritional relationships are not known.

Eyes

Thickened conjunctivae may give a porcelainlike appearance, obscuring the vascularity of the conjunctiva. This has been associated with both vitamin A and riboflavin deficiency but may more often be caused by smoke, dust, sunlight and other traumatic factors.

Pingueculae are small raised yellow spots in the conjunctiva and are not known to be associated with any nutritional disease. However, Bitot's spots, which are often confused with pingueculae, are relatively specific for vitamin A deficiency. These are recognized as grayish-yellow, frothy, foaming, superficial patchy lesions seen most frequently on the exposed bulbar conjunctiva. The Bitot's spot is usually associated with a dryness of the conjunctiva called xerophthalmia, which produces photophobia, lacrimation and inflammation frequently followed by purulent exudate. This may be followed by softening of the cornea (keratomalacia) and, finally, scarring and blindness.

There may be some circumcorneal and conjunctival injection due to increased vascularity. The small branching capillaries appear to invade the cornea in a centripetal direction taking on the shape of arcades. This is said to be typical of riboflavin deficiency, but light, trauma or infection may produce conjunctival vascularity. If a diagnosis of riboflavin deficiency is correct, a patient giving symptoms of burning, itching eyes should respond rapidly to riboflavin supplementation.

Lips

Cheilosis begins as a pallor of the lips which is followed by fissuring and yellowish crusting at the angles of the mouth. The buccal mucosa appears to be extending onto the lips, giving an abnormally red line along the lip closure. There is also increased

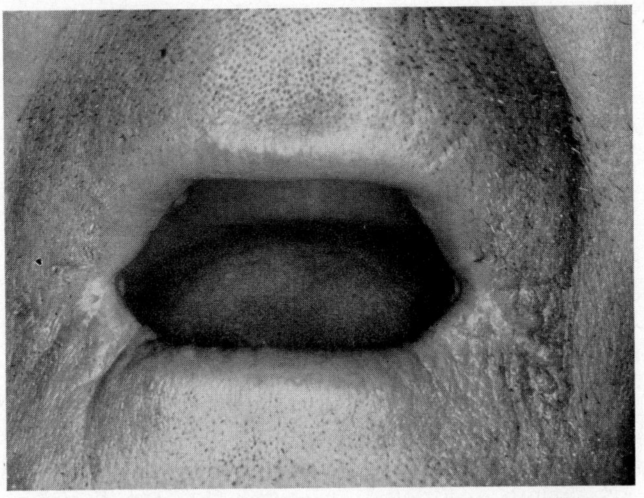

FIGURE 75. Angular cheilosis. (Courtesy, Dr. G. Shklar.)

vertical fissuring. The angles of the mouth present a picture of raw bleeding areas with crusts and scales (Fig. 75).

This is not specific for riboflavin deficiency but may be a sign of a nutritional imbalance of one or more of the following nutrients: riboflavin, iron, niacin, B_6, B_{12}, or folic acid. As in eye changes, some lip changes are associated with environmental trauma such as sunlight, allergies or reduced vertical dimension. There may be an excessive amount of free-way space due either to edentulism or faulty denture construction.

Tongue

The color changes and topographic differences noted in the dorsum, apex and lateral margins of the tongue are the two outstanding clinical signs. Color changes due to nutritional disease vary from a pallor to a strawberry red, beefy red or purplish magenta. The surface of the tongue may be smooth, pebbled, furrowed or hairy.

The filiform papillae, which are small and scattered over the dorsum and margin of the apical two-thirds of the tongue, first hypertrophy and then atrophy and disappear in the case of niacin deficiency or anemias, giving the tongue a smooth, slick appearance.

The fungiform papillae, which are above the general epithelial surface of the tongue, are scattered sparingly over the dorsum and apex of the tongue and are less numerous than the filiform papillae. Normally they are large in size and deep red in color. In riboflavin deficiency they will hypertrophy, giving a granular pebbly appearance and may give the tongue a purplish hue. With a continuation of the deficiency the fungiform papillae flatten out, fuse and atrophy.

In the first stages of pellagra, the tongue may appear swollen so that the pressure of the teeth against the anterior and lateral margins produces indentations and a typical beefy red appearance. It undergoes changes fairly rapidly to a dry, smooth, shiny red atrophic tongue. (See Fig. 66, p. 205.)

A pale tongue is usually the result of anemia such as results from deficiencies of iron, folic acid and vitamin B_{12} (Fig. 69, p. 221).

There are many non-nutritional conditions which may occur as, for example, black tongue; this is due to action of pigment-producing oral fungi on hyperkeratinized and hyperplastic filiform papillae, particularly during protracted antibiotic therapy. Furrows, fissures and serrations of the tongue have no recognized specific nutritional significance.

Gingivae

Several vitamin deficiencies have been associated with alterations in gingival health. Red, spongy, swollen interdental papillae

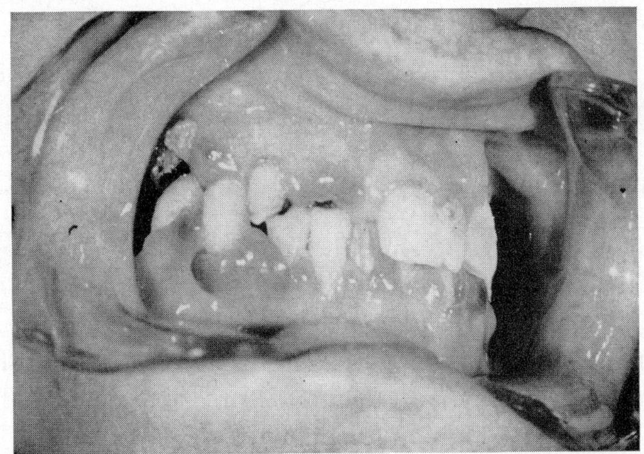

FIGURE 76. Scorbutic gingivitis. (Courtesy, Dr. G. Shklar.)

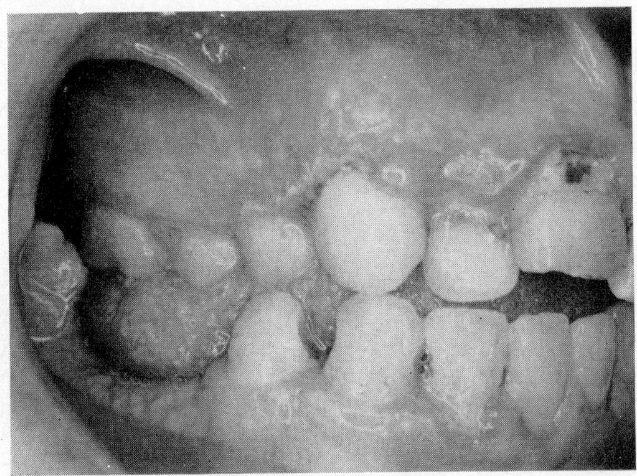

FIGURE 77. Acute necrotizing gingivitis.

and marginal gingiva which may hypertrophy to the point of almost completely covering the teeth are associated with scurvy (Fig. 76). Edentulous areas are never affected. Because the peridental membrane and supporting fibers undergo degenerative changes, the teeth lose their support and exfoliate. Unquestionably, the local irritating factors of calculus and bacterial infection are responsible for initiating the inflammatory changes, with ascorbic acid deficiency acting merely as the conditioning factor.

Niacin deficiency will lower the resistance of the gingiva so that it is secondarily invaded by Vincent's organisms. The punched-out interdental papillae covered with grayish pseudomembrane and gingival inflammation (Fig. 77) so characteristic of acute necrotizing gingivitis have been observed in acute pellagra.

Inflamed hypersensitive gingivae have been associated with vitamin A deficiency, which produces a metaplasia of the epithelium and may allow a secondary infection.

Buccal Mucosa

Pallor of oral mucosa, sometimes with vesicular eruptions, may suggest a hypochromic anemia due to iron deficiency. Of course, any severe anemia will result in pallor.

In many instances mucosal lesions are the result of the extension of a lip or gingival inflammation associated with various vitamin B complex or vitamin C deficiencies.

Teeth

Hypoplastic enamel which is characterized by pitting, grooving and total enamel loss may be characteristic of youngsters who were afflicted with rickets during the formation of their teeth (Fig. 78).

Mottled enamel may be found in persons who were exposed to

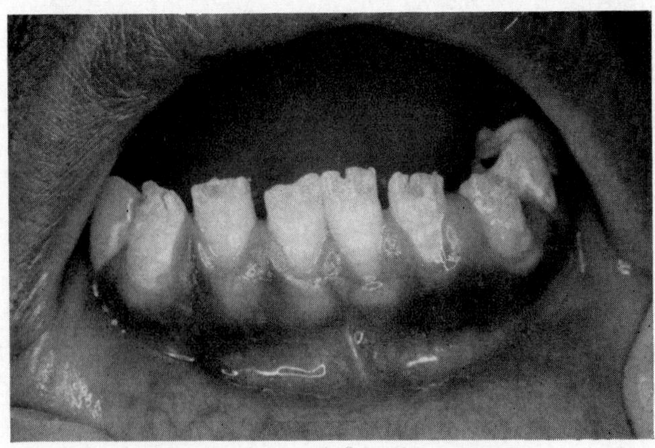

FIGURE 78. Hypoplastic enamel.

more than 2 ppm. of fluorine during the developmental period of their teeth. (See Fig. 43, p. 136.)

The importance of vitamin C in dentinal matrix formation, at least in guinea pigs, has been proved. The evidence for man that vitamin C deficiency can interfere with matrix formation is more presumptive than conclusive.

Dental caries is not a result of undernutrition but is influenced by an imbalanced diet. Moreover, the positive role of fermentable carbohydrates, which serve as a substrate for microbial growth, is undeniable. The effects of supplements of micro- and macronutrients to the dietary are under constant investigation. For example, calcium is essential for proper tooth formation and ultimate resistance to caries. Fluorine is a trace mineral which contributes greatly to the formation of caries-resistant teeth. It is quite possible that phosphates contribute to caries inhibition (p. 106).

Skin

Follicular hyperkeratosis produces a rough skin that has been likened to a permanent "goose flesh"; it does not disappear on

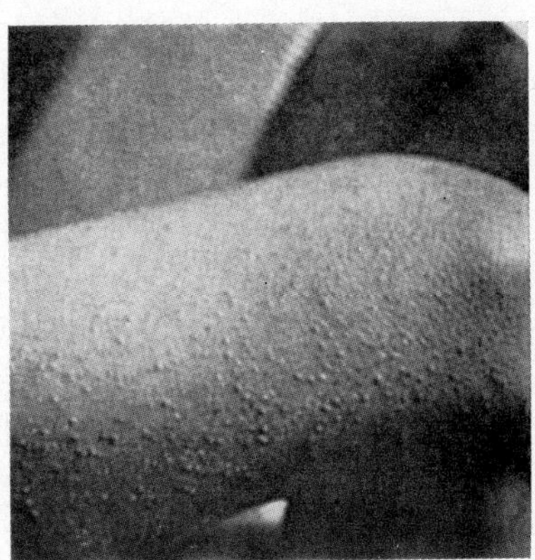

FIGURE 79. Early follicular hyperkeratosis resembling "goose flesh." (Jolliffe, N., Tisdall, F. F., and Cannon, P. R.: Clinical Nutrition. Paul B. Hoeber, Inc.)

rubbing (Fig. 79). The papillae are formed by keratotic plugs which project from the hair follicles and are surrounded by dry skin. It has been associated with both vitamin A and essential fatty acid deficiency. Perifolliculosis is a reddening around the pores which does not blanch upon pressure. It is usually limited to the hairy regions of the body, especially the legs. It has been associated with ascorbic acid deficiency.

Xerosis is a dryness of the skin which is very difficult to evaluate because it is closely related to bathing habits, personal cleanliness, etc. On the other hand, in a person with a clean skin, excessive dryness is often associated with vitamin A deficiency. The skin may even have an alligator-like, pseudo-plaque appearance.

Hyperpigmentation may be seen in protein deficiency. In pellagra, the skin exposed to sunlight, such as the neck and dorsum of the hands, develops hyperpigmentation, hyperkeratosis and desquamation. Acne has no clear relation to nutritional status.

Skeletal

In vitamin D deficiency, the thoracic cage may have a depressed sternum and beaded ribs. A bulging forehead and soft spots indicating delayed closure of the fontanelle, as well as slowly erupting teeth, enlarged wrists and bowed legs also occur in this nutritional disease.

Neurologic

There are clinical tests that deal with the neurologic system which the dentist would not be expected to perform. However, as a matter of knowledge, they are briefly discussed here.

There is calf muscle tenderness on applying pressure in the presence of thiamine deficiency. When an object is drawn over the bottom of the foot, a plantar hyperesthetic pain is elicited. There may be diminished vibratory sensation when tested with a tuning fork. In addition, if ankle or knee jerks are absent, a nutritional polyneuropathy may be responsible. Other signs of peripheral neuritis are burning sensations when the skin of the leg is stroked with an applicator, peculiar gait, and toe and foot drop as well as wrist drop.

In niacin deficiency there may be mental changes such as memory defects, disorientation, confusion and confabulation. There are also periods of excitement, depression, mania, delirium and paranoia. In beriberi, low blood pressure, electrocardiographic abnormalities, liver congestion, ascites and edema are likely to accompany the neuritic signs. Wernicke's disease, an involvement of the central nervous system as a result of B complex deficiencies (as in alcoholism), is characterized by encephalopathy, paralysis of the eye muscles and peripheral neuritis.

LABORATORY TESTS

Clinical appraisals are sometimes so nonspecific and so uncertain that confirmation from biochemical procedures is sought. Unfortunately, these are not always sufficiently reliable.

Mild protein deficiencies are not measurable by serum total protein or serum albumin, but these blood constituents are markedly lowered in severe protein deficiency. As for the blood levels of various essential vitamins, it is now recognized that these measure the post-absorptive state of an individual for materials in transit between less vital and more vital parts of the body. For example, it is possible to find a zero level of vitamin C in the plasma when the tissues are not seriously depleted. Blood levels of such vitamins as riboflavin, thiamine, vitamin C and niacin rise rapidly following a meal and decline during the fasting period.

It has been found that the determination of the B complex vitamins in blood plasma is not very useful. Even in obvious cases of riboflavin deficiency, for example, the blood plasma levels for this vitamin may be found within the normal range. In these instances, the blood is a transport mechanism where the nutrient is being drawn from less vital areas to the metabolically more essential tissues in order to maintain the integrity of these structures.

In population groups measurement of vitamins A and C in capillary blood by micro methods is commonly used to determine the existence of deficiency of these nutrients. These methods are not so reliable for the individual as they are for group studies. Ascorbic acid levels in tissues (or, for example, in leucocytes) are a more dependable biochemical measure of scurvy. For riboflavin and thiamine, load tests are a reliable index of tissue saturation and 24 hour urinary excretion measurements contribute good confirmatory evidence of the level of intake of these vitamins.

An elevation of serum alkaline phosphatase in children is strong presumptive evidence of active rickets. A prolonged prothrombin time is an indication of vitamin K deficiency.

An illustration of a very reliable laboratory procedure to determine a specific deficiency is the measurement of hemoglobin and hematocrit for the appraisal of anemias. The presence and also the type of anemia can be defined sufficiently well by using these two measurements for the information obtained to be extremely useful in determining the nutritional factor involved.

CONCLUSIONS

From this discussion it should be clear that the appreciation of the mechanisms that are involved in supplying nutrients to the tissue cells guides the assessment of the patient's nutritional status. This means that the clinician must not only consider a dietary history but also environmental factors and any systemic factors that might influence the ingestion, absorption, utilization and excretion of the nutrients. In addition to the subjective symptoms obtained from medical histories, objective clinical and functional signs as well as laboratory findings must be considered for the total appraisal.

Because neither primary dietary failure nor conditioning factors are limited to a single nutrient, every patient suspected of a nutritional deficiency is potentially a victim of multiple deficiency, with some few outstanding criteria that point to the most prevalent deficiency or deficiencies. For example, the finding in a child of edema, skin pigmentation, hair changes, apathy and anorexia would suggest severe protein deficiency (kwashiorkor), although concomitant deficiencies of vitamin A, vitamin C, iron, etc., might also be present. Similarly, the occurrence of pigmented lesions in areas of skin exposed to sunlight suggests a primary niacin deficiency as in pellagra, although experience has demonstrated that treatment with thiamine and riboflavin as well as niacin is usually necessary for satisfactory recovery. In fact, treatment with niacin alone will often precipitate signs of acute thiamine or riboflavin deficiency.

On the other hand, ascorbic acid deficiency characterized by gingival hyperplasia, perifolliculosis, painful muscle and subcutaneous swellings, etc., may be relatively unassociated with deficiency of other nutrients, and administration of vitamin C alone will generally bring prompt and full recovery. Beriberi, characterized in the adult by lassitude, muscle tenderness, edema and peripheral neuritis, may also respond fully to thiamine alone. Even in these two specific nutritional diseases, however, associated deficiencies requiring treatment are often present.

There are also many nutritional inadequacies that can be detected by the alert clinician even though they do not present themselves as acute florid pathognomonic deficiencies.

One of the prime purposes for doing a nutritional assessment is to detect primary or secondary nutritional inadequacy which can lower the resistance of tissues to infection. Proper correction of the deficiency can then be planned.

REFERENCES

1. Dreizen, S., Stone, R. E., and Spies, T. D.: Oral manifestations of nutritional disorders. D. Clin. of N. A., July, 1958, pp. 429–440.
2. Ershoff, B. H.: Conditioning factors in nutritional disease. Physiol. Rev., *28:*107, 1948.
3. Follis, R. H., Jr.: Deficiency Disease. Springfield, Charles C Thomas, 1958.
4. Interdepartmental Committee on Nutrition for National Defense: Manual for Nutrition Surveys. Washington, Superintendent of Documents, U. S. Government Printing Office, 1957.
5. Jolliffe, N.: Handbook of Nutrition, 25. Conditioned Malnutrition. J.A.M.A., *122:*299, 1943.
6. Kruse, H. D.: A concept of the etiological complex of deficiency states with especial consideration of conditions. Milbank Mem. Fund Quarterly, *27:*5, 1949.
7. Sinclair, H. M.: The assessment of human nutriture. Vitamins and Hormones, *6:*101, 1948.
8. Thompson, A. M., and Duncan, D. L.: The diagnosis of malnutrition in man. Nut. Abst. & Rev., *24:*1, 1954.

Chapter XIV

Dental Caries—Its Etiology and Techniques for Determining Its Activity

Before a rationale can be developed for applying dietetic and nutritional knowledge for the control of dental caries, some basic concepts in dental caries etiology need to be considered. The reason that a complete answer to the problem of caries control has not yet been found is that there are so many contributing variables and interrelated factors which produce and extend dental decay. However, in the light of present-day knowledge derived from controlled animal and human experiments, a few indisputable facts can be used as a foundation for developing practical clinical preventive and control procedures. These indisputable facts are (1) that the resistance of the tooth to decay is established during the period of development when the tooth matrix is forming, mineralizing and maturing and (2) that the attacking forces are the posteruptive local environmental factors, namely bacteria, fermentable carbohydrate foodstuffs and saliva.

GENETICS AND NUTRITION DURING TOOTH FORMATION

Genetics

Genetics is one of the pre-eruptive forces that has been suggested as influencing caries production, but there is need for much more investigative work to prove an absolute relationship. By progeny testing and inbreeding, Hunt, Hoppert and Erwin[19] have been able to produce caries-susceptible and caries-resistant lines of white rats. Hodge et al.[18] have reported some initial success in producing caries-susceptible and resistant strains of hamsters, but these lines could not be maintained due to a condition of sterility which may have been brought about by homozygosity. Klein[25] concluded after analyzing the dental records of 4416 white children that in humans, the "existence of familial resemblances in caries experience of siblings is definitely established." There are those who have investigated caries incidence in twins and have differed on the significance of heredity. According to Mansbridge,[31] after his investigation of dental caries in identical and fraternal twins, environmental factors are more important but genetic factors do contribute to caries etiology.

Carbohydrates

Carbohydrate restriction during the period of tooth formation seems to have some beneficial effect on the ability of the tooth to resist caries. For example, during the war years of 1939 to 1945 when the consumption of sugar was rationed in European countries there was also a progressive decrease in the incidence of dental decay. The carbohydrate restriction was at a maximum around 1941 to 1942, but the major reduction in dental caries did not occur until a few years afterwards. This lag period between the lowered intake of fermentable carbohydrates and reduction in dental caries was explained by Sognnaes[52] as due to development of an increased resistance in the tooth when the sugar intake was low. The possibility that there was increased intake of protective foods during this sugar rationing period has been suggested.[36] In Finland there was a reduction of sugar intake and nutritional conditions were poor during the war years, yet there was a reduction in caries.[62] Therefore, low sugar intake appears to be the more important factor.

The effects of a high sucrose diet fed during tooth formation on later caries incidence has been observed in animals. For example, if a stock diet consisting of natural foods was fed to hamsters, rats or mice during pregnancy and the lactation period and the young were fed a 67 per cent sucrose cariogenic diet post-weaning, the latter developed a low caries incidence. On the other hand, if a 67 per cent sucrose caries-producing diet was fed during the pregnancy and lactation periods as well as post-weaning, the caries incidence was much higher.[53] Similarly, in monkeys[54] it was shown that teeth that were developed on the natural jungle diet did not decay even though a highly cariogenic diet consisting of 73 per cent sucrose was fed for 4½ years. On the other hand, if the high sucrose cariogenic diet was started during the period of tooth development, caries developed 20 months after eruption.

Vitamins

Several investigations have pointed to the possibility that vitamin deficiencies during tooth formation may produce imperfections in the tooth, making the latter susceptible to decay. For example, Mellanby[35] in 1934 hypothesized that children who had a mild surface hypoplasia were more susceptible to decay than those who did not have this type of enamel defect. There are some investigators[1,8,34] who have confirmed this hypothesis and others who disagree.[32,57] Mellanby[37] has suggested that it is the absence of vitamin D that is responsible for producing the hypoplasia and, furthermore, if adequate amounts of vitamin D are given a growing child, the usual amount of dental decay will not be experienced.

Because deficiencies of vitamin A and C[63,64] have also been shown to produce pathological changes in the dentin and enamel during its formation, it has been suggested that these nutrients may be important in caries susceptibility. However, this has not been proved.

Minerals

In addition to the contributions that vitamins make in the formation and mineralization of the matrix, adequate amounts of the basic minerals calcium and phosphorus must not only be provided but must also be available for utilization. This means that systemic conditioning factors which in any way impair calcium absorption, such as low gastric intestinal acidity (achlorhydria) or improper ratio of calcium to phosphorus to vitamin D, as well as interfering food factors, such as excessive fats, oxalates or phytates, need to be considered. Furthermore, improperly functioning parathyroids or other interrelated endocrine glands may influence the rate of absorption of calcium and ultimately influence the amount available to the developing tooth.

By introducing into the experimental diets of hamsters either a natural ash supplement,[39] a salt mixture supplement[17] or a phosphate supplement[40] during the period of tooth development, dental caries incidence was reduced as much as 91 per cent. Others[55] have found significant cariostatic effects when an ash of a stock diet (Purina Laboratory chow) was added to a purified diet and fed to rats during the formation and mineralization of the tooth. Favorable results have been found when metaphosphoric acid was used as a source of assimilable phosphate in diets of hamsters starting at the eighth day of age. At this age the effect of the supplement can be considered for the most part a systemic or nutritional one rather than a local one.

If fluoride is ingested during tooth formation and mineralization it will make the enamel more resistant to decay than when no fluoride is ingested. This was shown when enamel samples of deciduous teeth of children who used a drinking water containing 1.2 ppm. fluoride were compared to samples of teeth of children who did not drink fluoridated water.[13] There are many other examples of the effects of different trace elements on the dental caries incidence in the developing tooth which have been reviewed in the chapter, Trace Elements.

Even after the matrix of the tooth has become mineralized, the quality of the newly erupted tooth continues to be influenced. There appears to be a rather active exchange between the chemistry of the oral environment and the chemistry of the tooth. This has been demonstrated by the use of radioactive isotopes.[56]

ORAL ENVIRONMENT AFTER TOOTH ERUPTION

Within the last decade experiments with (1) germ-free animals,[41] (2) feeding rats by stomach tube[24] and (3) feeding one animal in parabiotic rats[21] have provided convincing evidence of the local intraoral postdevelopmental factors in dental caries etiology. No dental caries was found in caries-susceptible experimental rats who were fed a caries-producing ration under germ-free conditions. Caries did not occur in even one of thirteen caries-susceptible experimental animals fed a high-sugar diet by stomach tube; whereas their litter-mates, who were fed the same type of cariogenic diet through the usual oral route, all developed some dental caries. In the parabiont fed dextrose there was a high incidence of decay, indicating a local carious and systemic effect, whereas in the other parabiont in which the dextrose action was only systemic, caries was not present or was at a minimum.

When a dental plaque which consists of mucin, bacteria and food debris is bathed in a glucose or sucrose solution, it will drop from a *p*H of 7 to a *p*H of 5 within 1 or 2 minutes and take about an hour to return to normal.[58] Lactic acid is formed by a stepwise degradation of phosphorylated glucose. One of the intermediate products of this oxidation is pyruvic acid and, as has already been described in the chapter on intermediary metabolism, this pyruvic acid can give rise to many different acids through a cyclical sequence of reactions called the Krebs cycle (Fig. 29, p. 82). Whether it is lactic acid or any other organic acid that causes the decalcification of enamel is not important. The important feature is that if a *p*H of 5.5 or lower is produced on the tooth surface, dental caries will be initiated.

From all this it appears that there are three important factors that must be considered in the local etiology of dental caries, namely carbohydrate foods, bacteria and saliva.

Carbohydrate Food Factor

In experimental animals it has been shown that carbohydrate-free diets fed to caries-susceptible animals were not effective in producing decay.[49] It has also been demonstrated that glucose and sucrose in a diet will produce decay more rapidly than other carbohydrates.[48] For example, if dextrin or starch was used in the place of granulated sugars as the carbohydrate component of an experimental diet, there was a reduction in incidence and extent of tooth decay. Whether cooked starches in human foods can compare to the uncooked starches in animal feed as to their cariogenicity is a moot question.[20]

Many investigators agree that carbohydrates are involved in dental decay in man, but there are numerous dissidents. For example, Koehne et al.[26] and Collins et al.[6] have found that highly refined carbohydrates will have a deleterious effect on the teeth of children and adolescents. On the other hand, Brodsky,[3] Potgieter et al.[43] and Savara and Suher[46] found no relationship between sweets and dental caries. The problem in all these studies is that they were not well controlled. The precise amount, kind and frequency of eating the carbohydrates were not and could not be regulated in a population group that was not confined to a particular home or institution where surveillance of food intake could be made by competently trained individuals.

These contradictory results of the role of carbohydrates in dental caries prompted the design of an experiment with better controlled conditions by Gustafsson et al.[15] They carried out a long-term nutritional study on 436 mental patients with an average age of 32 who were confined, practically permanently, in an institution in Vipeholm, Sweden. Diets were carefully supervised as to preparation and nurses were able to insure the cooperation of the patient in following the experimental prescriptions.

The first year and a half was a combination preparatory and vitamin study in which a base line caries index was established when the patients consumed a diet of protective foods four times a day with no candy or chocolate.

The next four years consisted of the carbohydrate study period in which ten groups were fed the same basal diet with the same amount of sugar at meals, but they differed from each other in that some groups had increased amounts of sugar at the meal and others had increased amounts of sugar between meals. There were four main groups:

1. Basal diet.
2. Basal diet and additional sugar in solution at meals.
3. Basal diet and additional sugar in bread consumed at meals.
4. Basal diet and additional sugar in the form of sweets consumed between meals.

Those who were on the basal diet (the control group throughout the study) had a low caries activity. (See Fig. 8, p. 35.) In those groups that had as much as 300 grams of sucrose added to the meal in liquid form as a beverage or in food preparation, the caries activity was only slightly increased. The same slight caries activity increase was noted in the group that was given, at meals, bread which contained 50 grams of refined sugar. However, in all groups where the additional sugar supplement was eaten between meals there was a very significant increase in dental caries. Even if there was a small amount of additional sugar added, such as those that ate candy between meals, there was a marked increase in caries activity. However, when the sweets were withdrawn from between-meal periods, the caries activity decreased to the level of the initial preparatory period.

From this study they proved that an increase in sugar intake will cause an increase in caries activity, and a decrease in sugar intake by these same individuals will cause a corresponding decrease in caries activity. However, it should be pointed out that this conclusion did not apply to all participants for there were many individual variations. Results varied not only from one individual to another in caries incidence but also the caries incidence varied from one year to another in the same patient. For example, there were patients who experienced as many as 9 new cavities per year on a sugar-free, low-carbohydrate diet and there were others who consumed large quantities of sweets and had no new caries.

This study also proved that if sugar with only a slight tendency to be retained, such as sucrose solution, was ingested *at meals* or if sugar-rich bread which has a strong tendency to be retained was consumed *at meals*, the risk of increasing caries activity was least. However, when sugar with a strong tendency to be retained in the mouth, such as exhibited by sticky solid sweets like caramels and toffees, was eaten *between meals frequently* the risk of increasing caries activity was greatest.

Another conclusion was that "carious lesions may continue to appear despite the avoidance of refined sugar, maximum restriction of natural sugars and total dietary carbohydrates."

In addition to these clinical observations of increased caries activity and food retention, there is experimental evidence that the salivary glucose level is influenced by the form of the sweets. Stated differently, the rate of oral sugar clearance is influenced by the physical form of the sweets. Lundqvist[30] found that with an increased oral clearance time there was a tendency to increased caries activity. He measured the per cent carbohydrate in the saliva of seven study groups in the Vipeholm study. In Fig. 80 it is seen that the sugar clearance values in the control group, the sucrose group and the bread group at meals are all similar. Thus the amount of sugar at meals appears to be of no consequence. However, the sugar clearance is much less with the between-meal groups as is seen by the increased number and width of the peaks in Fig. 80 in the chocolate, 8 toffee, caramel and 24 toffee groups.

Volker[59] also proved that clearance of sugar is primarily dependent on its physical form and only secondarily concerned with the quantity ingested. By incorporating the same amount of glucose in different vehicles (gum base, cake, solution and wafer), he showed that a wafer maintained salivary glucose level four times higher than that of a solution at the end of 2 minutes. Even at the end of 16 minutes the wafer caused a five times greater salivary glucose level than the solution. It was not the sugar content that

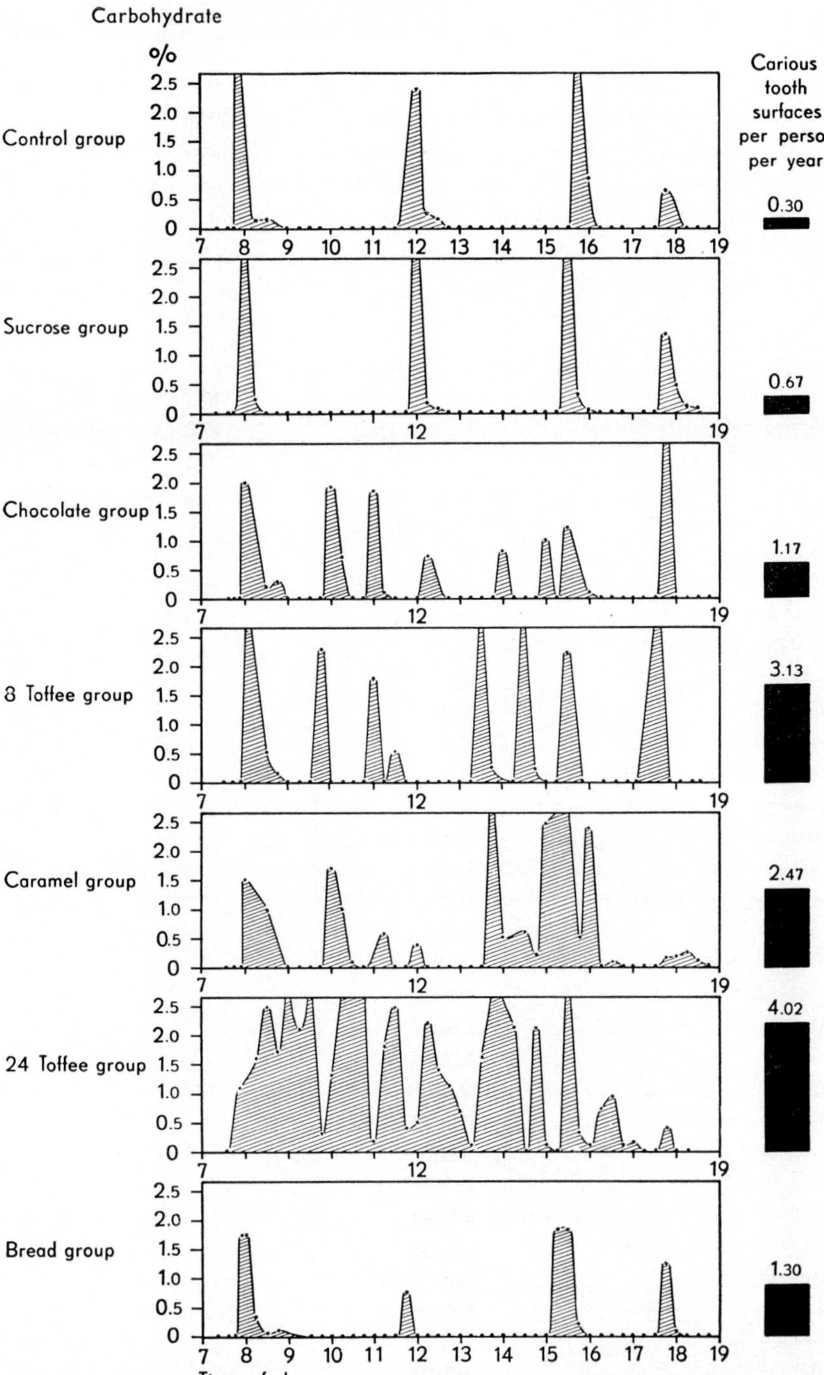

FIGURE 80. Sugar clearance in day-series in different study groups. One individual series in agreement with each group's average value is chosen. The caries activity is expressed as an average value for each group within which clearance determination has been performed. (Lundqvist, C.: Odontologisk Revy, Vol. 3, Suppl. 1, 1952.)

caused this difference but the mechanical retention of the hard wafers in contrast to the quick clearance of the solution.

In another large scale study,[23] 243 institutionalized children in two groups which were observed for two years received 11 oz. and 22 oz. of sugar per week per individual. The sweets were consumed at random but for the most part were used at meals. At the end of two years the caries incidence in both groups was the same. This

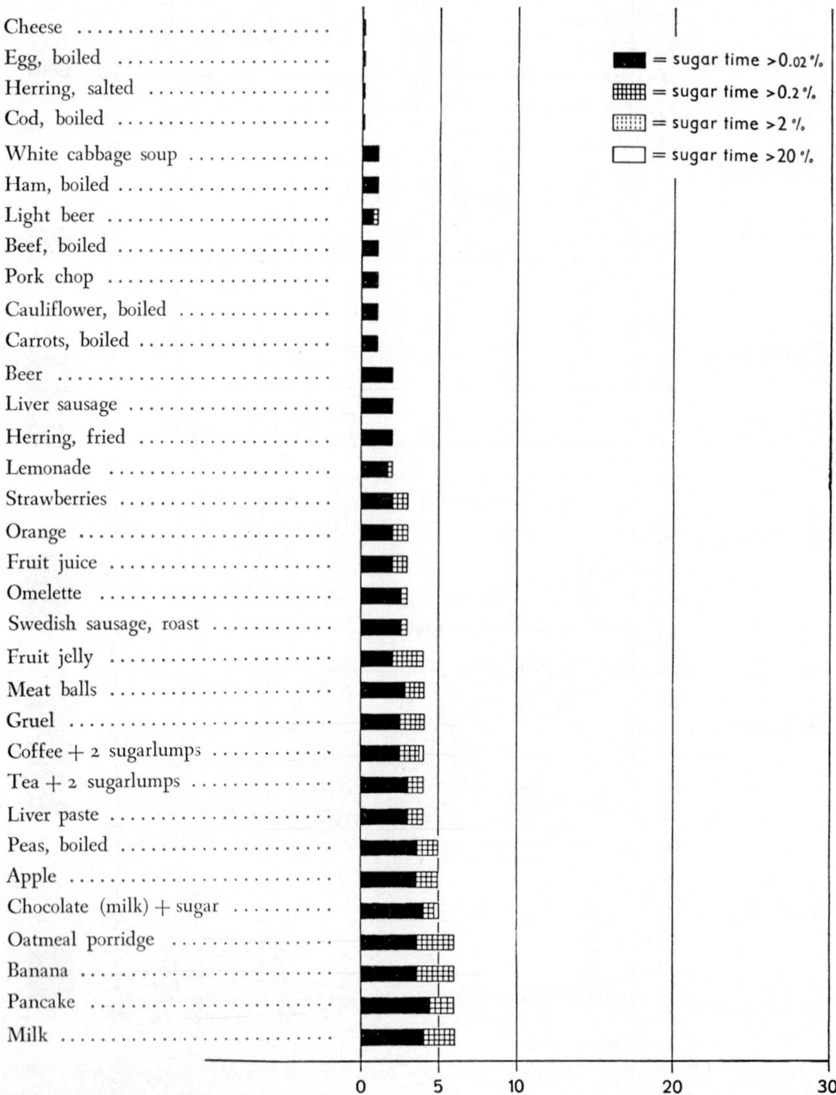

FIGURE 81. Survey of different food substances graded after caries potentiality index. The length of the columns represents the sum of the duration of

confirmed the fact that increased sugar at meals did not significantly influence caries incidence.

Caries-Producing Potential of Different Carbohydrate Foods

From these studies one might conclude that all carbohydrate foods may not be equally harmful and perhaps the more innocuous

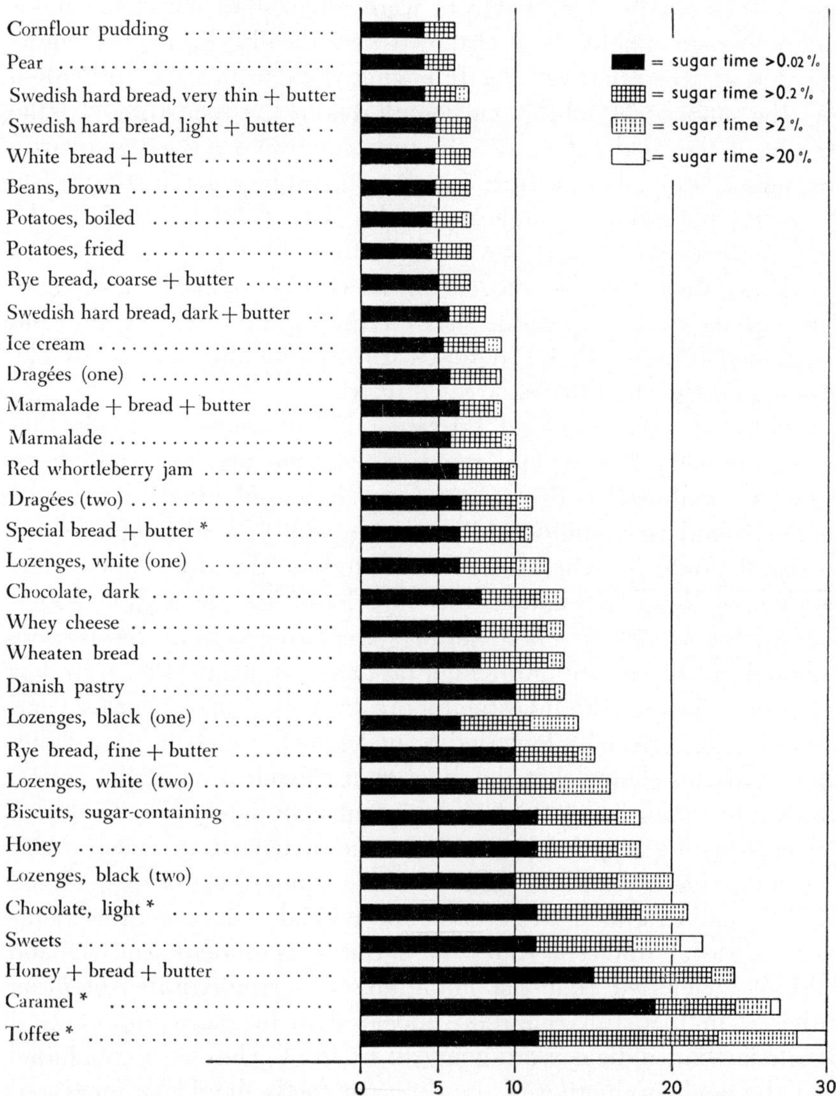

the sugar concentrations above stated levels. (Lundqvist, C.: Odontologisk Revy, Vol. 3, Suppl. 1, 1952.)

* Tested in the Vipeholm Study.

ones might be substituted for the harmful ones. To this end a grading of foodstuffs has been proposed in terms of their "caries-producing potentiality" or "decalcification potential."

Lundqvist[30] rated the "caries potentiality" of nine fluid products and fifty-seven solid foodstuffs or combinations of foodstuffs. He used representative foods from the bread-cereal group, milk and egg groups, meat group, fish group, fruits and berries, vegetables, honey and candy. Two subjects were allowed to chew the foods and saliva specimens were obtained periodically during the chewing period. He obtained the following data from each individual (a) the amount of soluble carbohydrates in the foodstuff, (b) the weight of the food eaten, (c) the total sugar and reducing sugar in the saliva, and (d) the time for demonstrable sugar in the saliva. A "caries potentiality" suggested index was given for each of the sixty-six foods which was based on the time during which the saliva contained sugar and on the maximum concentration of the sugar. The results of this grading showed that candy bars, honey and sweetened bread had the highest caries potentiality and foods like cheese and eggs had the least. See Fig. 81.

Bibby et al.[2] compared the amounts of ninety-six foods that were retained after several mouthfuls of the test food had been chewed, swallowed and cleansed from the mouth. Washings of the retained food were multiplied by the amount of acid the particular foodstuff produced when it was incubated in saliva for 4 hours. The product of these two figures was called the "decalcification potential" of the foodstuff. Their findings were that starchy foods were retained but those containing high fat or salt concentration were less retentive. Because the investigators realized that there were several variables that must be included to make such a classification valid, they made no claims that this be a final classification of the caries-producing potential of food. Subsequent experiments[28] with 4 or 5 subjects testing fifty foods proved to the investigators that a retention index has value, but even the same sample would be retained to different extents by the same individual when measurements were made at different times. In a third experiment Ludwig and Bibby[29] concluded that the milligrams of carbohydrate retention rather than foodstuff retention appeared to be more important if decalcification indices were going to be used. They also concluded that the acid production of the different foods should be measured in the dental plaque or cavities after eating, not in the washing or rinsings from the mouth. Table 18 shows the theoretical caries-producing potential of different foodstuffs which were used as tests in the Lundqvist,[30] Bibby et al.[2] and Ludwig and Bibby[29] studies. Recently Caldwell and Bibby,[5] in an attempt to determine whether there was a variation in activity of different foods to expand established cavities, reported that foods like crackers, figs, cookies, candy bars and ice cream caused a rise in cavity *p*H rather than a drop as they had expected. They explain that the rise in *p*H must have been due to the higher *p*H of the food than the cavity and the buffering capacity of the food.

TABLE 18. COMPARISON OF CARIES-PRODUCING POTENTIAL OF DIFFERENT FOODS

Lundqvist[30]		Bibby et al.[2]		Ludwig and Bibby[29]	
Food Product	Caries Potential Index	*Food Product*	Decalcification Potential	*Food Product*	CHO Retained (MG)
Toffee and bread	30	Cookie (fig)	814	Cookie (fig)	560
Honey and butter	24	Date	811	Date	393
Light chocolate	21	Chocolate	777	Toffee	250
Biscuits containing sugar	18	Ice cream	677	Salted cracker	240
Lozenges, black	14	Cookie (shortbread)	481	Cracker (oil sprayed)	220
Danish pastry	13	Danish pastry	434	Cookie (shortbread)	220
Marmalade	10	Cracker (salted)	408	Milk chocolate	185
Ice cream	9	Caramel	394	Chocolate pudding	105
Potatoes	7	Chocolate pudding	390	White bread	92
Banana	6	Cracker (oil sprayed)	372	Ice cream	72
Milk	6	Toffee	346	Apple	40
Apple	5	White bread	338	Pineapple juice (canned)	39
Coffee, 2 lumps sugar	4	Potato (boiled)	307	Orange juice (canned)	27
Orange	3	Cola drink	237	Cola (carbonated)	25
Fruit juice	3	Apple	228	Orange soda (noncarbonated)	24
Carrots	1	Orange soda	219	Cola (noncarbonated)	24
		Orange juice	212	Orange soda (carbonated)	23
		Potato chips	116	Grape soda (carbonated)	23
		Carrot (fresh)	88	Orange juice (fresh)	15
		Carrot (cooked)	3	Carrot (fresh)	7

Lanke[27] measured the ability of different foodstuffs to produce salivary sugar. He compared the salivary sugar levels of potatoes and bread, the two most common foodstuffs in the ordinary Swedish diet which contain starch. Potatoes gave an increased salivary sugar level for only about ⅓ the time of that of different breads. In fact, he found that bread gave a more prolonged salivary sugar curve than such sweets as toffees, but not chewing gum. He also found that even though the amount of sugar is small in lozenges, "chain eating" will produce a salivary sugar level which will be maintained at high enough level to produce considerable acid. Another conclusion was that there were significant differences in salivary sugar in different persons eating the same foodstuff. The variation between individuals on different foodstuffs was found to be even greater than when the same person tested different foodstuffs (Table 19).

TABLE 19. TIME THE FOODSTUFF IS RETAINED IN THE MOUTH AND CHEWING FREQUENCY IN DIFFERENT INDIVIDUALS

Subject	*Caramel*		*Chocolate*		*Bread*	
	Secs.	Peaks/Mins.	Secs.	Peaks/Mins.	Secs.	Peaks/Mins.
E	85	97	59	103	42	100
M	89	74	51	92	44	84
H	97	80	70	80	52	82
U	92	71	86	82	61	82
A	79	71	49	79	47	69
D	248	58	107	68	66	66
Mean	109	72	78	79	56	81

(Representative samples adapted from Lanke, L. S.: Influence on salivary sugar of certain properties of foodstuffs and individual oral conditions. Acta Odont. Scand., Vol. 15, Supplement 23, Page 131, 1957.)

Bacterial Factor

Even prior to W. D. Miller's[38] chemico-parasitic theory of dental caries etiology in 1890, acids and filamentous bacteria were associated with tooth decalcification. However, the idea that microorganisms were acid producers as well as proteolytic agents belongs to Miller. He proved by in vitro experiments that, in the presence of carbohydrate foods, the bacteria of the saliva can produce sufficient acid to decalcify teeth. There are other theories about dental caries etiology besides the decalcification theory. One is that proteolytic bacteria[42] are responsible for initiating caries by attacking the organic matrices of enamel and dentin first. Another theory is called the proteolytic-chelation theory,[47] which suggests that the action of salivary organisms on organic matter of the teeth can form complexing substances which will decalcify the teeth without acid formation. Whichever theory one accepts, the one indisputable fact is that bacteria are necessary for caries etiology. There is even some recent evidence[22] that dental caries in hamsters may be transmissible. The sudden change in "susceptibility" in some of these experimental animals is said to be due to the establishment of a "cariogenic" flora in the alimentary canal of the mothers and its transmission to their young.

If one accepts the chemico-parasitic theory of dental caries etiology as well as the more recent findings on the importance of local action of bacteria on teeth, then it becomes necessary to understand more about the oral microbiology. One aspect would be the nutrition of the oral bacteria. The microorganisms of the mouth derive their nutrition from the salivary secretions and from the dietary residues around the teeth. Of the two, the dietary residues provide the more likely means for providing rapid growth and acid production, because Lundqvist[30] has shown that saliva does not contain any free sugar. Even in hyperglycemia there is no transfer of sugar to the saliva.

Therefore, carbohydrates are found in the saliva only because they have been dissolved from the saccharide foods ingested. The greater the quantity of this substrate, the greater the number of bacteria which, in turn, means the greater the amount of acid produced. These are all measurable. The final step in deductive reasoning is that, without any overpowering resistant forces present either in the saliva or the tooth, caries will develop at the same rapid rate as the number of bacteria. Because new carious lesions cannot be seen before 4 to 6 months, number of bacteria or acid production have been used as the second best measurements of caries activity.

Measuring Caries Activity

The dentist knows that for any treatment procedure to be appreciated by the patient some objective sign of improvement must be shown. When the altered dietary regime produces some benefits, this will serve as an incentive for him to continue. For example, the obese patient who is on a weight-reducing diet will probably not be able to see any gross change in his appearance after the first week or two on his diet, but if he steps on the scale and sees the arrow point to a lower weight figure, he will be favorably impressed. By the same token, a patient with rampant caries for whom a diet is being prescribed needs some measurement of his progress. This will promote his continued cooperation.

In spite of the limitations of the correlations that either bacterial counts or acid production may have with the eventual development of new carious lesions, both the number of bacteria and the amount of acid they produce have been shown to be related to the amount of carbohydrate in the diet. This means that increased numbers of lactobacilli can be interpreted as an indication that a suitable substrate has been provided so that bacteria can produce sufficient acid to produce decay, if all other factors are favorable. This last part of the statement, "if all other factors are favorable,"

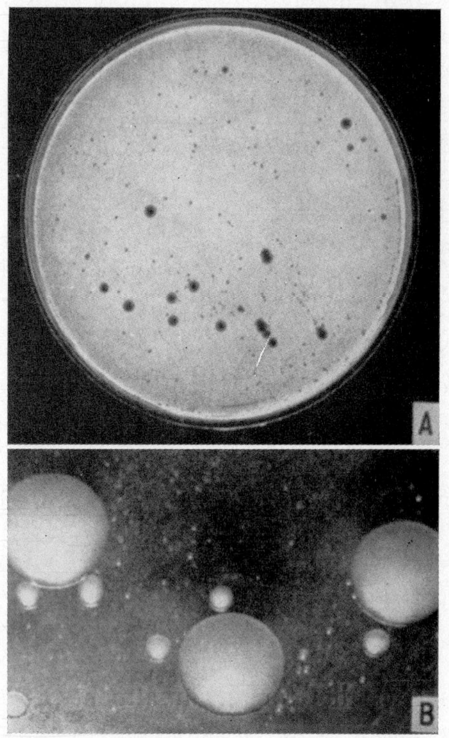

FIGURE 82. The use of tomato juice agar to determine the number of lactobacilli in human saliva as an index of caries susceptibility. The sample of saliva is spread upon the tomato juice agar plate after which it is incubated for four days at 37°C. (*A*) The tomato juice agar plate after incubation. (*B*) Typical colonial forms as they appear on the plate. The largest colonies are yeast, the medium size colonies are lactobacilli, while the small colonies are lactobacilli and streptococci. (Burnett, G. W., and Scherp, H. W.: Oral Microbiology and Infectious Disease. The Williams & Wilkins Co., 1957.)

is the contingency which has been overlooked by the adherents to the lactobacillus count as *the* index of caries susceptibility.

In reviewing the several laboratory tests that have been used to predict or assess caries activity, Brudevold[4] states that the relation between lactobacillus counts and caries is controversial for two reasons: (1) the procedures of the tests are not adequately standardized, and (2) the relation to dental caries exists only under certain conditions. He concludes, however, that laboratory tests should be included as an adjunct to clinical examination in the hope that some basic information of the dental caries mechanism will result.

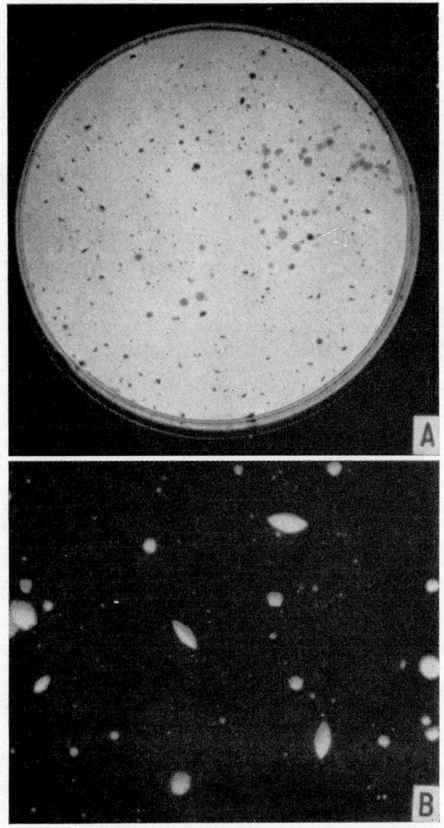

FIGURE 83. The use of Rogosa's Medium to determine the number of lactobacilli in human saliva as an index of caries susceptibility. The sample of saliva is added to melted agar and a poured plate is made and incubated for three days. (*A*) The plate at the end of the incubation period. (*B*) Surface and subsurface colonies, magnified. (Burnett, G. W., and Scherp, H. W.: Oral Microbiology and Infectious Disease. The Williams & Wilkins Co., 1957.)

Salivary Lactobacillus Counts. Rodriguez in 1930 developed a method for counting oral lactobacilli which were grown anaerobically in a horse serum agar.

Hadley[16] developed a medium consisting of nutrient agar and tomato juice which was adjusted to a *p*H of 5.0 with lactic acid. Oral lactobacilli were the predominating organisms that grew on this medium, but streptococcic yeasts, micrococci and staphylococci also grew. In this technique a sample of saliva is spread with a bent glass rod on the tomato juice agar plate and incubated at 37°C. for 4 days.

A slight modification of Hadley's basic tomato juice medium was made by Diamond[10] when he added 1:10,000 sodium azide. By this he inhibited such contaminants as yeasts and was able to produce a more selective medium for salivary lactobacilli. The bent rod technique for spreading the inoculum was also used here.

An improved medium for lactobacillus counts has been developed by Rogosa[44] in which only lactobacilli can grow. Instead of the spreading technique, a pour plate technique is used. The procedure for doing a lactobacillus count using the Rogosa medium is as follows:

Two or three specimens of saliva should be collected on successive mornings. The ideal time for collection of the specimen is upon arising in the morning before brushing, eating or rinsing. The patient is instructed to soften a piece of paraffin by holding it under running warm tap water and when it is completely moldable to place it in the mouth and chew. When saliva has increased perceptibly, the patient should expectorate each mouthful as it accumulates into a wide-mouth, screw-top, sterile bottle. Because the total volume of stimulated saliva may be a desirable measurement, the patient is advised that he should not swallow any of the saliva during the collection period but, instead, should expectorate as much as possible into the bottle. This procedure is usually continued for a full 15 minutes by the clock.

A nearby public health or dental school bacteriological laboratory is best equipped for performing the lactobacillus count. It is well for the dentist to write for mailing instructions and the collecting bottles that are preferred by the laboratory. If this is inconvenient and a local medical laboratory can perform this test, the following technique may be followed:

1. Materials used are S. L. Rogosa medium,[44] sterile petri dishes, sterile pipettes, 90 ml. sterile dilution H_2O, 9 ml. sterile dilution H_2O, incubator, water bath, sq. mm. paper for counting number of colonies.

2. Technique for quantitative dilution and making plate cultures is as follows:

a. Shake saliva sample for 2 min. and let paraffin, if present, settle to bottom.

b. Pipette 1 ml. of saliva and inoculate a dilution bottle of 99 ml. of sterile water.
c. Shake this dilution bottle vigorously to count of 20 and draw up 1 ml. of diluted saliva and discard. Draw up 1 more ml. and deposit in sterile petri dish.
d. Mark this petri dish 1/100.
e. Repeat steps c and d.
f. To make 1/1000, pipette up 1 ml. of the diluted saliva from the 99 ml. bottle and deposit in the 9 ml. of sterile water.
g. Shake this dilution bottle to the count of 20, draw up 1 ml. of the diluted saliva and discard. Draw up another ml. and deposit in sterile petri dish.
h. Mark this petri dish 1/1000.
i. Repeat steps g and h.
j. The S. L. Rogosa medium, which has been liquefied by heat and immersion in water bath at 42°C., is then poured into each of the petri dishes, covering the bottom 1/8″. As soon as the cotton plug is removed, the mouth of the flask is passed through a flame and inserted under the edge of the lifted petri dish cover and the medium is quickly poured out.
k. The saliva and medium are thoroughly mixed by swirling the covered petri dishes several times clockwise and counterclockwise.
l. Agar plates placed in the incubator after solidification should be inverted to avoid spreading of the growth through condensation of moisture on the surface of the medium.
m. Incubate for 4 days at 37°C.

3. Procedure for recognizing, counting and interpreting the clinical significance of the lactobacillus count.

a. *Lactobacillus acidophilus* has three principal colonial forms (Fig. 83):
   (1) Smooth grayish medium-sized colonies up to 1.0 mm. in diameter or larger.
   (2) Small rough colonies from 0.5 to 1.0 mm. in diameter.
   (3) Small smooth colonies generally less than 0.5 mm. in diameter.
b. If there are fewer than 30 colonies on the 1/1000 dilution, disregard these plates and count the colonies on the 1/100 dilution plates. Use the average of two plates as your lactobacillus count. If there are more than 300 colonies on the 1/100 plates, disregard these plates and count the colonies in the 1/1000 dilution plates.
c. The average number is multiplied by the dilution to give the number of organisms present per ml. of saliva.

The interpretation of the count in terms of soluble carbohydrate retention is as follows:

Number of Organisms per cc.	**Soluble Carbohydrate Retention*
0–1000	little or none
1000–5000	slight
5000–10,000	moderate
10,000–over	excessive

* This may be also interpreted as a suggested degree of caries activity.

Snyder's Test. To overcome the objections of the complex problems that may be encountered in the average dental office with many suggested caries activity tests, some simple colorimetric tests have been devised. These use a solid bacteriological culture medium which is inexpensive and can be purchased already prepared from a pharmaceutical supply house or local medical laboratory. One of these is Snyder's medium.[50] In addition to the medium, the equipment necessary to perform the test includes pipettes graduated in tenths of mililiters and a small incubator.

This colorimetric test measures the acidogenic potential of the total oral flora. By the use of a solid agar medium there is good dispersion of the colonies. The medium is made up of 1000 ml. of infusion broth, 20 grams of glucose and 50 ml. (0.04 per cent aq.) of bromocresol green, which is adjusted to *p*H 5.0 with lactic acid, and then 20 grams of agar is added. The resulting blue-green medium is poured into individual screw-capped tubes which can be autoclaved and kept indefinitely in a refrigerator.

The technique for performing this test is as follows:

1. Snyder test solid agar medium in a tube is immersed in a hot water bath and boiled until liquid.
2. After the medium is completely liquid the tube is removed from the water bath and cooled to about 50°C. by rolling the tube between the palms of the hands.
3. Using a tenth milliliter calibrated sterile pipette, 0.2 ml. of original saliva sample, which has just previously been shaken, is drawn up.
4. The cap is unscrewed, the mouth of the tube is flamed; saliva is deposited; the mouth of the tube is flamed; cap is rescrewed.
5. It is incubated at 37°C. for 3 days.
6. Color changes are observed at 24, 48 and 72 hour intervals.

The color changes in the medium represent acid formation which results from the degradation of a substrate by the enzymes liberated from the oral bacteria. The rate of acid formation which can be observed daily is directly proportional to the number of bacteria present in the salivary specimen. The higher the bacterial count, the more rapid will be the color change. This color change will appear sharper and can be better discerned if the tubes are held against a white background and examined with reflected light. The indicator is a deep blue-green at *p*H 5.4 and a pure green at *p*H 4.6. From this color it will change to a yellow as a *pH* of 4.2 to 3.8 is approached. A positive color change in 24 and 48 hours is indicative of marked to moderate caries activity. Little or no change in 48 to 72 hours is evidence of slight or negative caries activity (Fig. 84).

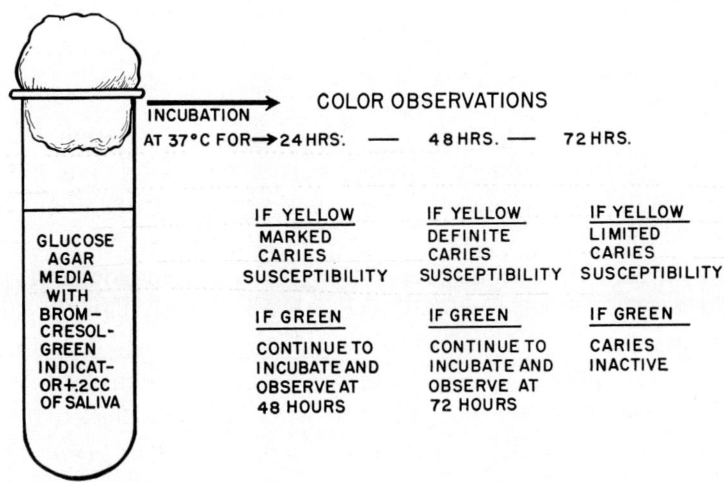

FIGURE 84. Snyder test and dental caries susceptibility. (From Snyder and coworkers, J. D. Res., 35:332–343, 1956.)

On the basis that this test measures the capacity to produce acid, Snyder[51] suggests that the change in colorimetric medium could be used as a measure of the effectiveness of diet therapy by noting whether there is a delay in occurrence of positive tests to 48 or even 72 hours.

A more selective colorimetric medium for lactobacilli has been suggested by Rogosa and Wiseman[45] in which alizarin red S is used as an indicator in a tube of S.L.R. (modified) medium. The colors vary from purple-red at *p*H 5.6 to purple and orange at *p*H 4.7 and, finally, to a yellow at *p*H 4.2. This medium is specific for lactobacilli and does not measure the acid production of other organisms. In comparing the rate of color or acid formation of this medium with Snyder test agar, no essential difference was found.

Recently, investigators[7] established that there was a positive relationship between lactobacillus counts, Snyder tests and subsequent incidence of dental caries in 584 patients. However, neither the number of bacteria nor the speed of color change in the Snyder's medium in any way predicted the number of carious lesions. The mere fact that a positive count or a positive Snyder test resulted was sufficient. These tests really did not prove themselves as reliable a clinical tool as one would like for predicting caries incidence but they were invaluable as an aid in dental health education and in encouraging patients to adopt a program of preventive dentistry.

Salivary Factors

Salivary Flow. The rate of salivary flow or secretion may be significant in the etiology of dental caries because if it is low the acid-producing organisms and carbohydrate foodstuffs will be retained on the teeth. Convincing proof that impairment in salivary flow will increase caries has been shown in sialadenectomized rats.[61]

In humans with xerostomia it has been shown that all permanent teeth can become cariously involved in the short period of only one year after eruption. In fact, in a survey of students which was designed to determine the effect of salivary flow with the amount of decay developed it was found that 49 per cent of the students with less than average rate of salivary secretion developed decay compared to only 30 per cent of the students with more than average salivary flow.[32] There may be congenital or inflammatory lesions on the orifices of the salivary glands which mechanically interfere with flow. On the other hand, there may be psychosomatic factors that subsequently affect the chemistry of the secretory glands. If either psychological or anatomical factors are operating for any length of time so that the low secretion of saliva persists, tooth breakdown is inevitable.

McDonald[33] has suggested that measuring the salivary flow in the individual patient with rampant caries might be one procedure that would be worthwhile. Certainly if the patient has a low rate of salivary secretion, some specific measures should be taken to deal with it.

The following is the procedure for determining and increasing the salivary flow:

1. Patient should collect in the morning upon arising all the saliva he can stimulate by chewing on paraffin. This chewing of paraffin and expectoration of saliva should be done over a full 15 minute period.
2. Transfer the saliva from the collecting bottle to a graduate and measure the cubic centimeters of saliva.
3. Calculate the theoretical normal flow from the following formula: $0.78 \times \text{age} + 5.6$.
4. Compare the actual with the theoretical normal.
5. If the amount of saliva collected appears to be much less than desirable, at least two steps can be taken to remedy this situation:
   (a) Suggest that the patient chew on paraffin at the end of each meal.

(b) Suggest that the patient take a few drops of pilocarpine in water at the beginning of each meal. In about twenty minutes the saliva will flow profusely. The following prescription for pilocarpine may be used:

℞ Pilocarpine hydrochloride	0.3 gm.
Aq. dist.	15.0 ml.

Sig: Drink a glass of water containing 5 drops at beginning of meals. Increase the dose each day by one drop until 8 to 10 drops per dose is used.

Other Factors. Other salivary factors that have been suggested as contributing to dental caries etiology are enzymes. Correlating dental caries with amylase activity has not proved too convincing, but more recently measuring aldolase activity has been suggested

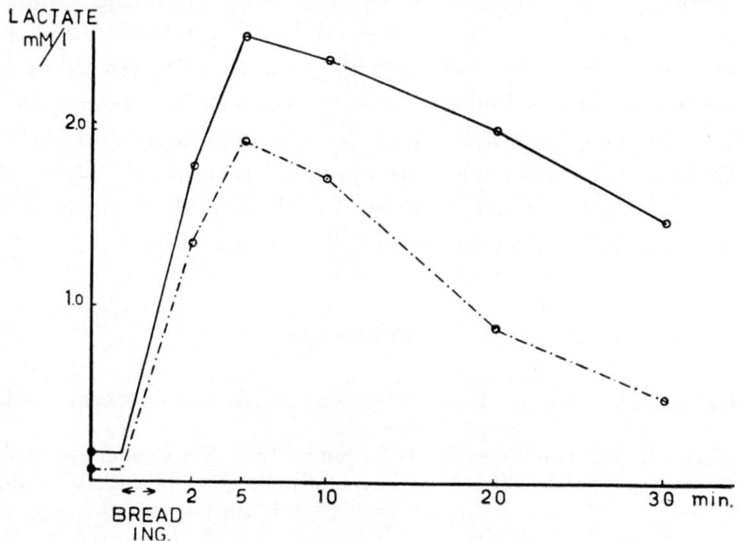

FIGURE 85. Average salivary lactate values for susceptible group (——) and resistant group (—·—). (Ericsson, Y., Hellstrom, I., Jared, B., and Stjernstrom, L.: Investigations into the relationship between saliva and dental caries. Acta Odont. Scand., *11*:179, 1954.)

by Bramstedt (at the A.D.A. centennial meeting) as a yardstick for caries activity which may have some merit. Aldolase is an enzyme which splits fructose 1-6 diphosphate. He found that when he measured the aldolase activity of the first 4 milliliters of unstimulated fasting saliva, caries-resistant patients had a higher aldolase content than caries-susceptible ones. Bramstedt also advocated measuring the oxygen uptake in saliva as an effective test for caries susceptibility. Caries resistance was correlated with high oxygen consumption and rampant caries with a low oxygen uptake.

Ericsson et al.[12] found that there was a relation between salivary glucose and lactate levels and between both these factors and the incidence of dental caries (Fig. 85). He found that the caries-susceptible group had a higher average sugar and lactate level in the saliva a half hour immediately after the ingestion of bread. This finding, he feels, is a confirmation of the fact that intra-oral sugar time and acid production are most important in the etiology of dental caries. Furthermore, it is this individual difference in ability to clear one's mouth of sucrose which is important in caries susceptibility.

In addition to these components in the saliva that have been measured and correlated with caries activity, there has been consideration of such factors as salivary *p*H,[60] buffering capacity,[11] ammonia, calcium and phosphorus content,[14] physical properties of saliva such as viscosity[7] and bacterial inhibitors. However, for every investigator who has found a positive correlation between the particular salivary component which he was measuring and caries activity, there is another who has found no correlation. There seems to be no single test that is suitable for all individuals because there are so many different factors involved in caries etiology.

REFERENCES

1. Bibby, B. G.: The relationship between microscopic hypoplasia (Mellanby) and dental caries. J. D. Res., *22:*218, 1943.
2. Bibby, B. G., Goldberg, H. J. V., and Chen, E.: Evaluation of caries-producing potentialities of various foodstuffs. J.A.D.A., *42:*491, 1951.
3. Brodsky, R. H.: Factors in the etiology and arrest of dental caries. (Diet) J.A.D.A., *20:*1440, 1933.
4. Brudevold, F.: Comments on the use of laboratory procedures in clinical testing of dental caries preventives. Chicago, Amer. Dent. Asso., 1955.
5. Caldwell, R. C., and Bibby, B. G.: The effect of foodstuffs on the *p*H of dental cavities. J.A.D.A., *57:*685, 1958.
6. Collins, R. C., Jensen, A. L., and Becks, H. J.: Study of caries-free individuals. II. Is an optimum diet or a reduced carbohydrate intake required to arrest dental caries? J.A.D.A., *29:*1169, 1942.
7. Davies, G. N., King, R. M., and Collins, A. A.: The relationship between lactobacillus counts, Snyder tests and the subsequent incidence of dental caries. Archive of Oral Biol., *1:*74, 1959.
8. Davies, J. H.: An investigation into the relationship between dental structure and dental caries in children attending public elementary schools. Brit. Dent. J., *67:*66, 1939.
9. Dewar, M. R.: Laboratory methods for assessing susceptibility to dental caries. II. Correlation of results obtained by clinical examination and by standardized laboratory methods. D. J. Australia, *22:*24, 1950.

10. Diamond, B. E.: A selective medium for lactobacilli counts from saliva. J. D. Res., *29:*8, 1950.
11. Dreizen, S., Mann, A. W., Cline, J. K., and Spies, T. D.: The buffer capacity of saliva as a measure of dental caries activity. J. D. Res., *25:* 213, 1946.
12. Ericsson, Y., Hellstrom, I., Jared, B., and Stjernstrom, L.: Investigations into the relationship between saliva and dental caries. Acta. Odont. Scand., *11:*179, 1954.
13. Finn, S. B., and Demarco, C.: The effect of artificial water fluoridation on the solubility of enamel. J. D. Res., *35:*185, 1956.
14. Fosdick, L. S., Hansen, H. L., and Epple, C.: Enamel decalcification by mouth organisms and dental caries. A suggested test for caries susceptibility. J.A.D.A., *24:*1275, 1937.
15. Gustafsson, B. E., Quensel, C. E., Lanke, L., Lundqvist, C., Grahnen, H., Bonow, B. E., and Krasse, B.: The Vipeholm dental caries study: effect of different levels of carbohydrate intake on caries activity in 436 individuals observed for five years. Acta. Odont. Scand., *11:*232, 1954.
16. Hadley, F. P.: A quantitative method for estimating bacillus acidophilus in saliva. J. D. Res., *13:*415, 1933.
17. Harris, R. S., Nizel, A. E., and Gardner, D. S.: Effect of food ash and trace minerals upon dental caries in hamsters. Proc. IV, International Congress of Nutrition, p. 195, 1957.
18. Hodge, H. C., Johansen, E., and Hein, J. W.: Third report on the breeding of caries-immune and caries-susceptible strains of Syrian hamsters. J. D. Res., *34:*757, 1955.
19. Hunt, H. R., Hoppert, C. A., and Erwin, W. G.: Inheritance of susceptibility to caries in albino rats. J. D. Res., *23:*385, 1944.
20. Jenkins, G. N.: Dental caries in relation to nutritional environmental effects. Proc. of Nut. Soc., *18:*85, 1959.
21. Kamrin, B. B.: Local and systemic cariogenic effect of refined dextrose solution fed to one animal in parabiosis. J. D. Res., *33:*824, 1954.
22. Keyes, P.: Dental caries in the Syrian hamster. VII. The induction of rampant caries activity in albino and golden animals. J. D. Res., *38:*525, 1959.
23. King, J. D., Mellanby, M., Stones, H. H., and Green, H. M.: Effect of sugar supplements on dental caries in children. Medical Res. Council, Special Report Series, No. 288. London, Her Majesty's Stationery Office, 55 pp., 1955.
24. Kite, O. W., Shaw, J. H., and Sognnaes, R. F.: Prevention of experimental tooth decay by tube feeding. J. Nut., *42:*89, 1950.
25. Klein, H., and Palmer, C. E.: Studies on dental caries. V. Familial resemblance in the caries experience of siblings. Pub. Health Rep., *53:*1353, 1938.
26. Koehne, M., Bunting, R. W., and Hadley, F. P.: Review of recent studies of cause of dental caries. J. Am. Diet. Assoc., *9:*445, 1934.
27. Lanke, L. S.: Influence on salivary sugar of certain properties of foodstuffs and individual oral conditions. Acta. Odont. Scand., *15:*Suppl. 23, 1957.
28. Ludwig, T. G., Dewar, M. R., and Bibby, B. G.: Further observations upon the caries-producing potentialities of various foods. Proc. I.A.D.R., J. D. Res., *32:*665, 1953.
29. Ludwig, T. G., and Bibby, B. G.: Acid production from different carbohydrate foods in plaque and saliva. J. D. Res., *36:*56, 1957.

30. Lundqvist, C.: Oral sugar clearance: its influence on dental caries activity. Odont. Revy, *13:* suppl. 1, 1952.
31. Mansbridge, J. N.: Heredity and dental caries. J. D. Res., *38:*337, 1959.
32. Marshall-Day, C. D., and Sedwick, H. J.: The fat-soluble vitamins and dental caries in children. J. Nut., *8:*309, 1934.
33. McDonald, R. E.: The Clinical Management of Rampant Dental Caries, in Muhler and Hine, Symposium on Preventive Dentistry. St. Louis, The C. V. Mosby Co., 1956.
34. Mellanby, H.: Dental hypoplasia and caries among children of Finnish Lapps. Brit. Med. J., *1:*682, 1940.
35. Mellanby, M.: Diet and teeth: An experimental study. Part III. The effect of diet on dental structure and disease in man. Med. Res. Council Special Rep., Series No. 191. London, 1934.
36. Mellanby, M., and Coumoulous, H.: The improved dentition of 5 year old London school-children. Brit. Med. J., *1:*837, 1944.
37. Mellanby, M., and Mellanby, H.: The reduction in dental caries in 5 year old London school-children (1929–47). Brit. Med. J., *2:*409, 1948.
38. Miller, W. D.: The Microorganisms of the Human Mouth. Philadelphia, S. S. White Dent. Manuf. Co., 1890.
39. Nizel, A. E.: The cariogenic properties of similar foodstuffs grown in high- and low-caries areas. I. The influence of trace elements. Thesis, Tufts Univ. School of Dent. Med., 1952.
40. Nizel, A. E., and Harris, R. S.: Effect of different dietary levels of metaphosphoric acid on hamster caries. J. D. Res., *38:*686, 1959.
41. Orland, F. J., Blayney, J. R., Harrisson, R. W., Reyniers, J. A., Trexler, P. C., Wagner, M., Gordon, H. A., and Luckey, T. D.: Use of germfree animal technic in the study of experimental dental caries. I. Basic observations on rats reared free of all microorganisms. J. D. Res., *33:*147, 1954.
42. Pincus, P.: The study of caries: Attack on enamel without acids. Dent. Record, *59:*615, 1939.
43. Potgieter, M., Morse, E. H., Erlenbach, F. M., and Dall, R.: Food habits and dental status of some Connecticut children. J. D. Res., *35:*638, 1956.
44. Rogosa, M., Mitchell, J. A., and Wiseman, R. F.: A selective medium for the isolation and enumeration of oral lactobacilli in saliva. J. D. Res., *31:*470, 1952.
45. Rogosa, M. L., and Wiseman, R. F.: A colorimetric test for relative abundance and acidogenic potential of lactobacilli in saliva. J. D. Res., *31:*470, 1952.
46. Savara, B. S., and Suher, T.: Dental caries in children one to six years of age as related to socioeconomic level, food habits, and toothbrushing. J. D. Res., *34:*870, 1955.
47. Schatz, A., and Martin, J. J.: Some perspectives of dental caries research: microbiological and biochemical considerations. Ann. Dentist., *17:*1, 1958.
48. Schweigert, B. S., Shaw, J. H., Phillips, P. H., and Elvehjem, C. A.: Dental caries in the cotton rat. 3. Effect of different dietary carbohydrates on the incidence and extent of dental caries. J. Nut., *29:*405, 1945.
49. Shaw, J. H.: The effect of carbohydrate-free and carbohydrate-low diets on the incidence of dental caries in white rats. J. Nut., *53:*151, 1954.

50. Snyder, M. L.: A simple colorimetric method for the estimation of relative numbers of lactobacilli in the saliva. J. D. Res., *19:*349, 1940.
51. Snyder, M. L., Suher, T., Porter, D. R., Claycomb, C. K., and Gardner, M. K.: Evaluation of laboratory tests for the estimation of caries activity. J. D. Res., *35:*332, 1956.
52. Sognnaes, R. F.: An analysis of a war-time reduction of dental caries in European children, with special regard to observations from Norway. Am. J. Dis. Child., *75:*792, 1948.
53. Sognnaes, R. F.: Caries conduciveness effect of a purified diet when fed to rodents during tooth development. J.A.D.A., *37:*676, 1948.
54. Sognnaes, R. F.: Is the susceptibility to dental caries influenced by factors operating during the period of tooth development? In Taber, L., ed.: Sugar and Dental Caries Symposium. Supplemental Issue, J. Calif. Dent. A., *26:*37, 1950.
55. Sognnaes, R. F., and Shaw, J. H.: Experimental rat caries. IV. Effect of a natural salt mixture on the caries conduciveness of an otherwise purified diet. J. Nut., *53:*195, 1954.
56. Sognnaes, R. F., Shaw, J. H., and Bogoroch, R.: Radiotracer studies on bone, cementum, dentin, and enamel of Rhesus monkeys. Am. J. Physiol., *180:*408, 1955.
57. Staz, J.: Hypoplastic teeth and dental caries. J. D. Res., *23:*220, 1944.
58. Stephan, R. M.: Changes in hydrogen-ion concentration on tooth surfaces and in carious lesions. J.A.D.A., *27:*718, 1940.
59. Volker, J. F.: Etiology of Dental Caries, in Finn, S.B.: Clinical Pedodontics. Philadelphia, W. B. Saunders Co., 1958.
60. Wach, E., Kesel, R. G., Hine, M. K., and O'Donnell, J. F.: Testing caries activity by acid production in saliva. J. D. Res., *22:*415, 1944.
61. Weisberger, D., Nelson, C. T., and Boyle, P. E.: The development of caries in the teeth of albino rats following extirpation of the salivary glands. Am. J. Ortho. and Oral Surg., *26:*88, 1940.
62. Wilska, A.: En fysiologs syn pa Kariesproblement. Odont. Tidskr., *54:*296, 1946.
63. Wolbach, S. B., and Howe, P. R.: The effect of scorbutic state upon the production and maintenance of intercellular substances. Proc. Soc. Exper. Biol. & Med., *22:*400, 1925.
64. Wolbach, S. B., and Howe, P. R.: The incisor teeth of albino rats and guinea pigs in vitamin A deficiency and repair. Am. J. Path., *9:*275, 1933.

Chapter XV

A Step-by-Step Technique for the Nutritional Guidance of Patients with Rampant Caries

Two types of dietary regimes are in common usage for the control of rampant caries. There is one that was originated by Jay et al.[2] and has been used by them and others[4] successfully for many years. They emphasize the use of an adequate diet but rigidly restrict the total carbohydrate intake to 100 grams for an initial two week period as a means of lowering the *Lactobacillus acidophilus* count. This is designated Plan I. Thereafter, increased starches (Plan II), sugar with one meal (Plan III), and unrestricted diet (Plan IV) are allowed, depending on the *Lactobacillus acidophilus* count.

A second regime, which will be described here in a step-by-step fashion, provides for a normal adequate diet without any restrictions in total carbohydrate but a definite restriction in retentive fermentable types of carbohydrate. Caries activity tests are performed and have been found to serve as an excellent stimulus for patient education and cooperation. The limitations of these tests must be recognized, however, as their relation to dental caries exists only under certain circumstances. A vital part of this regime is a consideration of the motivating factor for the selection of the diet or, as it is referred to here, the *why* of the diet.

BASIC CONCEPTS

It must be clearly understood that diets are not recommended as a method of treating dental caries. Only by operative and restorative procedures can teeth be repaired. However, proper selection and assimilation of food can act in a prophylactic capacity against the initiation or extension of decay. Accordingly, the term "nutritional guidance" rather than "nutritional therapy" is used.

It has been established through controlled animal experiments that food[5] and bacteria[6] must be in contact with the tooth to initiate a carious lesion. Furthermore, the foods that proved to be the best substrates were the readily fermentable carbohydrates, the monosaccharides and disaccharides.[8] More complex carbohydrates such as polysaccharides were found to be, comparatively, much less cariogenic.[7] From this and from human clinical studies such as the one conducted in Vipeholm[1] it would appear that restriction of fermentable carbohydrates in the daily diet would be advisable.

From clinical experience it appears that a sound and practical approach to the control of rampant caries is the provision of an adequate diet which restricts only the fermentable carbohydrates but not carbohydrates in general. In our experience, it has been exceedingly difficult for patients to follow a restriction of carbohydrates even for short periods. This is probably due to the fact that carbohydrates constitute such a large part of our daily diet and are physiologically desirable.

Consideration must also be given to the physical nature of the food as well as the frequency of eating. Food retention is as damaging to tooth structure as local irritants are to the periodontium. In periodontal problems, removal of local irritants is a primary consideration for the restoration of periodontal health. Likewise, to realize effective caries control, the local factor, food retention, must be eliminated. This can be accomplished through the usual restorative and oral hygiene procedures. Limiting the eating periods to three a day, if possible, and using foods that are detergent can also serve as valuable adjuncts in maintaining oral hygiene.

Nutritional guidance to be successful must not only consider how to improve *what* the patient eats but it must also concern itself with *why* the patient has been selecting and eating his past and present foods. The why of the diet involves a consideration of the patient's childhood diet, present and past ability to digest, absorb and utilize foods, food cravings, food habits, and cultural, religious and family attitudes toward food. In short, the technique to be described deals with the total nutritional problem, not diet per se.

The word "technique" is used advisedly because it implies objectivity rather than abstract philosophical discussion. By a methodical step-by-step procedure, a diagnosis is made and a guidance program suggested. In other words, the patient can see by analysis of his diet that there are specific amounts of foods missing or used in excess. Vague terms like "too few vegetables," are replaced in this technique by, "According to an evaluation of your diet, you are eating two portions less of the green or yellow vegetables per week than is recommended." If all other factors are favorable, the effect of the retained fermentable carbohydrate on the oral environment can also be determined in an objective fashion (lactobacillus count, Snyder test, etc.). These tests serve as a valuable, psychological, visible aid for patient cooperation. In addition, when we present the treatment plan to the patient, it is done as a written dietary prescription.*

PATIENT SELECTION

Unquestionably all dental patients would benefit from a nutritional guidance program, but this is not feasible. A detailed dietary service such as will be described here is most profitable for those patients who have not been able to control the progress of their dental decay through periodic routine dental mechanical procedures. This is usually a patient with rampant caries.

Rampant caries is a condition characterized by a decaying process that is more extensive and more rapid than would normally be expected, and it occurs in otherwise caries-immune, free-cleansing tooth surfaces. This extensive caries susceptibility can occur even in clean, well-cared-for mouths. It is not unusual for the patient to state that all the necessary restorative dentistry had been completed no longer than six months previously. The usual clinical picture is the occurrence of ten or more surfaces of decay in the interproximal surfaces of the lower anterior teeth and on the smooth buccal and lingual cervical surfaces. Grossly, the cervical lesions appear as erosive, chalky white and diffuse areas of decalcification.

* Diet prescription as used here and in succeeding pages means prescribing a total dailv food intake, a meal plan and menu rather than specific amounts of carbohydrate, protein and fat.

A second group of patients who need definitive dietary guidance is those undergoing orthodontic treatment. The bands and appliances that are a necessary part of orthodontics also serve as excellent food retainers and, subsequently, tend to promote caries. To minimize this, diets with low caries-producing potential from a biochemical and physical standpoint should be recommended.

FIRST VISIT

If the patient falls into either of the above two categories, the interview might begin with an explanation of the carious process and factors which contribute to it. For example: "The acid formed from the action of bacteria on certain types of foods will 'eat away' the tooth enamel. This allows bacteria to penetrate and 'dissolve' the inner portion of the tooth, the dentin. The process of dental decay is actually not quite so simple as this, and there are other theories that have been proposed, but this explanation has been the one accepted by the profession as being quite reasonable." It can be further explained that once the tooth is completely formed, the innate caries susceptibility cannot be altered because fully matured teeth do not accept new nutrients in any significant amounts. Thus, the only rational approach for effecting caries control is to deal with the local oral environment, namely, the oral bacteria in the saliva and in the dental plaque as well as the food that remains lodged in and around the teeth.

The patient will listen attentively and then probably counter with the statement that he eats no differently than his brother or sister, yet he develops many more cavities. Why? Your answer might be that dental caries, like other diseases, depends, in part, on the resistance of individuals which differs even in brothers and sisters. An example of individual differences is shown in diabetes. The diabetic eats no more sugar than the next person, but his inability to metabolize it makes him different. The diabetic's sugar tolerance is low. Similarly, the teeth of the caries-susceptible patient have a lower resistance to acid formation. In short, caries susceptibility may, in part, be a manifestation of individual metabolic differences.

STEPS IN ARRIVING AT DIAGNOSIS

The why of the diet, as the word implies, gives the reasons for food selection. Its determination is made by delving into personal and social matters that sometimes cannot be tactfully ascertained at the very first visit. However, when rapport has been established during subsequent visits, even without direct questioning a few chance remarks about home life, living conditions, etc., may give clues as to why certain foods such as sweets, for example, are used in excess. When questioning does start, diplomacy, empathy and a manner which conveys understanding are necessary. Although

TABLE 20.

Date *1/8/60*

Name	Age	Sex	Occupation	Desirable Weight	Nationality	Marital Status
John Doe	*15*	*M*	*School*	*140 lb.*	*American*	*Single*

Address *26 West Street*

General Appearance: *Well developed*

Chief Complaint and Present Illness: *Several new "brown spots" were seen between the lower anterior teeth. These have appeared within the last few months.*

Past History:

1. Food intake during: (a) pregnancy, (b) lactation, (c) infancy, (d) childhood, (e) pre-adolescent, (f) adolescent periods.
   No Vitamin D supplements as a child.
   Always liked and ate excessive sweets.
   Had a good appetite and found that he had to eat between-meal snacks.
2. Systemic Nutritional Conditioning Factors during Childhood.
   No allergies

Family History:

1. Food habits, special diets, and mealtime in the household.
   Mealtimes are not regular. Everybody helps himself whenever he feels like it.

Personal and Social History:

1. Allergies, gastrointestinal disturbances and others.
   None.
2. Occupational tensions; domestic discord; economic problems.
   Some difficulty has been encountered from a financial standpoint. Father is out of work.

Diet Evaluation:

1. The number, the form and the frequency of caries promoting foodstuffs eaten daily.
   Total sugar intake equivalent to 19 teaspoonful.
2. Adequacy in type and amount of food groups.
   Low in milk and vegetable-fruit group.
3. Balance of meals, menus and frequency of eating.
   Poor meal balance. No variety to menus. Too many between-meal snacks.
4. Consistency and detergency.
   Soft diet.

Objective Signs:

1. Skin Lesions.
   None.
2. Amount and location of caries; tooth arrangement, morphology and salivary characteristics.
   Twenty carious surfaces, some cervical erosion, lower anterior interproximal caries, crowding of teeth, saliva appears thick and ropy.

Laboratory Tests:

Snyder test; salivary flow.
Yellow reaction to Snyder test in 24 hours. Salivary flow below normal.

Impressions:

Excessive sweets and inadequate diet due to lack of knowledge and low economic status.

typical questions will be suggested here, it should be made clear that these are intended only as a guide. There is no stereotyped form. Avoid using a check-off system from a printed form because the resultant answers will be a mechanical "yes" or "no" devoid of incidental voluntary coloring and comment. The incidental matters that patients are prone to relate often provide the most important clues to a diagnosis.

As in all histories, the complaints, the pertinent present history, as well as the past history, make up the symptomatic portion of the diagnostic work-up. Before questioning starts on the chief complaint, the usual vital statistics of name, address, age, sex, marital status, occupation, nationality, height and weight are noted on a history form similar to the one shown in Table 20.

A. History

1. Chief Complaint and Present Illness. The patient with rampant caries will often complain about the brown spots that "keep cropping up" between his teeth. He also may complain of sensitivity to sweets or to cold and hot foods around the gum line areas of his teeth.

The clinician notes on cursory examination that the patient has numerous carious lesions and asks, "When did you last see the dentist?" The answer usually is: "Only six months ago. I was all fixed up and was told that I had no more cavities." "Isn't it rather soon to have so many new cavities?" the patient asks. The clinician agrees that there has been a rapid rate of recurrence and that perhaps the patient requires more than the routine dental reparative services, namely an improved dietary regime.

2. Past Nutritional History. After the patient has elaborated on his chief complaint and present illness, he, or in the case of an adolescent or a child, the parent, is questioned about the past nutritional history from the time the patient was born to the present. Curiously enough, recollections about food and food habits of a child are usually quite vivid.

What is the dental significance of the history of the childhood nutrition? It reveals how nutrition influenced tooth quality. It indicates whether or not adequate amounts of nutrients such as calcium, phosphorus and vitamin D were available for mineralization of the developing tooth matrix. Since tooth formation starts 6 weeks after conception and mineralization of ground substance occurs during the last trimester of pregnancy, the diet of the mother while she was pregnant is the period about which the questioning should start. For instance: Were you able to eat well during your pregnancy? Did nausea and vomiting interfere with your appetite or your food intake? What dietary supplements did your physician prescribe? Did you use them? Were you able to take milk? How much per day? Did you have any craving for sweets, cakes and pies? Did you avoid any foods like vegetables, fruits, meat, etc.?

Was the child a full-term or premature baby? The answer to this question will tell whether the maternal nutritional influence was operative during the critical last few months of fetal tooth formation or whether, due to premature birth, the unerupted tooth was dependent on the type of nourishment the infant received from sources outside his mother's body.

At what age were sources of vitamins C and D such as orange juice and cod liver oil supplements started? When were solid foods such as cereals, fruits and vegetables introduced?

Having completed the nutritional history of infancy, we proceed to questions concerning eating habits during childhood. What frequently happens is that the child's desire for food decreases noticeably about the age of 18 to 24 months. This is natural because the rate of growth has slowed down after the early, rapid, spurt growth of infancy. This sharp contrast in lowered food intake is sometimes misinterpreted by the parent as being abnormal.

Some typical questions you might ask of the mother are: At what age did your child's appetite begin to diminish? What did you do about it? Were you concerned to the point that you allowed and even encouraged his eating candy and sweets as long as he ate? Did you flavor his milk with some sweetening agent to make it acceptable? How much milk did he drink? Did you try to appease him by giving him cakes, pastries, sweets, etc.? Did he eat between meals?

In addition to the type and amount of food that the child ate, we are interested in knowing if there were any systemic problems that might have influenced the assimilation of the food. For example, did he tend to be constipated? Was mineral oil ever used excessively? (It will interfere with absorption of vitamins A and D.) Was there ever any suggestion by a pediatrician that a condition of achlorhydria (lack of gastric hydrochloric acid) might have been present? This might indicate a diminution of calcium absorption. Was there any history of hypothyroidism? This endocrine disturbance has been related to caries susceptibility.

3. ***Family History.*** The family history is most important because it gives clues to the environmental factors that influence food selection and meal patterns.

What is the father's occupation? In a household where the father is a baker, grocer, caterer or sweet-shop proprietor the retentive types of fermentable carbohydrate foods are usually found readily available in the refrigerator and cupboards.

Are there any members of the family on special diets? For example, a patient on a gallbladder diet probably eats less fat and more carbohydrates such as sweets and jellies. Does everybody in the household eat the same menu as the person on the special diet?

Are there any religious, cultural or regional customs that might influence the use of sticky sweets? For example, many New Englanders feel that a meal is incomplete without pie or cake for dessert.

4. ***Food Habits.*** Food habits are formed as a result of daily routine. If the patient is a late riser, he may skimp on or even omit breakfast. Does the patient rise early enough to enjoy a good breakfast? How important is mealtime to him? Is food just a means of keeping alive and satisfying hunger or is it a pleasurable experience? Does he just "grab a bite" when he can? Does he have a mid-morning or mid-afternoon snack of coffee and doughnuts? Additional questions to patients who smoke might be: Are you in the habit of using Lifesavers to overcome bad breath? Are you a chain cough drop user? Are you working under tension during the day and do you chew gum or nibble sweets during periods of nervousness?

5. ***Personal Oral Hygiene Habits.*** Retention of food particles, as already stated, is one of the most damaging factors in caries production because the food particles serve as a substrate for acid production by oral bacteria. Therefore, questions on toothbrushing and mouthwashes are important. Some suggested questions might be: Do you have facilities for brushing your teeth after each meal? Do you make any other conscious effort to clear your mouth of food, such as rinsing, flossing, etc.?

6. ***Systemic Conditioning Factors.*** If there is a known history of a systemic upset such as food allergy or gastrointestinal disease, the diet may of necessity be highly selective and omit protective nutrients.

In adolescence the rate of growth is a clue to the food requirements. How many inches have you grown in the last 6 months?

How is your appetite? Do you get enough to eat at mealtimes or do you have to supplement your meals with snacks? If so, what do you eat between meals?

7. Social History. Through the social history, information is elicited about the patient's attitudes and behavior as well as about his socio-economic status.

Some of these attitudes may be expressed objectively in the overuse of or abstention from food. Food may be used to compensate for lack of other satisfactions in daily living. This is sometimes the basis for obesity. Similarly, in patients with rampant caries the excessive intake of sweets may have a psychological basis. The habit of excessive intake of sweets may have started during childhood when sweets were used as rewards or as expressions of affection.

Direct questioning is difficult in this area, but an alert interviewer may perceive strained relationships, if present, between child and parent. Rather than direct questioning, allow parents or patient to discuss their personal problems voluntarily. Some of the more common problems are (a) overprotective parents, (b) adolescent rebellion, (c) sibling rivalry, (d) domestic discord and (e) lack of parental guidance.

Economic status of patients can often be detected by observation of the patient's attire or from the conversation that he will volunteer about his personal financial problems.

B. Clinical Observations

Although the clinical examination is usually performed after the history has been taken, the clinician usually consciously or subconsciously begins his examination as soon as he sees his patient.

From the general appearance and facial expression may be gathered an impression of good or poor health, obesity or emaciation, and normal or abnormal skeletal development.

While the history is being taken, personality traits, unusual mannerisms, mental alertness or dullness, and even expressions of anxiety and emotional instability can be noted.

From a practical standpoint frank deficiency disease is rarely seen. However, changes in the color and texture of the skin suggestive of nutritional inadequacies may be seen.

Fortunately for the dentist, the mouth is one of the most sensitive indicators of a patient's nutritional status. Oral signs that may be suggestive of nutritional inadequacy are: (a) peculiar odor to the breath, (b) lesions or color changes in the lips, (c) color changes and atrophy of the mucosae of the tongue, palate and cheek, (d) change in color, tone and texture of the gingivae, (e) the accumulation of detritus and calculus, and (f) the incidence, location and extent of dental caries. Another significant factor may be the amount of saliva, its mucinous qualities as wel' as its ropy, serous, free-flowing characteristics.

C. Recording Food Intake

Actual food intake is not adequately ascertained by direct questioning about the usual eating patterns and meal practices. Important details may be omitted or inaccurate because remembering the kinds, amounts and preparation of foods is difficult. The parent will often comment on how well her child eats and how infrequently he partakes of sweets. This sort of information should be gratefully received but should be countered by the comment that specific amounts of each food must be recorded so that a meaningful diet evaluation can be made.

The preferred method for recording food intake is to use a specific diary form similar to the one shown in Table 21. On this diary are printed instructions on what and how to record the information about foods eaten at mealtime and between meals. It is kept for at least five days with a week-end day or a holiday as one of these days. Recording food intake during a week-end day or a holiday is desirable because there is usually a considerable difference between meals on those days and ordinary weekdays. Both types of days should be taken into consideration to arrive at a true representation of a food intake pattern. Usually the responsibility of keeping the diary is assigned to the parent unless the patient is old enough to be relied on. It is also important to instruct the patient that no change be made in the customary meals. The patient should not change or "improve" his diet during the period the food diary is being kept. If he does, this will prevent a true and accurate evaluation of his usual food intake pattern.

The patient should record every type of food or beverage that is consumed during the day and evening, no matter where it is eaten—at home, at work, at school, at play, at the corner "sweet shoppe," while watching television or movies or while reading.

For each meal or between-meal snack, instruct the patient

TABLE 21.

FOURTH DAY

Food: Quantity: Prepared:

BREAKFAST:

None

10:00 A.M.

LUNCH:
2 glasses milk
2 Baloney sandwiches
(4 slices white bread)
(4 slices baloney)

3:00 P.M.
1 coca-cola
1 egg & olive sandwich
(2 slices white bread)

DINNER:
2 servings roast turkey
1 serving mashed potatoes
1 serving boiled carrots,
olives, cranberry jelly
2 glasses milk

EXTRAS:
Bedtime
1 peanut butter sandwich
(2 slices whole wheat bread)
1 glass milk
1 glass raspberry tonic
1 glass orangeade tonic
2 glasses grape tonic
3 pieces sugar-covered
jelly candies

FIFTH DAY

Food: Quantity: Prepared:

BREAKFAST:

None

10:00 A.M.
1 piece toast
1 glass grape juice
1 glass milk

LUNCH:
2 glasses milk
1½ turkey sandwiches
(3 slices bread
3 slices turkey
2 leaves lettuce
1½ tsp mayonnaise)

3:00 P.M.

DINNER:
2 servings pork chops
1 serving mashed potatoes
1 serving string beans
1 glass milk
1 black & white cookie

EXTRAS:
1 glass orangeade tonic
1 peanut butter sandwich
(2 slices whole wheat bread)
1 glass milk

FOOD INTAKE DIARY

Of: John Doe

FOR THE FIVE DAYS (include one WEEKEND DAY or a HOLIDAY)

INSTRUCTIONS

1. Record every type of food consumed, solid or liquid, at mealtime, between meals, at the soda fountain, while watching television. Record also, candies, Lifesavers, gum, cough drops or syrups.

2. For each meal, list the food, preparation, (fried, boiled, etc.) and amount in household measures (1 t., 1 T., 1 cup (8 oz.), 1 4 oz. glass, no. of pieces).

3. For fruits and vegetables, record whether raw, fresh, frozen or canned.

4. Record amount of sugar or sugar products and cream or milk added to cereal, beverages or other foods.

5. Record foods in the order in which they are eaten.

6. Particular information on extras is most important to us. Do not leave out the smallest detail.

to record all foods and mixed dishes, the amounts in household measures (teaspoons, tablespoons, servings, cups), and their preparation (fried, boiled, baked, broiled).

Fruits, vegetables, bread, meat and cheese should be described according to their physical nature. They may be described as raw, refined, whole, chopped, hard, soft. The method of preparation, whether fresh, frozen, dried or canned, is useful information and should be included.

The sequence of foods as eaten should be accurately recorded to help establish the detergency of the diet.

Patients should also note the amount of sugar added to foods and beverages; the amount of fats and dressings added to vegetables and salads; and the amount of butter, margarine, jam or jelly spread on bread.

Any between-meal snacks such as cookies, cakes, chewing gum, lozenges, cough drops and cough syrup are as important to record as the main course of any meal.

In order to make clear the kind of detail that is desired in this diary, it is best to demonstrate by actually recording the patient's previous 24 hour food intake. The questioning usually begins with the meal or snack that the patient ate just prior to his office visit. For example, if your patient sees you at 1:30 P.M., the first meal to record is the noonday meal.

The questioning may be along the following lines: What did you eat at lunch today? (The patient might answer, "A sandwich and milk." This is an incomplete answer and the patient should be advised that the type of detail that is desired must be more descriptive.) What was the filler for the sandwich? What kind of bread? Rye? Soft, white? Toasted? Was there mayonnaise or butter spread on the bread? What did you have as a beverage? If milk, was it plain or flavored? Were the sandwich and milk consumed together or was the entire sandwich eaten first and the meal finished with milk? What did you have for dessert? If cookies, how many? What kind?

What did you eat between luncheon and breakfast? (The patient might answer, "A cup of coffee and a piece of cake at 10:00 A.M.") Did you use sugar in the coffee? How much? Was it coffee cake, layer cake or frosted cake? Was it large, medium or small? Did you chew any gum or suck on any Lifesavers this morning?

How about breakfast? ("Just juice, toast and coffee," the patient answers.) Is this the sequence in which you ate the foods? What kind of juice and how much? How many cups of coffee and how many teaspoons of sugar with each one?

The patient is next asked to recall what he ate at bedtime as well as during the evening. A record of nibbling while watching television or snacks before retiring, particularly when not followed by toothbrushing, is important information that should not be overlooked.

As for the dinner meal, it is sometimes difficult for the patient to recall immediately all the specific foods eaten. However, by allowing a little time for concentration, the patient usually recalls the main course first and then the side dishes. It may take a little suggestive reminding: Did you have potatoes with your meal? Did you put butter on your potatoes? What kind of salad did you have? Was there dressing on it? What did you have for dessert? Was a beverage taken with the dessert?

The last eating period that is inquired about and which will complete a 24 hour intake is the midday or after-school snack. Did you stop and eat something at the corner drugstore or soda fountain on the way home from school? What kind of snack did you find at home?

This demonstration of diary keeping will give the patient a much clearer idea of the detailed information that is expected of him. The 24 hour intake that has just been recorded can be used as the first day. For the next four days an attempt should be made to record each meal and snack as it is eaten. The patient should not trust his memory or his good intentions to record this information later. Keeping this diary properly is one of the first indications of the type of cooperation that can be expected when a diet prescription is given. Actually, the diagnosis and treatment plan can be only as accurate and as useful as the information on which it is based.

D. Collecting the Salivary Sample

The patient should be provided with a sterile, wide-mouth, screw-top bottle and a piece of paraffin for the collection of his saliva. It is desirable that a caries-activity test be done before a diet prescription is given. About 3 or 4 days before the second visit, the patient is instructed to collect a salivary sample. This collection procedure is done immediately upon arising in the morning before smoking, eating, drinking, mouth washing or brushing of the teeth. A bite-size piece of paraffin is held under running warm water until soft. After the paraffin has softened so that it is a uniform ball, it should be chewed vigorously to stimulate the flow of saliva. As the mouth fills with saliva, the patient should expectorate into the collecting bottle. He should try not to swallow any of the saliva. This chewing procedure and expectorating should continue for 15 minutes by the clock. In view of the fact that this is a bacteriological procedure, the patient should be cautioned against touching the inside of the collecting bottle or the inside of the cover. After the collection period, the paraffin is discarded and the jar is securely closed by the screw-top cover. The sample should be refrigerated until it can be delivered and is taken to the dental office on the same day or as soon after the collection as is practical. The test should be carried out that day.

E. Performing Caries-Activity Tests

Testing more than a single saliva specimen is better science, but is not always feasible. The dentist should select the one salivary test that can be most conveniently performed. If the *Lactobacillus acidophilus* count can be done by a local bacteriological laboratory, it might be the test of choice. A count of over 10,000 per milliliter of saliva indicates a high caries activity.

The Snyder colorimetric test has proved eminently satisfactory as a means of determining acid production from a sample of the patient's saliva. This is a simple test that can be performed in any dental office. If the blue-green color is reduced to yellow in 24 hours, the patient is classified as caries active. Another simple measurement that can be readily done in the office is that of the rate of salivary flow. The technique and the interpretation of the findings have already been described (Chapter XIV).

SECOND VISIT

In order to allow the patient to complete his 5 day food diary, this visit is scheduled for at least one week after the first. We are going to attempt at this second visit to do four things: (1) fill in any data in the patient's personal history that may have been omitted in the previous visit, (2) evaluate the patient's food intake (3) interpret the salivary caries-activity test, and (4) arrive at a diagnosis and give the patient a diet prescription.

In evaluating the diet of a patient with rampant caries, we look for three things: (1) the fermentable carbohydrate intake, (2) the detergent qualities of the diet and (3) the adequacy of the total diet.

A. Tallying the Fermentable Carbohydrate Intake

The patient is requested to go carefully through each meal or between-meal snack and pick out and circle in red the foods that

TABLE 22.

SWEETS INTAKE

FORM	When Eaten	1st Day	2nd Day	3rd Day	4th Day	5th Day	Total No. Exposures
Sugar in solution	During meal	✓					1
	End of meal		✓✓				2
	Between meals			✓	✓✓		3
Retentive sweets	During meal						
	End of meal	✓		✓	✓✓	✓	5
	Between meals		✓✓✓			✓✓	5
Solid sweets	During meal						
	End of meal						
	Between meals	✓✓			✓✓		4
						Grand Total	20

CLASSIFICATION OF SWEETS AS TO FORM

SUGAR IN SOLUTION	RETENTIVE SWEETS	SOLID SWEETS
Cough medicines (sweetened)	Cakes	Candy
Soft drinks, pop, tonic	Sugar-coated chewing gum	Cough drops
Sweetened condensed milk	Cookies	Frosting
Sweet sauces – chocolate, butterscotch, etc.	Doughnuts	Lifesavers
	Dried fruits	
	Fruits cooked in sugar	
	Ice cream	
	Jams	
	Jellies	
	Marshmallows	
	Muffins	
	Pies	
	Pastries	
	Puddings	
	Sugar-coated cereal	
	Sweet rolls	
	Vegetables glazed with sugar, e.g., candied sweet potatoes	
	Vegetables cooked with sugar or molasses, e.g., Boston baked beans	

contained refined sugars. Also to be circled are dried fruits like figs, dates, prunes, apricots and raisins. Each of these circled sweets is tallied on a "Sweets Intake" chart such as shown in Table 22. This chart classifies the sweets into three forms, namely, sugar in solution, retentive sweets and solid sweets. A list of sweet foods that can be described by one of these three terms is shown in this same chart. The table subdivides the day into periods to show when the sweets were eaten in relation to other foods in the meals: during the meal, at the end of the meal or between meals. The rest of the chart is divided into columns for each of 5 days, from which can be derived final totals and grand totals.

The simplest method of tallying sweets is in terms of number of times the tooth is exposed to sweets for 5 minutes or less. Regardless of the size or the amount of sugar eaten, as long at it took no more than 5 minutes to consume it, a single check mark (✓) is tallied. For example, if a cookie is eaten at 2:00 P.M., and a half hour later another cookie is eaten, two check marks (✓✓) would be the proper tally. But if two cookies were eaten within a 5 minute period, only a single check mark (✓) would be recorded.

A second method of tallying sweets is in terms of teaspoons of sugar. The number of teaspoonfuls of sugar in one serving of the common fermentable carbohydrate foods is shown in Table 23. The arabic figure representing the teaspoons of sugar can be inserted in the appropriate column. Here, too, separate tallies (in this case the individual arabic figures) are made for each sweet eaten in 5 minutes or less.

As an example of how both these methods are used, a brownie eaten at 10:00 P.M. and another eaten at 10:30 P.M. would be recorded as:

RETENTIVE SWEETS	During meal		
	End of meal		
	Between meals	3, 3 or ✓ ✓	

After the sweets have been classified according to (1) their form, (2) when they were eaten and (3) the teaspoons of sugar or the number of times the tooth was exposed, a total is calculated and inserted in the appropriate column of the sweets intake chart. An additional interesting and impressive result will be the grand total of these figures.

TABLE 23. NUMBER OF TEASPOONS OF SUGAR IN ONE SERVING OF SOME COMMON FERMENTABLE CARBOHYDRATE FOODS

The approximate refined carbohydrate content of popular foods expressed in amounts equivalent to teaspoonfuls of sugar: 100 grams sugar (20 teaspoonfuls)—½ cup—3½ oz.—400 calories.*

	Amount	*Sugar Teaspoonfuls*
Cake		
Chocolate cake	2 layer, icing (1/12 cake)	15
Angel cake	1/12 of large cake	6
Sponge cake	1/10 of average cake	6
Cream puff (iced)	1 average, custard filled	5
Doughnut, plain	3″ diameter	4
Candy		
Chocolate bar	average size	7
Chocolate cream	average size	2
Chocolate fudge	1½″ sq.	4
Chocolate mints	1 medium	3
Butterscotch	1″ × 1″	1
Chewing gum	1¢ stick	½
Sweet lozenge	1 usual size	⅓
Cooked Fruits		
Peaches, canned in syrup	2 halves, 1 tbs. juice	3
Sweet cider	6 oz. glass	4
Rhubarb, stewed, sweetened	½ cup	8
Apple sauce, unsweetened	½ cup	2
Prunes, stewed, sweetened	4–5 med., 2 tbs. juice	8
Cookies		
Macaroons	1 large or 2 small	3
Gingersnaps	1 medium	1
Molasses cookies	3½″ diameter	2
Brownies	2″ × 2″ × ¾″	3
Custards and Puddings		
Custard, baked	½ cup	4
Brown Betty	½ cup	9
Gelatin	½ cup	4
Cornstarch pudding	½ cup	3
Dried Fruits		
Apricots, dried	4–6 halves	4
Prunes, dried	3–4 medium	4
Dates, dried	3–4 stoned	4
Figs, dried	1½–2 small	4
Raisins	¼ cup	4
Currants, dried	2 tbs.	4
Ice Cream		
Ice cream	⅛ quart	5–6
Water ice	⅛ quart	6–8

TABLE 23. *Continued*

	Amount	Sugar Teaspoonfuls
Milk Drinks		
Chocolate	1 cup, 5 oz. milk	6
Cocoa	1 cup, 5 oz. milk	4
Cocoa malt	1 glass, 8 oz. milk	4
Eggnog	1 glass, 8 oz. milk	4
Pie		
Apple	1/6 med. pie	12
Cherry	1/6 med. pie	14
Custard, coconut	1/6 med. pie	10
Raisin	1/6 med. pie	13
Pumpkin	1/6 med. pie	10
Sauce		
Chocolate sauce	1 tbs., thick	4
Marshmallow	1 average	1
Soft Drinks		
Sweet, carbonated beverage	1 bottle, 6 oz.	4
Ginger ale	6 oz. glass	3
Spreads		
Jam	1 tbs. level	3
Jelly	1 tbs. level	2
Marmalade	1 tbs. level	3
Syrup, maple	1 tbs. level	2
Honey	1 tbs. level	3

* (Adapted from Dental Caries Control Manual Procedures and Technic of Caries Control Through the Use of a Low Carbohydrate Diet. Division of Dental Health, Tennessee Department of Public Health, Nashville, Tennessee. Journal of the Tennessee State Dental Association, January, 1956.)

B. Determining the Detergent Qualities of the Diet

Detergent qualities of the diet are judged by the kinds of foods that will help to clear the mouth of debris. The presence of at least one raw fruit or raw vegetable in a meal, as the last food eaten, will tend to accomplish clearance. This determination is very simply made by circling in blue every dessert that is made up of a raw fruit (apple, pear, orange, grapefruit) or raw vegetable (carrot, celery, etc). Total these blue-circled foods and record the number at the bottom of Table 24, Diet Evaluation Summary.

C. Technique for Evaluating Food Intake

The diet evaluation technique described here is based on an analysis of food groups rather than of nutrients. The plan used is the Daily Food Guide, "Food for Fitness," published by the U. S. Department of Agriculture in 1958 as a means of interpreting the Recommended Dietary Allowances of the Food and Nutrition Board of the National Research Council.

Using food groups has been found to be a simple, effective and adequate means of teaching good nutrition to patients with rampant caries. The value of analyzing a diet in terms of nutrients is recognized for conditions that warrant it. However, for the patient with rampant caries the simpler procedure has proved to be satisfactory.

The food groups are classified into four broad categories, the 4 Food Groups, and are used as a basis for an adequate diet. They are (1) milk group (milk and cheese), (2) meat group (meat, fish, poultry, eggs, dried beans and peas and nuts), (3) vegetable-fruit group (dark green and deep yellow vegetables, citrus fruits, and other fruits and vegetables, including potatoes), and (4) bread-cereal group (whole grain, enriched or restored breads, cereals and flour products). Foods which contain only calories and very few other nutrients, such as fats, oils, sugars and unenriched cereal foods, are not emphasized in this daily food guide.

The "Diet Evaluation Summary," Table 24, lists the 4 Food Groups in the left-hand column. The six columns across the top of the chart are one for each of 5 days and one for an average of the 5 days. For purposes of comparison, the next three columns record the recommended amounts of standard servings for children, adolescents and adults. The last column can be used to show the difference between the actual intake and the recommended intake.

A valuable aid in nutritional education is the procedure of allowing the patient to tally his own food intake in the appropriate columns. As the tallies are recorded the patient will undoubtedly begin to appreciate the difference between the types of foods he *thought* he was eating and the types he *actually* consumed.

By referring to Appendix III, p. 410, which lists the foods in the food groups, the amounts of food which constitute a serving and food equivalents in mixed dishes, we can readily transpose the information from the patient's food diary to the diet evaluation summary chart. Each average serving or portion is credited as a single unit and is recorded as a chit mark (/) in the appropriate column. Five servings would be recorded as 𝍸.

One-half portions are recorded as (½). For example, two eggs are considered one serving. If the patient ate one egg, the tally is ½ in the meat column. When a leaf of lettuce and a slice or two

TABLE 24.

DIET EVALUATION SUMMARY

FOOD GROUPS	1st Day	2nd Day	3rd Day	4th Day	5th Day	Ave. per Day	Recommended Amounts Child	Adol.	Adult	Differ-ence
MILK GROUP	/	//	///	/	//	2	3-4 serv.	4 or more serv.	2 serv.	child −2 adol. −2 adult none
MEAT GROUP	//	/	0	//	/	1+	2 or more servings			−1
VEGETABLE-FRUIT GROUP Total No. Serv. (Including those rich in Vitamin C* & Vitamin A**)	//	/	///	𝍸	0	2	4 or more servings (Including ----- ----- 1 serving --1 serving every other day----)			−2
BREAD-CEREAL GROUP Enriched or Whole grain	𝍸	𝍸 //	////	𝍸 /	///	4	4 or more servings			none

* Fruits and vegetables rich in vitamin C include:
citrus fruits (grapefruit, lemon, orange) cantaloupe, guava, mango, papaya and raw strawberries.

** Fruits and vegetables rich in vitamin A include the dark green and deep yellow ones:
broccoli, carrots, chard, collards, cress, kale, pumpkin, spinach, sweet potato, turnip greens and other dark green leaves and winter squash.
Also apricots, cantaloupe, mango, and, persimmons.

Note: A fruit or vegetable which is a good source of both vitamin C and vitamin A may be counted as a serving of both vitamin C-rich and vitamin A-rich fruits and vegetables but it will be counted as only one serving in the total number of fruits and vegetables.

DETERGENCY OF THE DIET

Number of detergent foods eaten 5

of tomato are included as part of a sandwich, this is tallied as a ½ portion in the vegetable-fruit column.

A specific example of how the tallying technique is applied can be demonstrated as follows:

A lunch composed of a tuna fish sandwich on enriched toasted white bread with butter, a wedge of lettuce with mayonnaise, a cup of milk and an apple would be tallied thus:

The tuna fish is entered as a single serving in the MEAT GROUP. Two slices of bread were used for the sandwich; therefore, two chit marks are entered in the BREAD GROUP. A wedge of lettuce and the apple are recorded in the VEGETABLE-FRUIT GROUP as two chit marks, and the cup of milk as one chit mark in the MILK GROUP.

FOOD GROUP	1st Day
MILK GROUP	/
MEAT GROUP	/
VEGETABLE-FRUIT GROUP	//
BREAD-CEREAL GROUP	//

The average intake is calculated by dividing the sum of the units by 5 and recording the number in the average column. Then the average is compared to the recommended amounts and the difference is recorded in the "Difference" column as plus (+) or minus (—) or none.

FOOD	1st Day	2nd Day	3rd Day	4th Day	5th Day	Av.	Rec. Amts. Ch.	Rec. Amts. Adol.	Rec. Amts. Ad.	Diff.
MILK	//	//	/	//	//	2	4	4	2	None

This completes the diet evaluation procedures.

D. Explaining the Significance of the Caries Activity Tests

In evaluating the salivary test, the rate of acid production (yellow in 24 hours signifies high caries activity) or the lactobacillus count (10,000/ml. of saliva signifies high caries activity) is used as a means of explaining to the patient his caries activity status. Details on interpreting the salivary test have been discussed in Chapter XIV. It is explained that the number of organisms and the acids they produce will, in most instances, reflect the amount of fermentable carbohydrate present in the mouth.

E. Making a Diagnosis

With the information that we have obtained on some of the possible predisposing factors that may have resulted in the patient's caries susceptibility, and with information on what the patient eats and why he selects these foods, a provisional diagnosis can be made. This may be one of the following:

1. Inadequate diet due to a lack of nutritional knowledge or poor socio-economic condition.
2. Excessive sweets intake due to home environment.
3. Use of sweets as a reward food by parents, grandparents, etc., or as countermeasure for an unpleasant situation (overprotective parent, sibling rivalry, frustration, tensions, etc.).
4. Conditioned malnutrition suggested by an uncontrolled medical problem.

STEPS TAKEN IN MANAGING THE "WHY" AND THE "WHAT" OF THE DIET—THE DIET PRESCRIPTION

A. Managing the "Why" of the Diet

A fundamental concept of the management of any disease is to remove the cause or factor which conditions it. From the list of some of the typical impressions just given, we can see that there may be secondary conditioning factors such as systemic disease (e.g., allergy), psychological problems or social problems that are the basis for the poor diet. Therefore, we have to deal with these first. If these secondary factors are ignored, the time spent in devising a new diet may have been wasted because the patient may find it impossible to cooperate if these are not brought under control first. In practice, the dentist can only recognize that such conditions exist and refer the patient to the physician, psychiatrist or social worker (whichever is indicated) for actual management. Fortunately, there are very few cases that need this special type of management. Most patients present superficial problems. A few typical problems which the dentist should be able to cope with and some suggested solutions are presented here:

Problem. One of the most common environmental factors that influences food selection is cost.

Solution. To cope with this problem there are several suggestions that can be made. Expensive cuts of meat are not more nutritious; they are more palatable with less preparation. But with present-day meat tenderizers and condiments even the less expensive cuts can be made tasty.

Expensive protein foods may be stretched by making mixed dishes; for example, meat and vegetable casseroles, ragouts and curries. Leftover foods can be put to good use by concocting interesting recipes. Some suggested low cost menus are given in Table 25. Nonfat milk powder is considerably less expensive than

TABLE 25. SAMPLE ECONOMICAL MEALS TO AID IN CARIES CONTROL

	Breakfast	
Scrambled egg Whole wheat toast and margarine Milk—children and adolescents Coffee, unsweetened—adults Whole orange	Shredded wheat with milk, no sugar Toast with margarine Milk Coffee, unsweetened Grapefruit, fresh	Hot oatmeal, milk Toast with margarine Milk Coffee Orange juice
	Lunch or Supper	
Corn chowder Crackers or biscuits with margarine Milk Tea, unsweetened—adults Apple	Egg salad sandwich with lettuce Milk Tea, unsweetened Crackers and cheese Celery curls	Grilled cheese and tomato sandwich Dill pickles (if desired) Milk Pear
	Dinner	
Braised pork chops and potatoes Scalloped tomatoes Raw cabbage salad Rolls, margarine Sliced peaches with cream Milk Tea or coffee, unsweetened	Baked fish fillets Baked potato with sour cream and chives Green beans, margarine Hard rolls, margarine Melon Milk Tea, unsweetened	Italian spaghetti with meat balls Tossed green salad Crusty bread, margarine Orange-banana fruit cup Milk Tea or coffee, unsweetened

fluid milk; its use is highly recommended. Margarine is nutritionally equal to butter and costs about one-third as much. A good cookbook will give suggestions for making appetizing dishes from lower cost foods.

Problem. Citizens of foreign birth usually have a dual problem; they are often in a low income group and consequently are financially unable to purchase their traditional foods because they are more expensive in this country. Because of this they buy the most available and least expensive foods, which are usually breads, cereals and sweets.

Solution. People of every nationality have dishes and foods that are composed of each of the basic food groups. The dentist, with a knowledge of food habits of other nationalities, can suggest the good points of the national diet. For example, to Italian patients cheese may be a more acceptable food from the milk group than fluid milk. Encouragement in use of domestic cheeses wherever possible rather than the more expensive imported ones will help the food budget. For the orthodox Hebrew, the generous use of fish which is classified as "parve" (meaning neutral), and which is usually cheaper than Kosher meats, may be encouraged. It is equal to meat in protein value and it does not preclude the use of milk at the same meal.

Problem. Adverse working conditions and hours as well as daily routine may limit daily menus to frequent snacks rather than a few complete meals.

TABLE 26. SUGGESTED BETWEEN-MEAL SNACKS FOR A PERSON WITH RAMPANT CARIES

FRUITS:	Raw: apple, fresh apricots, melons (watermelon, cantaloupe), cherries, grapefruit, grapes, oranges, peaches, pears, pineapple, tangerines. Fresh fruit juices (unsweetened).
VEGETABLES:	Raw: cabbage, cauliflower, carrots, celery, cucumbers, lettuce and other salad greens, radishes, tomatoes, turnips. Tomato juice.
MILK:	Unsweetened
CHEESE:	All kinds—cheddar, cottage or cream
NUTS:	All kinds
COMBINATIONS:	Apple slices with cheddar cheese
	Cream cheese balls rolled in chopped nuts
	Celery stuffed with cottage cheese and chives
	Baloney slices spread with cream cheese and cut in wedges
	Shrimp on toothpicks with tomato cocktail sauce made without sugar
	Deviled eggs
	Pear halves spread with cream cheese and sprinkled with chopped nuts

Solution. Suggest better sleep habits so that the patient can arise in time for more balanced breakfasts. Although most people who have to carry their noonday meal from home use sandwiches, these can have a nutritious filling of meat, fish, cheese or egg. It is quite possible that salads and even some mixed dishes can be taken to work in plastic containers. Good meals will increase the quality and satiety value of the diet so that snack eating will be less necessary. If snacks are needed, they may be selected from Table 26.

Problem. Use of sweets to overcome psychological tension.

Solution. The pleasant taste of sweets is sometimes subconsciously used to overcome unpleasant situations and frustrations. The dentist, in a nondirective manner, can suggest that the patient or the parent consider the factors that might affect this excessive craving for sweets. For example, the parent may be asked how the patient gets along with friends or members of the family. The parent may reveal that the child is having social difficulties. The dentist may then inquire whether this may have anything to do with the eating pattern. In many cases the parent may quickly grasp the relationship between the child's social problem, his unhappiness or his temporary emotional disturbances and the eating of candy. At this point, there is usually no difficulty in arriving at some practical recommendation.

Problems which emanate from such temporary situations are amenable to manipulation. There are others that are of a more profound and permanent nature. The dentist should never attempt to break through any serious level of resistance nor should he offer a diagnosis which may be strongly resisted by the patient. In these latter cases, professional psychiatric advice should always be sought.

Case histories describing superficial emotional problems are briefly recounted here.

1. A 15 year old boy who had recently lost his parents and had had to move to a new city to live with relatives developed rather peculiar eating habits. Four or five times a week he went to the movies in the afternoon because he was lonely and had not made any new friends. While at the movies he ate 4 to 6 bananas, 5 candy bars, etc. This had been going on for several months before he was seen. His relatives were advised of the boy's need for companions of his own age. It was suggested that he might join the local Y.M.C.A. or community center where supervised athletics and other social activities were available.

2. Twin girls about 7 years of age, one of whom had rampant caries and the other a much lower caries incidence, were referred for consultation by the pediatrician. According to the pediatrician, the disturbing feature was that the child with the caries problem was the healthier of the two. The sickly child had required almost constant medical care from birth and would have been the one expected to be more caries susceptible. After interviewing the parent, it became evident that the healthy child did not receive

even the average amount of maternal attention. Catering to the sick child had been so demanding, the mother just had no time for the other twin. To compensate for this deficiency the grandparents took over and showed their affection for and attention to the healthier child by giving her generous amounts of sweets. Obviously, this excess of sweets, a result of the misdirected good intentions of the grandparents, was the cause of the decay.

3. A 19 year old boy who had recently become more aware of the opposite sex was concerned about his "bad breath." To offset this, he indulged in chain eating of cough drops or Lifesavers (2-3 packages a day). He was reassured that he could not develop "bad breath" if his teeth were restored and cleaned and if he would carry out proper oral hygiene at home. Toothbrushing instructions were given, and mouthwashes and a diet of protective foods with emphasis on detergency were advised.

B. Managing the "What" of the Diet

Having pointed out some of the contributing factors to poor diet selection, we are now ready to consider diet improvement. Not only what you advise the patient but how you present the advice is important. A good approach to the problem is a diet prescription (Table 27). Patients accept a prescription more readily than they do verbal admonishments. Furthermore, they do not have to depend on memory. They can always refer to the written prescription or instructions whenever questions arise as to which foods they may include or must avoid.

There are three components to the diet prescription: (1) advice about sweets intake, (2) advice about detergency of the diet, and (3) a diet, meal and menu plan.

1. Advice about Sweets Intake. The total amount of sweets or number of exposures to sweets is transposed from the sweets intake chart to the diet prescription. It is pointed out from the chart how frequently retentive and solid sweets were eaten. Stress is placed on this latter finding. The statement can be made that in a controlled clinical study it was determined that the form and frequency of sweets intake was found to be more important from a caries-producing standpoint than the amount of sugars.[1] It was discovered that even though the total amount of sugar was the same in several test groups, those who used liquid sucrose had much less caries than those who used toffees.

To dramatically emphasize the amount of sweets consumed the

TABLE 27.

DIET PRESCRIPTION FOR CONTROL OF RAMPANT CARIES

I. Total Sweets Intake 35 tsp. per week

Recommended Substitutes: Nuts, milk, hard cheese

II. Number of Detergent Foods Used 4 per week

Improve by Increasing: Celery stalks, Carrot sticks

III. a) DIET

FOOD GROUPS	Actual Intake	Recommended Intake	Improve by + Increase	Improve by - Decrease
MILK GROUP	1	2	1	
MEAT GROUP	2	2		
VEGETABLE-FRUIT GROUP	0	4	4	
BREAD-CEREAL GROUP	8	4		4

b) MEAL PLAN

Recommended Typical Meal Plan		Patient's Typical Meal Plan	Recommended Improvements
Breakfast			
Meat or Milk	- 1 serv. or more	Bread	Milk Fruit
Bread-Cereal	- 2 serv. or more		
Vegetable-Fruit	- 1 serv.		
Lunch			
Bread-Cereal	- 2 serv. or more	Bread	Vegetable
Meat	- 1 serv. or more	Meat	Milk
Vegetable-Fruit	- 2 serv. or more	Fruit	
Milk	- 1 serv.		
Dinner			
Meat	- 1 serv. or more	Meat	
Vegetable-Fruit	- 2 serv. or more	Vegetable	Fruit
Bread-Cereal	- 1 serv. or more	Bread	
Milk	- 1 serv.	Milk	

c) MENU PLAN *

BREAKFAST	LUNCH	DINNER
Toast and Butter Milk Raw orange	Tuna fish sandwich Milk Raw carrot stick	Chicken Potato, string beans Raw salad Milk Raw apple

* Use Exchange List of Foods (Appendix IX) as a guide in designing menus to suit individual tastes.

patient might count out and place in a pile the number of lumps of sugar equivalent to the teaspoons of sugar ingested from fermentable carbohydrate foods. Almost invariably the patient will state, "I never realized I ate so much sugar, but I do need the sugar for energy. What other foods can I use?" The answer may well be, "Use increased amounts of foods from the 4 Food Groups or additional amounts of fat unless contraindicated."

A common question is, "Must I omit fruits?" The answer is that only dried fruits like dates, figs, prunes, raisins and apricots and fresh fruits like bananas which are sticky and retentive need be omitted. Encourage the use of citrus fruits and raw detergent fruits.

In general, then, the prime factor is to restrict all refined and some natural sugar products. To the question, "Isn't it difficult to stop eating sweets if you have been using them for a long time?" the answer is, "No, if you wean yourself completely rather than gradually." In fact, the taste for sweets can even become distasteful once one has learned to abstain. It is much like giving up cigarettes or the excessive food or drink habit. It is merely a matter of will power. Dr. Joliffe, in treating his obese patients, feels that they can learn to reduce and stay reduced if they educate their appetite-regulating mechanism, which he calls "appestat," to accept lower amounts of food.[3] The same procedure has been found effective in managing sweets intake for rampant caries patients.

However, there are individuals who do not have the will power to abstain from consuming sweets. In these cases, artificial sweeteners such as saccharine or a cyclamatic product (Sucaryl) can be condoned. Saccharine is sweeter than Sucaryl and less expensive. Saccharine develops a bitter taste when cooked whereas Sucaryl does not.

As will be seen in a typical sweets intake chart, most sweets are consumed at the end of a meal or between meals. If substitutes for sweet desserts or sweet between-meal snacks are suggested, this may help the patient to learn to abstain from sweets. A list of permissible snacks can be given the patient. Table 26 lists suggestions that may be used.

2. Advice on the Detergency of the Diet. Detergent foods, like a toothbrush, help to keep the teeth clean and free from debris. However, such foods should be used only as adjuncts to toothbrushing and not in its place.

By pointing out the paucity of detergent foods in the patients'

TABLE 28. GENERAL SUGGESTIONS FOR FOODS TO BE INCLUDED AND AVOIDED AT EACH MEAL

	Include	*Avoid*
Breakfast		
Eggs	Any style (bacon or sausage if desired) French toast with butter or margarine	Syrup on French toast
Bread (with butter) or Cereal	Whole grain or enriched toast or hard variety (dark rye, Ry-Krisp) Cereal, cooked, with butter and milk	Dried cereals with sugar, syrups, jams, jellies, buns, pastry or sweet rolls
Fruit, citrus	Whole fruit, fresh, (orange, grapefruit, melon) Frozen or unsweetened canned juice	Adding sugar to fruit
Milk	Plain or buttermilk	Chocolate or other flavored and sweetened milk
Beverage	Coffee, tea, water, as desired	Sugar
Lunch		
Soups, juice	Fresh or canned soups, vegetable juice or unsweetened fruit juice	
Sandwich	Toasted or dark bread—Meat, fish, fowl, egg or cheese fillings	Raisin or cinnamon bread, jam, jellies or honey filling
Salads	Any combination of fresh fruits or vegetables, raw carrot or celery sticks	
Milk	Plain or buttermilk	Any flavored milks or soda pop
Desserts	Raw apples, oranges, tangerines or other fruits in season	Cakes, cookies, pies, pastry, bananas, ice cream, raisins, figs, dates or other dried fruits
Water	As desired	
Dinner		
Soup, juice	Fresh or canned soups, vegetable juice or unsweetened fruit juice	
Meats, fish	Beef, lamb, pork, veal, fowl or fish (liver at least once a week)	
Vegetables	1 or 2 portions, especially green or yellow, and potatoes	Candied sweet potatoes or glazed vegetables
Salad	Any combination of fresh fruits or vegetables, raw carrot or celery sticks	
Desserts	Raw apples, oranges, tangerines or other fruits in season	Same as lunch
Milk	Plain or buttermilk	Any sweetened milk
Beverage	Coffee, tea, water, as desired	Soda pop

present diet and suggesting that every meal, even breakfast, end with a detergent fruit or vegetable, a significant step will have been taken towards caries control.

The commonest and simplest detergent foods are raw fruits and vegetables. For example, instead of drinking orange juice at the beginning of the meal, eating a whole orange or half a grapefruit at the end will help to clear the mouth of debris. Finishing lunches and dinners with an apple, pear, celery or carrot sticks, etc., is a procedure highly recommended for assuring detergence.

Although water is not a detergent food, liberal use of it at the end of meals will help to clear the mouth of retained food.

*3. **Diet, Meal and Menu Plan.*** From the diet evaluation summary chart the actual intake and recommended intake can be filled in for each of the 4 Food Groups in the diet prescription. The difference between these two columns should be recorded in the improvement column.

The patient should now have been made aware of how much of the 4 Food Groups he has been eating and how much he should be eating. His next step is to pay particular attention to increasing his consumption of the foods that he has habitually been using in less than recommended amounts.

To distribute the recommended total food intake properly throughout the day, a suggested typical meal plan should be followed. (Such a plan is shown in Table 27.) A meal plan expressed in terms of food groups serves as a basis for the menu planning. It allows the patient to plan his meals to meet his individual needs through the use of food exchanges.

The technique for determining the patient's actual meal plan is to choose from his food diary one day which represents his usual food intake. Beside each food note the food group that it represents. By this procedure the patient's typical meal plan may be determined and recorded in the proper column in the diet prescription. By comparing the patient's typical meal plan with the recommended one, the improvements that the patient needs to make are easily determined and recorded.

The menu is the conversion of food groups into specific foods. To improve the patient's usual menu, we start with his typical breakfast and suggest, not drastic changes, but slight modifications. Emphasis is placed on quality improvement rather than quantity. If the patient says, "I just don't have any appetite when I get up," it is unrealistic to prescribe a full-course meal. Liquids are

TABLE 29. A SAMPLE DIET FOR A 6 YEAR OLD CHILD

1. *Recommended food intake for a day:*

Milk group	3 or more servings
Meat group	2 or more servings
Vegetable-fruit group	4 or more servings
Bread-cereal group	4 or more servings

(Additional foods from the above groups plus fats may be used to meet individual's energy needs.)

2. *Meal Plan*

Breakfast:

Milk or meat group—1 serving
Bread-cereal group—2 servings
Vegetable-fruit group—1 serving

Lunch:

Meat group—1 serving
Bread-cereal group—2 servings
Milk group—1 serving
Vegetable-fruit group—1 serving

Dinner:

Meat group—1 serving
Vegetable-fruit group—2 servings
Bread-cereal group—1 serving
Milk group—1 serving

3. *Menu*

Breakfast:

Wheat flakes, milk
Toast, butter
Milk to drink
Whole orange

Lunch:

Egg salad sandwich—consisting of
  whole wheat bread
  hard cooked egg
  lettuce
  butter or mayonnaise
Milk
Apple and cheese strips

Dinner:

Hamburg patties
Scalloped potatoes
Buttered green beans
Bread, butter
Milk
Celery and carrot strips
Peach

TABLE 30. A SAMPLE DIET FOR A 9 YEAR OLD CHILD

1. *Recommended food intake for a day:*

Milk group	3 to 4 cups
Meat group	2 servings or more
Vegetable-fruit group	4 servings or more
Bread-cereal group	4 servings or more

(Additional servings of any of the above food groups plus fats may be eaten to meet energy needs.)

2. *Meal Plan:*

Breakfast:
- Meat group—1 serving
- Bread-cereal group—2 servings
- Milk group—1 serving
- Vegetable-fruit group—1 serving

Lunch:
- Meat group—1 serving
- Bread-cereal group—2 servings
- Milk group—1 serving
- Vegetable-fruit group—1 or 2 servings

Dinner:
- Meat group—1 serving
- Bread-cereal group—1 serving
- Milk group—1 serving
- Vegetable-fruit group—2 or more servings

Between meals:
- Milk group
- Vegetable-fruit group

3. *Menu*

Breakfasts:	
Fried egg	Shredded wheat with milk and sliced fresh peach
Toasted English muffin with butter	Toast and butter
Milk	Milk
Grapefruit (fresh)	Orange juice
Lunches:	
Macaroni and cheese	Egg salad sandwich with lettuce and mayonnaise
Grilled frankfurter	Dill pickles
Milk	Milk
Roll and butter	Salted peanuts
Cabbage-pineapple salad	
Dinners:	
Broiled liver	Hamburg patties
Mashed potato	Creamed potatoes
Broccoli, butter	Carrot and celery strips
Tossed salad	Corn on the cob
Bread, butter	Bread, butter
Fresh pineapple	Fruit gelatin mold
	Milk

TABLE 31. A SAMPLE DIET FOR A 13 YEAR OLD GIRL

1. *Recommended food intake for a day:*

Milk group	4 or more servings
Meat group	2 or more servings
Vegetable-fruit group	4 or more servings
Bread-cereal group	4 or more servings

(Additional foods from the above groups plus fats may be used to meet energy needs.)

2. *Meal Plan*

Breakfast:

Meat or milk group—1 serving
Bread-cereal group—2 servings
Vegetable-fruit group—1 serving

Lunch:

Meat group—1 serving
Bread-cereal group—2 servings or more
Vegetable-fruit group—1 serving or more
Milk group—1 serving or more

Dinner:

Meat group—1 serving
Vegetable-fruit group—2 servings
Bread-cereal group—1 serving
Milk group—1 serving

Bedtime:

Milk group—1 serving

3. *Menu*

Breakfast:

Scrambled eggs
Toast, butter
Milk
Grapefruit (fresh)

Lunch:

Tuna fish casserole
Cole slaw
Milk
Crackers and cheese
Pear (fresh)

Dinner:

Meat loaf
Buttered carrots
Tossed green salad
Crusty rolls
Milk
Strawberries and cream

Bedtime:

Milk
Popcorn

TABLE 32. A SAMPLE DIET FOR A 15 YEAR OLD BOY

1. *Recommended food intake for a day:*

Milk group	4 or more servings
Meat group	2 or more servings
Vegetable-fruit group	4 or more servings
Bread-cereal group	4 or more servings

(Use additional servings of the above food groups and fats to meet energy needs.)

2. *Meal Plan*

Breakfast:
- Meat group—1 serving
- Bread-cereal group—2 to 4 servings
- Milk group—1 serving
- Vegetable-fruit group—1 serving

Lunch:
- Meat group—1 serving
- Vegetable-fruit group—2 servings
- Bread-cereal group—2 to 4 servings
- Milk group—1 serving

Dinner:
- Meat group—1 serving
- Vegetable-fruit group—3 servings
- Bread-cereal group—2 servings
- Milk group—1 serving

Bedtime or snack:
- Milk group—1 serving
- Bread-cereal group—1 serving
- Vegetable-fruit group—1 serving

3. *Menu*

Breakfasts:

Fried eggs, with bacon if desired
Toast, butter
Milk
Orange

Scrambled eggs
Whole wheat toast, butter
Milk
Grapefruit

Lunches:

Hamburgers
Cole slaw
Milk
Cheese and crackers
Apple

Corn beef sandwiches on rye bread (with lettuce)
Milk
Cheese and crackers
Pear

Dinners:

Pot roast
Mashed potatoes with gravy
Carrots
Tossed salad
Rolls, butter
Watermelon

Pork chops
Rolls (hard)
Baked potato
Green beans
Carrot strips
Plums

Bedtime or snacks:

Popcorn
Milk

Milk
Apples

easy to swallow, so suggest a glass of orange juice or a cup of milk to start. The following week, instead of having one or the other, he may accept both liquids. From there the next step of adding toast and butter will not be too difficult, and ending the meal with a raw orange rather than using orange juice at the beginning of the meal may be acceptable.

The same procedure of gradual changes is used for lunch. If the patient's lunch has been a jelly sandwich and coffee, don't prescribe vegetable soup, tuna casserole, raw salad, bread and butter, milk and fruit. Merely suggest that, instead of jelly, he use tuna fish for a filler and include milk as a beverage along with coffee or tea without sugar plus some carrot strips for a final food. Let that be sufficient for the first change. In the weeks that follow, a gradual build-up of quality and variety can be attained by using the Exchange List of Foods in Appendix IX. The ultimate goal is to have the patient include and avoid foods at each meal as suggested in Table 28. Sample diets, depending on the age, sex, size and activity of the patient, are shown in Tables 29, 30, 31 and 32.

SUBSEQUENT VISITS

A follow-up visit should be scheduled about 8 weeks after the treatment plan is instituted. Prior to this visit the salivary specimen bottle and food diary should have been mailed to the patient. He is advised to complete the 5 day food diary in the same manner as he did the first one. He also should collect a salivary specimen on the morning of his office appointment in the same manner as before.

The food diary is re-evaluated for fermentable carbohydrates, detergency, and diet adequacy. The results of this evaluation are compared to the original plan to note whether recommendations have been followed. Misinterpretation, misunderstandings and problems that have arisen during this 8 week period are discussed. Menu changes are recommended, if necessary. Salivary tests are repeated to see if there is any noticeable change in the oral environment.

If there is no improvement, further questioning may reveal some factor that the patient felt was insignificant. For example, one patient who seemed to be following dietary advice still showed no significant reduction in oral acid production. By coincidence, she mentioned that she had been constipated and, rather than use a laxative, had been nibbling on "some natural dried fruits that do not contain refined sugar." Unfortunately, the patient did not realize that natural dried fruits are just as cariogenic as sugar and sugar products. She was advised to increase her roughage and bulk with cellulose foods and eliminate the dried fruits. Subsequent tests were more favorable.

After the 8 weeks, if there is improvement, follow-ups can be done at 3 to 4 month intervals. However, if there have been adverse findings, more frequent counselling may be necessary. Continuous follow-up, even by phone, is very helpful in maintaining patient cooperation. The personal interest that the clinician gives these patients is rewarded in many ways.

REFERENCES

1. Gustafsson, B. E., Quensel, C., Lanke, L., Lundqvist, C., Grahnen, H., Bonow, B., and Krasse, B.: Vipeholm dental caries study: effect of different levels of carbohydrate intake on caries activity in 436 individuals observed for five years. Acta Odont. Scand., *11:*232, 1954.
2. Jay, P., Beeuwkes, A. M., and Benson, H. M.: Dietary Program for the Control of Dental Caries. Ann Arbor, The Overback Co., 1955.
3. Joliffe, N.: Reduce and Stay Reduced. New York, Simon & Schuster, 1957.
4. Kitchin, P. C., and Permar, D.: Results of an eight-year study of the effectiveness of carbohydrate restriction in reducing salivary lactobacillus counts. J. D. Res., *34:*89, 1955.
5. Kite, O. W., Shaw, J. H., and Sognnaes, R. F.: The prevention of experimental tooth decay by tube feeding. J. Nut., *42:*89, 1950.
6. Orland, F. J., Blayney, J. R., Harrison, R. W., Reyniers, J. A., Trexler, P. C., Ervin, R. F., Gordon, H. A., and Wagner, M.: Experimental caries in germ-free rats inoculated with enterococci. J.A.D.A., *50:*259, 1955.
7. Shafer, W. G.: The caries-producing capacity of starch, glucose, and sucrose diets in the Syrian hamster. Science, *110:*143, 1949.
8. Shaw, J. H.: The effect of carbohydrate-free and carbohydrate-low diets on the incidence of dental caries in white rats. J. Nut., *53:*151, 1954.

Chapter XVI

Fluoridation Vehicles—
Water Supplies, Foods and Supplements

INTRODUCTION

The use of fluorides for preventing or retarding dental decay has been suggested in addition to rapid oral clearance of retentive foods and the regulation of the intake of fermentable carbohydrates. In the earlier part of this text a brief review of the chemistry, physiology, general pathology and dental pathology of fluorides was given. A historical review was also included on the relation of fluorides in excessive amounts to mottled enamel and fluorides in optimal amounts to lowered caries incidence. Possible mechanisms for the decay preventive action of fluorides were suggested as: (1) its ability to decrease acid solubility when incorporated in enamel; (2) its ability to inhibit acid production of the oral microorganisms; and (3) its ability to reduce the number of lactobacilli in the saliva.

ARTIFICIAL FLUORIDATION OF WATER SUPPLIES

As a result of the epidemiological surveys of Dean,[7] which correlated low caries and optimal fluoride levels in communal water supplies, Cox[6] suggested that optimal amounts of fluorides be added to public water supplies that were low in or free of fluorides.

In view of the various climatic conditions that would be encountered in different areas, Cox further suggested that the concentration of fluoride levels should depend on several factors: (1) the water consumption of normal children, (2) the mean temperature and (3) the humidity of the geographical area. In addition to these factors, it was also important to appreciate that the maximal effect of fluorides was on the enamel structure during its formation and calcification. Therefore, to properly evaluate artificial fluoridation of water supplies, its dental effects had to be studied: (a) in children, for at least ten years while their teeth were being mineralized; and (b) in areas where optimal fluoride concentrations in water supplies could be easily regulated. Hutton,[10] in Brantford, Ontario, in 1942, and Ast,[1] in New York in 1943, proposed an experiment which consisted of studying the effects of artificially fluoridated water on residents in two nearby communities that were similar in socio-economic, cultural and environmental factors. Both of these communities would have, at the outset, fluoride-free water. After base line medical and dental examinations, the drinking water supply of one community would be artificially fluoridated so that 1.0 ppm. of fluoride would be present. This would constitute the experimental group. The control group would be the other community, which would continue to use the usual fluoride-free water supply. In 1945 three sets of communities embarked on an artificial fluoridation experiment. These communities were Grand Rapids, Michigan, as the experimental group and Muskegon, Michigan, as the control; Newburgh, N.Y., as the experimental and Kingston, N.Y., as the control; and Brantford, Ontario, as the experimental and Sarnia, Ontario, as the control. Soon after these studies were started other cities (Southbury, Connecticut, Sheboygan, Wisconsin, Marshall, Texas, and Ottawa, Kansas) fluoridated their water supplies.[14]

After ten years the three original experimental cities reported lower dental caries experience in their children compared to the children of the control cities. The Newburgh-Kingston[2] study showed that the 6 to 9 year olds whose teeth had been under the influence of fluoride during the entire formative period (in utero, during lactation and postweaning) had approximately 57 per cent less decay than their controls in Kingston (Fig. 86). In older age groups there was also less caries but at a lesser percentage differential. For example, the per cent difference in 10 to 12 year old groups was 52 per cent, in 13 to 14 year old groups it was 48 per cent, and in the 16 year olds it was 40 per cent. Evidently, the more immature the tooth the greater the opportunity to develop a higher caries-resistant quality in the presence of fluorides.

Observations were made on gingival disturbances and enamel opacities. No difference was observed in gingival disease. There was no disfiguring mottled enamel as a result of the 1.0 ppm. fluoride addition to the Newburgh water supply, but there were a few cases of questionable, mild and very mild fluorosis. However, the fluoride-free Kingston children had significantly greater numbers of non-fluoride enamel opacities than the Newburgh children.

The medical examination[12] given by qualified pediatricians showed no significant differences in height, weight, bone density,

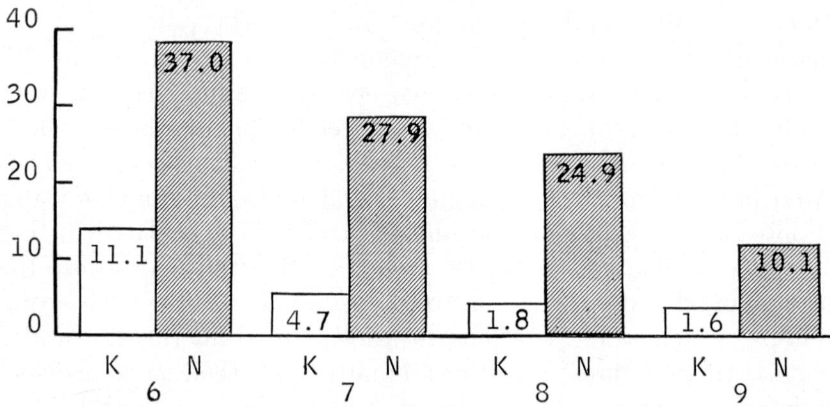

FIGURE 86. Percentage of children ages six to nine with all their deciduous molars present and caries free. (Modified from Ast, D. B., Smith, D. J., Wachs, V. B., and Cantwell, K. F., in J.A.D.A., 52:314, 1956.)

bone age, eye and ear examinations and routine blood and urine examinations.

In a study which compared the caries incidence of children living in cities whose water supplies were either artificially fluoridated (Brantford) or naturally fluoridated (Stratford) compared to a control city that was fluoride free (Sarnia), it was shown that the children from the first two cities had 50 per cent less decay than the third. Furthermore, the caries experience in the group of 6 to 8 year old children from both fluoridated cities was about the same, which meant that artificial fluoridation of water supplies was an effective caries-preventive public health measure.

Other fluoridation studies have shown similar favorable reductions in dental caries. Hill et al.[9] reported on the caries incidence after eight and a half years of fluoridation at Evanston, Illinois.

They found a reduction of 80 per cent in the caries incidence of permanent teeth of 6 year olds. These children were exposed to fluorides at conception. Milan, Tennessee, Madison, Wisconsin, Maysville, Kentucky, Marshall, Texas,[8] and Athens, Georgia,[13] all report significant favorable reductions in dental decay. Recently Knutson reported at the centennial meeting of A.D.A that 35,738,-842 people in 1830 communities in the United States were drinking fluoride-treated water as of August, 1959. Another 7,000,000 had natural fluoride in their drinking water.

The adjustment of water supplies so that the fluoride content is at 1.0 ppm. is recommended by the most important agencies and organizations concerned with health in the United States, e.g., American Dental Association, American Medical Association, National Research Council, United States Department of Health, Education, and Welfare, Public Health Service, etc.[14]

ENRICHING FOODS WITH FLUORIDES

In view of the fact that only about 110,000,000 people drink from community water supplies and 174,000,000 people constitute the total population of this country, some procedure other than artificial fluoridation of communal water supplies must be used to provide fluoride dental benefits to the other 64,000,000 people. Fluoridation of bottled water, addition of fluorides to table salt and the taking of fluoride pills or fluoride drops are possible methods of artificial fluoridation. Before deciding on which of these alternate vehicles one might select, it is best to briefly review the amount of fluoride that is ingested from the various foods eaten each day. With the exception of sea foods and tea, the average amount of fluoride that would be ingested from all foods combined would probably not amount to more than 0.2 to 0.3 ppm.[11] An exceptionally heavy tea drinker would have to drink ten cups a day to obtain the same benefit as from a quart of drinking water fortified with 1.0 ppm. F. One would have to consume nearly 200 grams of fish to produce an equivalent of 1.0 ppm F in the water supply.

Enriching foods such as bread, cereals or milk with fluorides appears undesirable because the intake of these staples varies so for different age groups, different activities, different physiological periods, etc.

Water intake is less variable and the benefits are more uniform when drinking water is used as a vehicle. Bottled water which contains measured amounts of fluoride appears to be a very reasonable vehicle. Its main disadvantage is its high cost. Sognnaes[13] suggests that other liquid vehicles that may merit attention are juices and soups. He feels that these vehicles have the advantage of being low in cost, contribute other valuable nutrients and are not consumed in excess. The disadvantage of adding fluoride to milk stems from the fact that the small distributor would have difficulty in controlling the addition of fluoride to small quantities of milk.

Salt has been suggested as a vehicle for fluoride. The disadvantages of this are: (1) uncertainty as to whether the fluoride would be uniformly distributed, and (2) the possibility that the fluoride might affect the hygroscopic properties of the product.

FLUORIDE SUPPLEMENTS AS PILLS OR DROPS

In prescribing supplements of dietary fluorides, the Council on Dental Therapeutics[5] suggests that in "selected instances where there is strong motivation on the part of the parent and a clear realization of the need for careful regulation of the daily intake," fluoride tablets can be prescribed. Those being recommended are sodium fluoride preparations (Fluoritabs and Karidium). Other fluoride tablets such as calcium fluoride or bone meal tablets are not recommended[4] for several reasons: (1) There is no adequately controlled clinical study that can demonstrate that either of these compounds is useful in caries control. (2) Chemically both these compounds are practically insoluble in the fluids of the mouth. (3) They have no systemic effect on the tooth or saliva because they are not readily absorbed through the intestinal tract. There are no published data on a controlled clinical study to prove the absolute effectiveness of sodium fluoride but there are some observations on children who were given these supplements and there is "suggestive evidence of the development of caries-resistant teeth"[5] without dental fluorosis.

By checking with the public health department, the fluoride content of local water supplies can be ascertained. The aim should be to provide 0.5 mg. of fluoride ion per day for children from two to three years of age and about 1.0 mg. per day beyond 3 years of age. Fluoride supplements are not recommended where drinking water has more than 0.7 ppm. fluoride. These supplements should be started as early in life as possible and maintained until 10 years of age. No more than 264 mg. of sodium fluoride should be dispensed at one time. The bottle should be labeled, "CAUTION: Store out of reach of children."

The following prescription is suggested:[5]

℞ Sodium Fluoride tablets 2.2 mg.
Dispense 100
Label: Use according to written directions
CAUTION: Store out of reach of children

Written directions should be provided according to the age of the child as follows:

(1) Before 2 years of age: Add one fluoride tablet to each quart of water used for drinking purposes and for the preparation of formulas and other food.
(2) From 2 to 3 years of age: *Every other day* add one fluoride tablet to an amount of fruit juice or drinking water which the child will consume at one time.
(3) After 3 years of age: Administer one tablet *each* day in an amount of fruit juice or drinking water that will be consumed at one time.

In communities where the water is fluoride-free or around 0.1 ppm., fluoride drops such as Luride can be recommended. (Each drop is standardized to provide 0.1 mg. fluorine as sodium fluoride). Five drops daily is suggested for children under 3 and 10 drops daily is used for children over 3. These drops are added to water or fruit juice.

The Council on Dental Therapeutics[5] suggests a fluoride solution in which 240 cc. contain 0.132 gm. of sodium fluoride. This is for communities which are devoid of fluoride in the drinking water. However, as previously stated, fluorides are prescribed where drinking water contains less than 0.7 ppm.

"The amount of fluoride may be adjusted downward by 10 per cent for each 0.1 ppm. of fluoride ion in the drinking water. Thus when the level in the drinking water is 0.6 ppm., the amount of fluoride in the prescription will be reduced by 60 per cent, that is, to 0.053 Gm. Similarly at a level of 0.4 ppm. the amount of sodium fluoride would be 0.079 Gm. and at a level of 0.2 ppm., the prescription would specify 0.106 Gm.

℞ Sodium Fluoride	0	132
Distilled water, to make	240	0

Label: Use according to written directions
CAUTION: Store out of reach of children

Written directions should be provided according to the age of the child as follows:

(1) Before 2 years of age: Add one teaspoonful to each quart of water used for drinking purposes and for the preparation of formulas and other food.

(2) From 2 to 3 years of age: *Every other day* add one teaspoonful to an amount of fruit juice or water that the child will consume at a time.

(3) After 3 years of age: Each day add one teaspoonful to an amount of fruit juice or water that the child will consume at one time."

REFERENCES

1. Ast, D. B.: The caries-fluorine hypothesis and a suggested study to test its application. Pub. Health Rep., *58:*857, 1943.
2. Ast, D. B., Smith, D. J., Wachs, V. B., and Cantwell, K. F.: Newburgh-Kingston caries-fluorine study. XIV. Combined clinical and roentgenographic dental findings after ten years of fluoride experience. J.A.D.A., *52:*314, 1956.
3. Chrietzberg, J. E., and Lewis, F. D., Jr.: An evaluation of caries prevalence after five years of fluoridation. J.A.D.A., *56:*192, 1958.
4. Council of Dental Therapeutics: Current status of dental uses of fluorides. J.A.D.A., *45:*468, 1952.
5. Council on Dental Therapeutics: Prescribing supplements of dietary fluorides. J.A.D.A., *56:*589, 1958.
6. Cox, G. J.: New knowledge of fluorine in relation to dental caries. J. Am. Water Works Assoc., *31:*1926, 1939.
7. Dean, H. T.: Endemic fluorosis and its relation to dental caries. Pub. Health Rep., *53:*1443, 1938.
8. Hill, I. N.: Fluoridation research and related developments. J.A.D.A. *54:* 454, 1957.
9. Hill, I. N., Blayney, J. R., and Wolf, W.: Evanston dental caries study. XVI. Reduction in dental caries attack rates in children six to eight years old. J.A.D.A., *53:*327, 1956.
10. Hutton, W. L., Linscott, B. W., and Williams, D. B.: The Brantford fluorine experiment; interim report after 5 years of water fluoridation. Canadian J. Pub. Health, *42:*81, 1951.
11. McClure, F. J.: Fluorine in foods: Survey of recent data. Pub. Health Rep., *64:*1061, 1949.
12. Schlesinger, E. R., et al.: Newburgh-Kingston caries-fluorine study. XIII. Pediatric findings after ten years, J.A.D.A., *52:*296, 1956.
13. Sognnaes, R. F.: Relative Merits of Various Fluoridation Vehicles; in Shaw, J. H., ed.: Fluoridation as a Public Health Measure. Washington, Am. Assoc. for Adv. of Sci., 1954.
14. Stadt, Z. M.: Resume of Dental Benefits of Fluorine Ingestion; in Shaw, J. H., ed.: Fluoridation as a Public Health Measure. Washington, Am. Assoc. for Adv. of Sci., 1954.
15. Volker, J. F.: The Prevention of Dental Caries with Fluoride; in Finn, S. B.: Clinical Pedodontics. Philadelphia, W. B. Saunders Co., 1957.

Chapter XVII

The Role of Diet and Nutrition in Etiology, Diagnosis and Management of the Patient with Periodontal Disease

DIET AND NUTRITION IN ETIOLOGY OF PERIODONTAL DISEASE

Periodontal disease, like most other diseases, is the resultant of two forces, namely, the destructive and the resistant ones; and each of these forces is influenced by local and systemic factors which are interdependent and never operate as single etiologic agents. However, the degree of participation of either local or systemic factors in producing the disease is an individual variable. It is obvious, then, that in management of periodontal disease the dentist should not emphasize the elimination of the local factor with total disregard for the systemic factor or vice versa.

Food as a Local Etiologic Factor

There are a number of local factors that may contribute to periodontal disease, such as calculus, trauma from occlusion, food impaction, faulty restorations, habit, missing teeth, occlusal neuroses, use of tobacco, mouth breathing and mechanical and chemical traumata. Of these, food may be involved in calculus formation and food impaction.

There are several theories of calculus formation—physicochemical, bacterial and systemic. The physicochemical theory advanced by Prinz[25] suggested that a foreign body nidus made up of food debris, bacteria and desquamated epithelial cells will attract calcium salts. Food debris is involved in Stanley's bacterial theory of calculus formation.[27] In animals, deficiencies of vitamin A[18] as well as of niacin and pyridoxine[5] have been associated with disposition to more rapid calculus formation. The lack of mastication due to soft diets has been suggested as a reason for accumulation of food debris with consequent formation of calculus.[18]

Food impaction is due not only to improper dental restorative or anatomic conditions such as poor contact points, improperly restored marginal ridges, and excessively deep fossae, but also to the physical nature of the food. The stringy, resilient type of fibrous meat is an example of a food that lodges between teeth; seeds from berries may also become impacted and serve as local gingival irritants.

Nutrition as a Systemic Etiologic Factor

Like all labile tissues, the periodontal tissues are affected by stresses of everyday living, of which diet and nutrition are one. Specific nutrients have been associated with maintaining the integrity of the epidermal, mesodermal and calcified tissues of the periodontium, e.g., vitamins A, B complex and C might affect epithelial and collagenous tissues, and calcium, phosphorus and vitamin D might affect bone.

More detailed discussions of how deficiencies or excesses of nutrients affect the periodontium have been given in the section on Basic Nutrition and elsewhere.[13] Most of our present knowledge on this subject deals with the experimental animal rather than man.

NUTRITIONAL DIAGNOSIS

If it is agreed that nutrition can contribute to periodontal health just as it does to the health of any other tissue, then assessment of the patient's nutritional status by the dentist should be considered an integral part of his diagnostic procedure in periodontal disease.

Furthermore, ascertaining the nutritional status of the patient should not be considered a separate discipline or an extra chore but rather one that is part of the over-all diagnosis and treatment.

The point that is often raised is that the average patient does not present himself with florid signs of a nutritional deficiency. This is true. Why, then, do a nutritional assessment? The reason is that primary or secondary conditioning factors (see Chapter XIII) may be of sufficient magnitude to deplete the nutrient reserve and thus produce a tissue depletion. It is the recognition of the possible presence of subclinical signs that is important and this is accomplished through a diagnostic procedure which includes a medical history, dietary history, general inspection and laboratory data.

Medical History

As the patient walks into the operatory and seats himself in the chair, the patient's stature, gait, vigor and general health can be noted. While the history is being recorded, the dentist may gain an impression of the patient's emotional attitude, alertness and intelligence. The complaints of local oral problems such as "bleeding gums," "bad taste," "itchy gums" may be also accompanied by systemic complaints of "tiredness," "no appetite," "upset stomach," "losing weight rapidly," and so forth.

Some symptoms that suggest nutritional problems are apathy, photophobia, visual disturbances at night, sore lips, sore tongue and ulcerated angles of the mouth, digestive disturbances, diarrhea, dyspnea, edema, paresthesia. These symptoms, of course, may occur in many other pathologic conditions that are not even concerned with nutritional deficiencies.

In all patients who are going to require periodontal treatment, a brief medical history is usually elicited. Some typical questions might be "Are you under a physician's care for any chronic illness? If so, for how long, and what type of therapy are you receiving?" Chronic illnesses such as gastrointestinal disease, liver disease and alcoholism are all secondary nutritional conditioning factors which can interfere with complete utilization of nutrients.

A brief family history should also be taken to determine the health of parents and siblings as well as the occurrence in present or former generations of diabetes, digestive or hematopoietic diseases (Table 20, p. 326).

Diet History

The next step is to acquire information about the patient's daily diet. This includes not only the kinds but also the amounts of food eaten. Of particular interest in the patient with periodontal disease is the consistency and detergency of the diet. By consistency we mean the degree of density or firmness, which indicates its stimulatory effect. Detergency is the ability of a food to clear itself from the mouth and also to cleanse the teeth. Detergent foods are usually fibrous and, therefore, are of firm consistency, but not all firm foods are detergent. This differentiation should be kept clearly in mind when we make an evaluation of the patient's diet.

A. Twenty-four Hour Food Diary and Cursory Evaluation. There are several methods of obtaining a dietary history. The simplest procedure is to ask the patient to recall his food intake at meals and between meals of the previous 24 hours. Next, find out whether or not these were the foods and types of meals that have been usually eaten. How long has this type of diet been going on? Are there particular environmental circumstances that have dictated the selection of these foods? The following example shows the correct and incorrect method of recording the diet.

Incorrect	*Correct*
a sandwich some milk and a piece of fruit	1 sandwich consisting of a slice of ham and lettuce, tomato, and mayonnaise, on 2 slices of white enriched bread 1 cup of milk 1 raw apple

If an immediate evaluation is necessary, as in the case of acute necrotizing gingivitis, the day's intake can be evaluated as to adequacy in terms of the 4 Food Groups. Foods from each of these food groups should be present in each meal. For example, a day's intake consisting of coffee and doughnuts for breakfast, a hamburg sandwich and cola drink for lunch, and spaghetti, pie and coffee for supper can readily be evaluated as being adequate only in the bread-cereal group but deficient in the meat, milk and vegetable-fruit groups.

B. Keeping a 5 Day Food Diary. A better method for obtaining dietary information is to provide the patient with a food diary form which has sufficient space to record each meal and between-meal snack for 5 days (Table 21, p. 332). One of the five should be a week-end day or holiday to obtain a representative dietary pattern. It is important to emphasize to patients that they should not conceal any information nor should they try to anticipate what the dentist may deem desirable and effect changes in their dietary intake during the period of diary keeping.

C. Evaluating Total Food Intake. The evaluation of the 5 day food diary consists of using the simple quantitative and qualitative standards known as "Food for Fitness—A Daily Food Guide," which consists of 4 Food Groups. If there is a particular indication or desire for details about nutrient intake, tables of food compositions can be used.[1] However, in the majority of cases the dentist will find the simple qualitative procedure adequate.

TABLE 33. TOTAL FOOD INTAKE CHART WITH SPECIAL CONSIDERATION TO THE PHYSICAL FORM OF THE FOOD

FOOD GROUPS	PHYSICAL FORM	1st Day	2nd Day	3rd Day	4th Day	5th Day	Average per Day	Recommended Intake	Diff.
MILK	Liquid, Soft	/	//		/	//	1½	2 Serv.	−½
	Hard		/		/				
MEAT	Soft, Chopped	/				/	2	2+ Serv.	0
	Solid		//	//	//	/			
VEGETABLE—FRUIT	Juice, processed			/		//	1+	4+ Serv.	−3
	Raw, Firm, Partly Cooked		/		//				
BREAD-CEREAL	Soft, Cooked	𝍸	𝍸	//	///	𝍸 //	5	4+ Serv.	+1
	Dry, Crusty Toasted		//		//				

A total food intake chart such as shown in Table 33 may be used, in which foods are grouped into the four classes: (1) milk group (milk, cheese), which provides protein, calcium, riboflavin, vitamin A and other nutrients; (2) meat group (meat, fish, poultry, eggs, dried beans and peas, and nuts), which provides primarily protein, B vitamins and iron; (3) vegetable-fruit group (dark-green and deep-yellow vegetables and potatoes), which provides most of the vitamins A and C, as well as other minerals and vitamins; and

(4) bread-cereal group (whole grain, enriched or restored bread, cereals and flour products), which furnishes B vitamins, iron, protein and food energy. Foods which contain only calories and very few other nutrients, such as fats, oils, sugars and unenriched cereal foods, are not emphasized in this daily food guide.

The procedure of evaluating the diet is to credit in the appropriate column with a chit mark each serving of food eaten. As a guide to what constitutes a single serving of a particular food and in which of the 4 Food Groups the food is classified, consult Appendix III. Mixed dishes are also found in this table. For example, a meal consisting of a serving of macaroni and cheese, a slice of bread and butter, 1 glass of milk and a few carrot strips would be tallied as follows: Macaroni and cheese is classified as 1 serving of bread-cereal group and ½ serving of milk group. Therefore, a single chit mark goes in the bread-cereal group and ½ credit in the milk. One slice of bread, one cup of milk and carrot strips are classified as single chit marks in the bread-cereal group, milk group and vegetable-fruit group.

FOOD GROUP	1st DAY
MILK	1½
MEAT	
VEGETABLE-FRUIT	1
BREAD-CEREAL	11

When all the transposing of the individual foods is completed, the total number of servings for each group is added and divided by 5 to arrive at an average which is recorded in the average per day column. This daily average is subtracted from the recommended amounts and the difference is recorded in the difference column in terms of servings.

If a person does not meet the recommended amounts of the standard, it does not necessarily mean that a nutritional deficiency exists. It merely suggests that the patient is consuming less than the amounts of nutrients which are considered desirable for maintaining good nutrition in healthy persons in the United States. These amounts represent goals to be strived for rather than requirements. By maintaining these standards the person is assured of not having a nutritional deficiency so long as there are no secondary conditioning factors to interfere with the utilization of the food.

D. Evaluating the Physical Form of the Diet. Each of the 4 Food Groups can be subdivided into two basic physical forms from a periodontal standpoint, the stimulatory and the nonstimulatory. The nonstimulatory types of foods would be the liquids, soft, chopped, processed and well cooked, whereas the stimulatory types would be the hard, solid, raw, slightly cooked and dry. A consideration of the different physical forms of the foods is given in the evaluation chart. As the foods from the dietary are being credited onto the evaluation chart, the marks should be inserted in the proper subdivision. For example, if the patient ate cream cheese this chit mark should be next to the "Liquid, Soft" subdivision of the milk group; on the other hand, if the patient ate American processed or Swiss cheese, the chit mark would be in the "Hard" subdivision of the milk group. In the other food groups whole portions of fish or chicken, meats that are baked, broiled or fried are considered hard; vegetables that are slightly cooked, like broccoli, carrots, and green beans, as well as potato skins, may be considered of firm consistency; crusty and toasted breads as well as dry cereals are also considered firm enough to produce some stimulatory effect on the periodontium.

If emphasis on lack of firm consistency is desired, this can be achieved by circling in red the chit marks in the subdivisions, "Liquid," "Soft," "Chopped," "Processed" and "Cooked."

The detergency or oral clearance of the diet is favorable if the dessert is a raw fruit like apples, apricots, cherries, grapefruit, grapes, melons, oranges, pears, peaches, pineapple and tangerines or a raw vegetable like carrots, cauliflower, celery, cucumber, peppers, radishes or combinations of these. If fluids like coffee, tea, milk, fruit and vegetable juices are used as a dessert alone, this is also favorable from an oral clearance standpoint. However, the combination of a bread-cereal group food with a fluid is undesirable because it will leave food debris. The favorable detergent foods may be circled in blue on the patient's diary.

E. Evaluating Food Habits. Other factors that need to be considered in a dietary history are environmental conditions that influence food selection and food habits. Food selection is influenced by such factors as restrictions for medical reasons, economic conditions, and cultural and religious beliefs. Some typical questions that may help elicit information about food selection are as follows: Are you eating a special type of prescribed diet which restricts certain foods? Is your diet restricted by any cultural or religious beliefs? How often do you eat in restaurants? Do you carry lunches from home? Do you have to prepare your own meals or does someone else do it for you? What are your cooking facilities?

Food habits are concerned with attitudes the patient has towards food. Does he feel that mealtime is a pleasurable and relaxed period of the day, or is eating considered a necessary chore? Does he omit meals? Does he have time to eat breakfast? Does he eat his meals at regular times during the day?

Inspection

Physical examinations usually include inspection, auscultation and percussion. However, the dentist through inspection alone can observe the presence of gross physical signs that might lead him to suspect a nutritional inadequacy.

It is easy, for example, to see whether a patient is fat or thin. The general appearance of apathy and pallor can be noted. The hair may have a dry appearance. The facial skin may show fine, scaly, greasy desquamation in the nasolabial folds, around the ears, and at the canthi of the eyes. There may be an excess of blackheads or whiteheads. The general skin may be dry and scaly, pebbled and pigmented or purpuric with petechiae. The palms of the hands may be excessively red and the nails may be brittle, ridged or spoon-shaped. The eyes may have circumcorneal injection or conjunctival injection. The lips may have a cheilosis accompanied by ulcerations at the angles of the mouth. The tongue may show papillary atrophy or hypertrophy and variations in color from pale pink to scarlet red to a magenta hue. The gingiva may show marginal redness and swelling. Numerous other physical signs which may be associated with malnutrition have been described in Chapter XIII.

Laboratory Aids[14]

A few laboratory tests have been found useful in determining the nutritional status of population groups; however, they are not always applicable to the individual. Table 34 shows some of the laboratory tests that a dentist might be interested in having performed for a patient with a periodontal condition that cannot be accounted for on the basis of local oral factors.

TABLE 34. LABORATORY TESTS AND NORMAL VALUES YIELDING INDIRECT EVIDENCE OF NUTRITIONAL STATUS

Nutritional Element	*Test*	*Normal Values*
Protein	Serum protein conc.	6–8 mg./ml.
	Serum albumin conc.	4–5 Gm./100 ml.
	Nitrogen balance	
Calcium	Serum Ca conc.	5.0 mg./liter
Vitamin D (infants)	Alkaline phosphatase	5–15 Bodansky units
	Serum phosphorus	2.5–3.6 in mEq./liter
Vitamin K	Prothrombin time	10–15 seconds
Iron	Mean corpuscular hemoglobin (from Hb. level, hematocrit and rbc)	32–34 per cent
Ascorbic Acid	Plasma ascorbic acid conc.	0.6–1.0 mg./100 ml.
	Ascorbic acid conc. in wbc-platelet layer.	20–30 mg./100 ml.

These four steps—medical history, dietary history and evaluation, general clinical inspection, and laboratory data—make up the necessary procedure for a nutritional diagnosis. From a practical standpoint, it will be found that laboratory procedures are seldom used, but the diet evaluation, medical history and clinical inspection are invariably considered.

DIET AND NUTRITION IN THE MANAGEMENT OF A PATIENT WITH PERIODONTAL DISEASE

If the nutritional diagnosis suggests that a medical condition exists which is interfering with food utilization, this is a systemic conditioning factor which the dentist need only suspect. His suspicions should be relayed to his medical colleague and the management of the systemic problem left to him.

However, if the nutritional diagnosis suggests that there is an inadequate food intake, then it is the dentist's responsibility to advise the patient how to acquire an adequate diet. In the sections to follow it will be shown how proper food has a beneficial local and systemic effect on the periodontium. It should be made clear that diet for periodontal health is not much different from that for general health, but emphasis is placed on food texture. Firm and detergent foods serve as adjuncts in carrying out proper oral physiotherapy, an indispensable factor for success in periodontal therapy.

Local Effects of Diet

There is some experimental evidence that firm foods will (1) promote periodontal health by their stimulating action, (2) decrease calculus formation, and (3) promote keratinization.

Foods of firm consistency require chewing and, therefore, keep the masticating apparatus in use. In all tissues, growth, development and maintenance depend on use. Disuse produces atrophy, degeneration and lowered resistance to infections. Chewing, by its mechanical action, produces a compression and expansion of the periodontal spaces around the teeth which, in turn, stimulates the removal of waste products through the venous system and lymphatics and the entry of nutrients to the periodontium via the arterial system.[23] Brekhus et al.[9] have shown that firm foods promote formation of a dense fibrous suspensory structure in the periodontal membrane by increasing circulation and fibroblastic activity. Coolidge[11] found that the width of the periodontal membrane was directly related to the intensity of masticating function. Gingival capillaries were increased in numbers, had a wider distribution, and were of better tone in experimental subjects who ate hard foods compared to those who ate soft foods, according to Pelzer[24] and Burwasser and Hill.[10]

The rate of calculus formation has been shown to be directly related to the detergency of the diet.[15,29] Foods that are fibrous rub against the teeth and actually mechanically cleanse them. They are, in a manner of speaking, a natural toothbrush. On the other hand, diets that are high in refined carbohydrates are usually retentive in nature and serve as a nidus for calculus formation. Furthermore, the fact that carbohydrate-rich diets do not provide adequate satiety leads to frequent snack eating, and this means that there will be an ever-present accumulation of food debris around the teeth. Choosing a better balanced diet and foods of firmer consistency will prevent food accumulation and slow down the rate of calculus formation.

The degree of keratinization of the stratified squamous epithelium which affords protection against trauma or other injurious agents is affected by the frictional qualities of the diet.[22,30] Nature reacts to mechanical irritation by increasing the thickness of the hornified layer of epithelium. Without this protection, chemical and bacterial irritants can make inroads into the gingival tissue and produce inflammation. This has been shown in an experiment[16] in which 4 out of 5 patients fed a diet of milk and honey for 30 days developed gingivitis. The importance of mechanical friction in preventing periodontal disease has also been shown in ferrets.[18] Three groups of ferrets were fed adequate diets of (1) bread and milk, (2) oatmeal and milk, and (3) raw meat with adequate vitamins and minerals. Despite the nutritional adequacy of the diet, in 8 to 12 weeks these animals developed periodontal disease. The periodontal disease in these ferrets was cured when they were provided short lengths of bone for gnawing and mastication.

Systemic Effects of Diet

The role of systemic effects of nutritional deficiencies on the periodontium has been ascertained from animal experiments and is well documented in other texts.[13] Its application to humans is, at present, merely theoretical and needs much further controlled investigation. Originally Boyle et al.[6,7] had suggested that diffuse alveolar atrophy was produced in animals by a vitamin C-deficient diet. However, Glickman[12] has shown that local irritants like food debris must be present to initiate gingival inflammation and that the vitamin C deficiency will then accentuate the destruction of the periodontal membrane and alveolar bone. Waerhaug[28] has also shown that vitamin C deficiency is a contributory rather than a causative factor in gingivitis and periodontitis.

A deficiency of protein also has an adverse systemic effect on the periodontium, producing its breakdown particularly in the presence of local irritants[26] and occlusal trauma.[20] Bradford[8] states that in tropical and subtropical areas where protein deficiency is endemic, periodontal destruction manifests itself in a youngster after the permanent teeth erupt and reaches an incurable state by the time he reaches maturity. More extensive investigations into the periodontal health of the inhabitants of these protein-deficient areas would be very illuminating.

Diets for the Patient with Chronic Periodontal Disease

The advice that the dentist should give the patient about diet consists of six points: (1) improve the quality and quantity of the total food intake so that the diet is an adequate one; (2) improve balance of meals; (3) choose a variety of foods for more interesting and better menu planning; (4) emphasize foods of firm consistency:

(5) stress detergent foods for desserts; and (6) include vitamin supplementation when indicated. This can be written out as a diet prescription such as Table 35.

TABLE 35

DIET PRESCRIPTION
FOR PATIENTS WITH PERIODONTAL DISEASE

I. Improve Total Daily Food Intake by:

Adding foods from the milk group.

II. Improve the Balance of the Meals as follows:

For Breakfast: Add more protein food

For Lunch: Add at least one more vegetable

For Dinner: Add some milk

III. This is a suggested Menu for you:

Breakfast:	Lunch:	Dinner:
Fried egg, bacon	Tuna fish salad, sandwich	Baked pork chops
Toast, butter	Wedge of lettuce	Baked potato
Coffee	Milk	Broccoli
		Tossed salad
Orange slices	Pineapple-strawberry fruit cup	Crusty bread, butter
		Milk
		Raw apple

IV. The following Foods of Firm Consistency should be emphasized in your Diet:

Broiled meats, raw fruits and vegetables

V. The following Detergent Foods should be used for Dessert and In-Between Meal Snacks:

Apples, pears, oranges and carrot strips

VI. The following Vitamin Supplement need be used only 2 Weeks:

Unicaps: Take one a day with water at the beginning of a meal.

1. To demonstrate to the patient which food groups have been deficient in his diet, show him the results of his diet evaluation. This is based on a comparison of the actual intake with the standard recommended amounts. Emphasis should be placed on those food groups which were shown to be deficient, and they should be increased to at least the recommended amounts. The two food groups most often found deficient are the milk group and vegetable-

fruit group. For example, if the patient is eating only one vegetable a day, say potatoes, then he should be advised that he ought to include at least one citrus fruit and one green or yellow vegetable as well as some other raw fruit or vegetable each day.

2. After the total intake is improved, foods from each of the 4 Food Groups should be advised for each of the three meals. This provides a balanced diet because all of the essential nutrients are provided at each meal. The areas of weakness in most meal planning are usually lack of a protein food for breakfast, the absence of a vegetable for lunch and inadequate sources of calcium for dinner in the evening. There may be some environmental factors, such as lack of facilities for preparing breakfast or lack of time, that must be taken into consideration when prescribing meals.

3. Menu planning is simply the interpretation of food groups into dishes and foods that are found in each of the food groups. To improve the patient's menus, suggest that a variety of different foods from the food groups be used. For example, if the vegetable for dinner one day is broccoli, the next day it could be corn and on the third day it could be cauliflower, and on the fourth day it could be carrots. Here again such environmental factors as cost must be taken into consideration. Menus can be made up that are high in nutritional value but low in cost.

4. The evaluation will show the general physical consistency of the diet, soft or hard. To improve it, one might suggest at least one food of firm consistency for each meal. Each of the food groups has firm as well as soft foods. For example, in the milk group there is hard cheese; in the meat group there are broiled steaks, chops and fried chicken on the bone; in the vegetable-fruit group, besides raw fruits and vegetables, corn on the cob and skins of baked potatoes can be suggested; in the bread group, crusty bread, melba toast and Ry-Krisp are excellent for providing a firm type of food.

5. From the diary the type of dessert will be noted as far as detergency is concerned. Substituting a raw fruit or vegetable for desserts like pie and coffee is usually all that is necessary. The following detergent fruits can be suggested: apples, apricots, cherries, grapefruit, grapes, melons, oranges, pears, peaches, pineapple and tangerines. Raw vegetables like carrots, cauliflower, celery, cucumbers, tossed salads and cole slaw should be used liberally, during the latter part of the meal if possible. Another suggestion might be the use of carrot strips or celery between meals.

Sample menus which may be used as a guide are shown in

TABLE 36. SUGGESTED MENUS FOR PATIENTS OF DIFFERENT NATIONALITIES WITH CHRONIC PERIODONTAL DISEASE

	Italian Patient	*Hebrew Patient*
Breakfast		
	Egg, soft boiled	Cottage cheese
	Italian bread	Bagel
	Coffee	Coffee
	Orange	Orange
Lunch		
	Lasagne, cheese	Salmon salad
	Salad greens	Pumpernickel bread
	Crusty bread, cheese	Carrot, celery curls
	Peach	Peach with sour cream
	Milk	Milk
Dinner		
	Antipasto, with cheese	Broiled chicken
	Scallopini	Broccoli
	Italian bread	Baked potato
	Watermelon	Tomato-cucumber salad
	Tea or coffee	Crusty bread
		Watermelon
		Tea or coffee

Tables 35 and 36. In these menus emphasis has been placed on the use of at least one food of firm consistency at each meal and a detergent fruit or vegetable at the end of the meal. Table 36 has suggested menus for patients of two nationalities, Italian and Hebrew.

6. Vitamin supplementation is rarely needed for the average adult if he is eating an adequate diet, because the government requires the enrichment and fortification of staple foods with B complex vitamins, calcium and iron. However, individuals who choose their menu according to the cost column rather than the food column may need supplemental vitamins. Patients whose food habits are bizarre or restricted due to a systemic condition (e.g., allergy, gastrointestinal disease) and have eaten an unbalanced diet over a prolonged period of time are also considered proper candidates for vitamin supplementation.[4] In other words, vitamin supplementation is not to treat the periodontal condition but rather to prevent the continuation of a nutritional deficiency which may interfere with restoring periodontal health.

The type of multivitamin preparation to advise depends on the circumstances. If the patient has been restricted from eating fats, a period of inadequate intake of fat soluble A and D vitamins is quite possible. Under these circumstances, prescribing the latter two vitamins would be in order. If there is inability to eat fruits and vegetables, then a combination of water-soluble vitamins B complex and C might be useful. If there has been a low intake in all food groups, it is quite possible that a combination of A, D, ascorbic acid, thiamine, riboflavin and niacin, with or without pyridoxine or calcium pantothenate, may be useful. Whichever vitamin preparation is prescribed, it should be done on a rational basis.

These preparations should contain one to one and a half times the Recommended Dietary Allowance. The Recommended Dietary Allowance[3] for each of these vitamins for adults is:

Vitamin A	5,000 units	Niacin	21 mg. equiv.
Vitamin D	400 units	Pyridoxine	1 mg.
Thiamine	1.6 mg.	Ascorbic acid	75 mg.
Riboflavin	1.8 mg.	Pantothenic acid	5 mg.

Many drug houses market multivitamin preparations under their own brand name. A list of these is given in Appendix IV and may be used as a reference when writing prescriptions. One capsule a day with meals usually meets the needs of the average patient. When the concomitant problem (lack of appetite, inability to chew, unusual food habits or limited food selection) is overcome, then these supplements may be discontinued.

Diets for the Patient with Acute Gingivitis or Acute Necrotizing Gingivitis

Acute gingivitis differs from chronic gingivitis in its intensity, velocity and duration. The signs and symptoms are more severe; the onset is usually sudden; and with proper treatment it is of short duration. In most instances, through the institution of proper local therapy, these acute symptoms subside. However, supportive nutritional therapy may be a necessary adjunct because of the patient's lack of appetite or previous unbalanced diet, as well as because of the possible etiotropic therapy of a nutritional supplement.

An evaluation of the 24 hour dietary intake as well as customary food habits will reveal the food groups that are lacking in terms of the standard diet based upon the 4 Food Groups. The foods that are most often lacking are protein foods and a source of vitamin C.

The advice that is given the patient about diets is as follows:

1. In view of the fact that your appetite is poor, eat only one or two foods at each meal. But eat 6 or 8 times a day, if possible, to meet caloric needs.

2. Emphasize protein foods from the milk and meat group. They

are milk, cottage cheese, ice cream, eggs, tuna fish, salmon, boiled chicken, chopped meat.

3. Pay particular attention to ingesting more than usual amounts of vitamin C-rich foods. If they cannot be eaten in their whole form they should be used as juices. In addition to fruits like orange, grapefruit and strawberries, cantaloupes, guava, mango, papaya, vegetables like cooked turnip greens, green peppers, tomato juice and baked potato can be used.

4. Plan your menu so that the general consistency of the diet is liquid and soft without spices or sharp-tasting foods during the acute period. The type of foods that are recommended should suit your individual tastes and economic status.

A typical menu might be:

Breakfast	*10 A.M.*	*Lunch*
1 cup of milk	1 glass of orange juice	1 slice of bread and butter
1 slice of bread and margarine or butter		Cottage cheese and peaches
		1 cup of milk

Supper	*Bedtime*
Cooked vegetable plate	Eggnog
Ice cream	

5. Use a multivitamin capsule that I am prescribing once a day prior to your breakfast meal.

There are some suggestions from laboratory and clinical studies that a niacin deficiency[17] may be a contributing causative factor in acute necrotizing gingivitis and ascorbic acid deficiency[19] in acute gingivitis. On the basis of this, as well as the fact that chewing raw fruits and vegetables rich in vitamins B complex and C is impossible because of the oral pain associated with this acute condition,[21] supportive vitamin therapy may be indicated for a few days or at most a week or two.

Most deficiency states involve multiple factors; therefore, the type of vitamin preparation to supply is a multivitamin one. Since fat-soluble vitamins A and D are usually stored well and are not readily depleted, it is not necessary to include these in the vitamin preparations.

The multivitamin preparation which is most often applicable is a combination of the B complex and C. The B complex vitamins are usually thiamine, riboflavin and niacin, with or without pyridoxine and calcium pantothenate. The therapeutically effective dosage that is recommended is 3 to 5 times[4] the Recommended Dietary Allowance. If the dentist will remember that the recommended allowance for riboflavin or thiamine under normal circumstance is about 2 mg., any multivitamin preparation can be considered a therapeutic one if it contains 6 to 10 mg. of each of these vitamins. The proper dosage of the other vitamins will be automatically included by the drug company. Different brand names of these vitamin preparations of therapeutic dosage are given in Appendix IV.

As soon as adequate amounts of foods from the 4 Food Groups can be ingested, vitamin supplementation can be suspended. In fact, the type of diet suggested as an adjunct in the management of chronic periodontitis should be adopted as soon as feasible.

Diets for Patients Who Undergo Gingivectomy

For the comfort of the patient and as an aid in promoting wound healing after gingivectomy, the proper diet should be prescribed. The dietary principles and specific high protein and high vitamin C diets suggested prior to and after oral surgery are equally applicable to patients who undergo gingivectomy. See Chapter XIX on diets for oral surgery patients.

REFERENCES

1. Anon: Composition of Foods—Raw, Processed, Prepared. Handbook No. 8. Washington, U. S. Department of Agriculture, 1950.
2. Anon: Food for Fitness—A Daily Food Guide. Leaflet No. 424. Washington, U. S. Department of Agriculture, 1958.
3. Anon: Recommended Dietary Allowances. Washington, National Academy of Sciences—National Research Council, 1958.
4. Anon: Vitamin preparations as dietary supplements and as therapeutic agents. Council on Foods and Nutrition, Am. Med. Assoc. J.A.M.A., *169:*41, 1959.
5. Becks, H., Wainwright, W. W., and Morgan, A. F.: Comparative study of oral changes in dogs due to deficiencies of pantothenic acid, nicotinic acid and vitamin B complex. Am. J. Orthodont. and Oral Surg., *29:*183, 1943.
6. Boyle, P. E., Bessey, O. A., and Wolbach, S. B.: Experimental alveolar bone atrophy produced by ascorbic acid deficiency and its relation to pyorrhea alveolaris. Proc. Soc. Exper. Biol. & Med., *36:*773, 1937.
7. Boyle, P. E., Bessey, O. A., and Wolbach, S. B.: Experimental production of diffuse alveolar bone atrophy type of periodontal disease by diets deficient in ascorbic acid (Vitamin C). J.A.D.A., *24:*1768, 1937.
8. Bradford, E. W.: Food and the periodontal diseases. Proceedings of the Nutrition Society, *18:*75, 1959.
9. Brekhus, P. J., Armstrong, W. D., and Simon, W. J.: Stimulation of muscles of mastication. J. D. Res., *20:*87, 1941.

10. Burwasser, P., and Hill, T. J.: The effect of hard and soft diets on the gingival tissues of dogs. J. D. Res., *18:*398, 1939.
11. Coolidge, E. D.: The thickness of the human periodontal membrane. J.A.D.A., *24:*1260, 1937.
12. Glickman, I.: Acute vitamin C deficiency and periodontal disease. I. The periodontal tissues of the guinea pig in acute vitamin C deficiency. J. D. Res., *27:*9, 1948.
13. Glickman, I.: Clinical Periodontology, 2nd ed. Philadelphia, W. B. Saunders Co., 1958.
14. Goldsmith, G. A.: Nutritional Diagnosis. Springfield, Ill. Charles C Thomas, 1959.
15. Haber, G. G.: The effect of the difference in the quality of bread upon nutrition and the development of dental caries and tartar in Germany and Switzerland. British D. J., *68:*142, 1940.
16. Haydak, M. H., Vivino, A. E., Bohfner, J. J., and Palmer, L. S.: A clinical and biochemical study of cow's milk and honey as an essentially exclusive diet of adult humans. A.J.M. Science, *207:*219, 1944.
17. King, J. D.: Nutritional and other factors in trench mouth with special reference to the nicotinic acid component of the vitamin B complex. Brit. D. J., *74:*113, 1943.
18. King, J. D., and Glover, N. E.: The relative effects of dietary constituents and other factors upon calculus formation and gingival disease in the ferret. J. Path. and Bact., *57:*353, 1945.
19. Linghorne, W. J., McIntosh, W. G., Tice, J. W., Tisdall, F. F., McCreary, J. F., Drake, T. G. H., Greaves, A. V., and Johnstone, W. M.: Relation of ascorbic acid intake to gingivitis. J. Canad. D. A., *12:*49, 1946.
20. Miller, S. C., Stahl, S. S., and Goldsmith, E. D.: The effects of vertical occlusal trauma on the periodontium of protein deprived young adult rats. J. Periodont., *28:*87, 1957.
21. Nizel, A. E.: Therapeutic nutrition for the periodontal patient. J. Periodont. *20:*203, 1955.
22. Orban, B.: Hornification of the gums. J.A.D.A., *17:*1977, 1930.
23. O'Rourke, J. T.: The relation of the physical character of the diet to the health of the periodontal tissues. A. J. Orth. and Oral Surg., *33:*687, 1947.
24. Pelzer, R.: A study of the local oral effects of diet on the periodontal tissues and the gingival capillary structure. J.A.D.A., *27:*13, 1940.
25. Prinz, H.: The origin of salivary calculus. Dent. Cosmos., *63:*231, 369, 503, 619, 1921.
26. Stahl, S. S., Sandler, H. C., and Cahn, L.: The effects of protein deprivation upon oral tissues of the rat and particularly upon the periodontal structures under irritation. Oral Surg., Oral Med., and Oral Path., *8:* 760, 1955.
27. Stanley, H. R., Jr.: The cyclic phenomenon of periodontitis. Oral Surg., Oral Med., and Oral Path., *8:*598, 1955.
28. Waerhaug, J.: Effect of C avitaminosis on the supporting structure of the teeth. J. of Perio., *29:*87, 1958.
29. Wallace, J.: The newer knowledge of hygiene in diet. J.A.D.A., *18:*1322, 1931.
30. Weinmann, J.: Keratinization of the human oral mucosa. J. D. Res., *19:* 57, 1940.

Chapter XVIII

Nutrition for the Patient with Full Upper and Lower Denture with Special Consideration to the New Denture Wearer

Earlier in this book, it was stated that one of the environmental factors that may condition a nutritional deficiency is the inability to chew properly due to broken or decayed teeth or ill-fittting dentures. That there is a correlation of proper mastication to proper digestion is undeniable.

The chief organ of digestion is the small intestine, which can be spared excessive strain if the food is properly prepared in the mouth by normal mastication. Masticating function is normal if "it is in harmony with proper food choices, the requirements of adequate nutrition, and the coordinated mechanical and chemical function of the alimentary tract."[4]

Chewing food well accomplishes several things. It makes available to the gastrointestinal tract for digestion nutrients that are encased in cellulose coverings, such as corn, beans, peas, raw fruits and raw vegetables. Through normal mastication the food is broken up into smaller particles so that there is greater surface area for the chemical action of salivary and gastric secretions. Chewing also stimulates a reflex action in the stomach and starts the flow of gastric juices which aid in digestion.

The cause of chronic gastritis is not precisely clear, but the dietary treatment usually advocates thorough mastication of food to make digestion as easy as possible. Therefore, for the patient with gastritis who wears dentures, consideration must be given to food texture.

One of the factors which may contribute to the development of peptic ulcer is the vigorous muscular action required of the stomach when it receives poorly masticated food. This again emphasizes why careful instruction about types of food to eat is important for the denture patient.

However, the evidence is not completely significant that masticatory insufficiency actually produces nutritive failure. There is an investigation by Greene et al.[1] in which the conclusion is drawn that "an intimate relationship exists between impaired masticating function (masticating insufficiency) and general nutritive failure." Alimentary tract disturbances of one nature or another were found in 84.7 per cent of the patients with masticating insufficiency compared to 73.3 per cent of the patients with well functioning dentures. The 11.4 per cent difference between the groups does not appear to be very large; at most, it shows a trend. From this it is evident that, with or without proper dentures, alimentary tract problems may arise. Nevertheless, one contribution that the dentist can make toward helping his denture patient minimize the possibility of future gastrointestinal disturbances is to recommend a diet that is not only nutritionally adequate but also in a physical form that the denture wearer is going to be able to manage.

The denture wearer may only be one-fourth as efficient in chewing food as persons who possess natural teeth, but it has been shown[2] that the ordinary modern American diet requires no more than 25 lbs. of biting force. This is an amount of force the average denture wearer can exert. However, the denture wearer will choose foods that require minimal incising and grinding forces and merely require swallowing. Therefore, he will eat more of the soft foods and less of such foods as sandwiches, raw vegetables and salads.

Patients appreciate specific advice on selection of foods and menus when new full dentures are delivered to them. In order to develop a rationale for recommending one food above others, a brief review of the processes of mastication and deglutition should be made. Actually, the new denture wearer must learn to coordinate his prosthesis with the movements of the mandible and associated structures. The discussion which follows will show why biting and chewing (mastication) are more difficult than swallowing (deglutition).

PROCESSES OF MASTICATION AND DEGLUTITION

Mastication[3]

Food is grasped (prehension) and torn or bitten (division), then chewed (mastication). The structures that are involved in the process of mastication are the temporomandibular joint, the primary muscles of mastication (masseter, temporal, internal pterygoid and external pterygoid), the secondary muscles of mastication (anterior belly of the digastric, stylohyoid, mylohyoid, and geniohyoid), the tongue, the palate, the cheeks, the lips and the teeth.

There are two fundamental movements of the mandible, a hinge action and a sliding action. These hinge and sliding actions work to open and close the jaw, to protrude and retrude the mandible, and to move the jaw in left and right lateral positions. By the contractions of the external pterygoid and suprahyoid muscles, the mouth is opened; and by the contraction of the masseter muscle, the mouth is closed. Lateral movements are produced by the alternate movements of the left and right external pterygoids. Protrusion is produced by the contraction of both external pterygoids together. Retrusion is the result of the combined action of the temporal and the hyoid group of muscles.

By the various voluntary movements of these muscles the food is pulverized between the teeth of the upper and lower jaw. From this pulverized mass a bolus is formed by the action of the tongue against the teeth. This bolus is moistened by saliva and placed on the dorsum of the tongue and is ready to be swallowed.

Deglutition

Deglutition takes place in three stages of which only the first is voluntary. The tongue with the bolus of food on it, by the action of the mylohyoid, the hypoglossal, the glossopalatine and the styloglossus muscles, is drawn backward and upward toward the hard palate and the pharyngeal fauces. Actually, the tip of the tongue is elevated toward the hard palate and the posterior portion is depressed, allowing for the collection of the food on the portion of the tongue that has become concave by the depression of the dorsum. By the pressure of the tongue against the teeth and palate the tongue curves backward and propels the bolus of food through the isthmus of the fauces into the pharynx. The second stage is an involuntary rapid reflex action in which the food is passed through the pharynx into the esophagus. In the third stage of deglutition the food passes from the esophagus into the stomach by a combination of peristaltic movements and gravity.

This brief discussion shows that mastication and deglutition of solid food are not simple muscular actions but rather a coordination of many muscles and anatomic structures. Other factors involved in chewing are the ability of the alveolar mucosa under the dentures to withstand pressures, the interocclusal relationship of the teeth, whether the teeth are porcelain or acrylic and the nature of the occlusal pattern. As complex as chewing solid foods may appear, biting into a food is even more complex. The ingesting action that is least complicated is the swallowing of liquids. There are no mechanical pressures necessary, thus sore spots from this source are minimized; there is no need of coordinating the many muscles of mastication. Therefore, although the sequence of eating food is first biting, then chewing and, finally, swallowing, it is much easier to learn these eating procedures in the opposite order; namely, swallowing, chewing and biting. Logically, then, foods of the proper consistency must be chosen so that these functions can be learned in this order.

DIET FOR THE FIRST DAY WITH NEW DENTURES

The patient with new dentures, for the first day, should select liquid foods which naturally require only swallowing. In a few cases it may be necessary to sacrifice nutritional adequacy for a day or two, but this should cause no concern in an otherwise well-nourished patient. However, if the liquid diet is continued over a long period of time, it can cause upsets owing to a lack of bulk, inadequacy and monotony. Comprehension by the patient of the meaning of a nutritionally adequate diet will help him in planning his food intake, regardless of the food consistency of the diet. If we plan such a diet from the 4 Food Groups, he can select foods from each food group which are essentially liquid. For example, he might use the following:

Milk group. Fluid milk may be taken in any form.

Meat group. For the first day or so eggs will be the food of choice in the meat group. They may be taken in eggnogs. Puréed meats (such as baby food meats) may be mixed with thin white sauce and used as a soup.

Vegetable-fruit group. These may be used as juices.

Bread-cereal group. For the first day or so thin gruels cooked in either milk or water may be used.

A Suggested Menu Using a Liquid Diet

Breakfast
Orange juice
Strained oatmeal gruel with milk or cream
Coffee—cream and sugar, if desired

10 A.M.
Eggnog

Lunch
Cream of tomato soup
Junket
Tea or coffee

3 P.M.
Ginger ale with ice cream

Dinner
Strained cream of chicken soup
Vanilla ice cream and orange sherbet
Tea or coffee

Bedtime
Cocoa or other milk drink

DIET FOR THE SECOND AND THIRD DAY

If no difficulty is encountered with the liquid diet, the next day the patient may use soft foods which require a minimum of chewing. This would mean he might add the following foods from each of the 4 Food Groups:

Milk group. Fluid milk as in the liquid diet.

Meat group. Tender meat, chicken or fish, such as finely chopped beef, ground liver, tender chicken or fish in a cream sauce. Eggs may be scrambled, or soft cooked. Dried peas may be used in a strained thick soup.

Vegetable-fruit group. In addition to fruit and vegetable juices, tender cooked fruits and vegetables may be used (skins and seeds must be removed). Vegetables such as the following may be chosen from this group: tender asparagus tips, cooked carrots, tender green beans, baked potato (no skins), chopped spinach or other greens, winter squash. The following fruits may be used, cooked or canned (no skins): applesauce, peaches, pears, apricots.

Bread-cereal group. Cooked cereals, such as Cream of Wheat or Wheatena, milk toast and softened bread may be used. Boiled rice, spaghetti, macaroni or noodles may also be used.

A Suggested Menu Using a Soft Diet

Breakfast
- Orange juice
- Scrambled eggs
- Oatmeal with milk or cream
- Buttered toast without crusts
- Coffee—cream and sugar, if desired

Lunch
- Cream of tomato soup
- Spinach soufflé with cheese sauce
- Bread (no crusts), butter
- Gelatin with whipped cream
- Tea or coffee

Dinner
- Ground beef patty
- Buttered noodles
- Diced carrots
- Bread, butter
- Milk
- Vanilla ice cream
- Tea or coffee

DIET FOR THE FOURTH AND SUBSEQUENT DAYS

By the fourth day, or as soon as all sore spots have healed, firm foods which do not require "biting into" may be added. Again referring to the 4 Food Groups, the following foods may be taken in addition to those mentioned under the soft diet. In most instances these foods should be cut into small pieces before being put into the mouth.

Milk group. Add cheddar-type cheeses as well as fluid milk and cottage cheese.

Meat group. Steak, chops, roasts, fish, eggs in all forms and cooked legumes may be eaten.

Vegetable-fruit group. All cooked and raw fruits except those which require biting into, such as apples and corn on the cob.

Bread-cereal groups. All except those with hard crust which require biting into, such as sandwiches, crusty bread and hard rolls.

A Suggested Menu Using a Firm or Regular Diet

Breakfast
- Orange slices or orange juice
- Oatmeal, cream or milk
- Toast, butter
- Coffee—cream and sugar, if desired

Lunch
- Cream of celery soup
- Crackers
- Welsh rarebit
- Lettuce salad, French dressing
- Soft rolls, butter
- Fruit gelatin
- Tea or coffee

Dinner
- Roast beef
- Mashed potatoes
- Buttered peas
- Tomato, lettuce salad
- Bread, butter
- Milk
- Vanilla ice cream with fresh peaches
- Tea or coffee

DIET AFTER SEVERAL WEEKS

After several weeks, solid foods which require biting may be allowed in addition to the foods in the diet plan just mentioned. However, the ability to manage foods such as sandwiches made with bread with hard crusts, raw apples, corn on the cob and raw celery is an individual variable. Theoretically, if all the mechanical, biological and psychological obstacles involved in denture wearing are overcome, the patient with full dentures should be able to manage foods of all textures, even those requiring prehension and division.

FOOD HABITS OF THE GERIATRIC PATIENT

Faulty eating habits are prevalent in older people, who make up the majority of the full denture patients. There are also the problems of ignorance of the principles of good nutrition, food fads, likes and dislikes carried over from younger days, limited food budgets and apathetic attitudes about food in general.

We should understand that changes take place in hunger, thirst and taste in older people. They develop an intolerance for certain foods because their digestive system becomes weakened. In general, they have poor appetite and tend to skip meals.

The calorie needs, according to the Recommended Dietary Allowances, decrease about 20 per cent between ages 25 and 65. This is due, no doubt, to the fact that as a person grows older his activity is lessened and his metabolic rate is lowered. This all adds up to the fact that he requires less energy-rich food than previously but his need for other nutrients is not reduced. His needs for protein, minerals and vitamins are as great as when he was younger. In other words, his diet needs to be decreased in quantity but not in quality. (See also Chap. XII, especially p. 269.)

Adequate water and soft bulk intake are vital both to promote proper urinary excretion and to avoid constipation. A total of about 2 quarts of liquids is recommended. For older people, drinking water in small amounts at frequent intervals is advised.

The inclusion of adequate amounts of protein foods may need special attention in discussing diets with older patients, especially those with dentures. Not only is meat the single most expensive food, but it requires more chewing. Chopped meat is as nutritious as steak but it is less expensive and easier to eat. Milk, another excellent source of protein, may be highly recommended for older people. If they are not willing to drink it, they may be encouraged to use it on cereals and in soups and puddings. An adequate intake of milk and/or cheese will help to protect the bones of older people against osteoporosis, as milk provides calcium as well as protein.

Another nutrient which has been found to be low in the diets of older people is ascorbic acid. Since ascorbic acid is found mainly in fresh fruits and vegetables, some planning is needed to include a rich source of vitamin C daily. Many canned juices are now being fortified with additional amounts of vitamin C. An older person may prefer tomato juice with his dinner to orange juice at breakfast. A discussion of the sources of this vitamin, which is necessary to the maintenance of intercellular tissues, may be very beneficial to the patient and his health.

In planning meals for the older person, it may be advisable to divide the total daily intake into five or six eating periods. Using smaller portions and providing snacks of milk or milk drinks, fruit and vegetable juice, and a cracker or two may be more acceptable. In general, diets should be individualized to suit the taste, habits, income and atrophic digestive apparatus of the older patient.

We as dentists can improve the patient's impaired mastication not only by proper mechanical denture construction but by prescribing balanced diets of the essential 4 Food Groups. The physical nature of the diet should be consistent with the patient's experience and ability to swallow, chew and bite with his artificial dentures.

REFERENCES

1. Greene, H. I., Dreizen, S., and Spies, T. D.: A clinical survey of the incidence of impaired masticatory function in patients of a nutrition clinic. J.A.D.A., *39*:561, 1949.
2. Howell, A. H., and Brudevold, F.: Vertical forces used during chewing of food. J. D. Res. *29*:133, 1950.
3. Langley, L., and Cheraskin, E.: Physiological Foundation of Dental Practice. 2nd ed. St. Louis, The C. V. Mosby Co., 1956.
4. O'Rourke, J. T.: Oral Physiology. St. Louis, The C. V. Mosby Co., 1951.

Chapter XIX

Diet in Oral Surgery

Nutritional deficiencies are not etiologic factors in producing the type of pathology which requires oral surgical treatment. Therefore, diet is often overlooked in the over-all management of the oral surgery patient. The dentist should look upon the diet as an adjuvant similar to analgesics and antibiotics which is a means of making the patient more comfortable and of speeding recovery. Some of the prime functions of adequate nutrition in oral surgery are: (1) to speed convalescence, (2) to promote wound healing, and (3) to increase the patient's resistance to infection.

BASIC CONCEPTS

Animal experiments[8] have shown that the principal nutrients that are involved in wound healing are protein, vitamin C, riboflavin and vitamin A. If these nutrients are present in the tissues in adequate amounts, the lag period for the wound to be restored to maximal strength is shortened. As yet there is no clear-cut evidence that the same nutritional factors that are important to wound healing in animals apply to man.[4,5] However, so much nutritional knowledge which has been developed from animal experimentation has been found applicable to man, it seems reasonable to assume that a positive relationship does exist between adequate nutrition and better wound healing.

Increased susceptibility to infection and decreased resistance to established disease may be brought on, in part, by undernutrition[2] since during a period of undernutrition there is decreased ability to manufacture antibodies.[9] Furthermore, malnourished bone marrow has a decreased capacity to form leucocytes.[1] It has been shown, for example, that protein-deficient animals are more susceptible to infection.[7]

These basic concepts of the role of diet and nutrition in wound healing and combatting infection are only a few of the reasons for the dentist to advise his patient on diet. Other reasons are: (1) inability to chew the usual foods before extractions due to broken down dentition or swelling; (2) inability to chew foods of firm consistency immediately after surgery because of painful and tender tissues; (3) the stress of increased temperature and infection in cellulitis or osteomyelitis which increases tissue requirements for nutrients, and (4) blood loss and excess excretion of nitrogen during extensive oral surgical procedures which, as in general surgery, may produce a negative nitrogen balance.

DIET PRIOR TO ORAL SURGERY

To assure an adequate tissue nutrient reserve, the dentist should evaluate the patient's nutritional status before surgery and particular attention should be paid to the adequacy of protein, ascorbic acid, riboflavin and vitamin A in the diet. The hematopoietic nutrients such as iron, B_{12} and folic acid deserve special consideration because blood loss from surgery may affect the level. It is true that in the great majority of instances the levels of these hematopoietic nutrients are not seriously affected by routine minor oral surgical procedures. Nevertheless, if the slightest advantage can be gained by providing in the diet adequate amounts of these nutrients and those which will promote wound healing, the attempt should be made.

The method of applying these principles to daily practice is to start dietary guidance at least a week prior to surgery. The advice should emphasize the importance of eating some complete protein foods, such as eggs, milk, meat, fish or poultry. Meat, especially the glandular types like liver and kidney, and heart, as well as fish, poultry and eggs not only provide protein but are also rich in iron and the B complex vitamins. Other food sources of these nutrients are green leafy vegetables, whole or enriched cereals and dried fruits. Liberal use of milk and cheese provides calcium, phosphorus and vitamin D for bone repair. Patients are prone to omit foods rich in ascorbic acid, which is so important in providing proper intercellular material and collagen for wound healing. For this reason a pint (two 8 oz. cups) of orange juice (equal to 200 mgs. of ascorbic acid or about three times the recommended amount) should be taken daily for at least a week preceding oral surgery. If there is any idiosyncrasy to orange juice, there are other combinations of fruit juices on the market which are fortified with vitamin C. Some contain acerola cherry juice, which is an exceedingly rich source of vitamin C. Other fruit juices such as cranberry juice have pure ascorbic acid added. If there is no difficulty in eating raw fruits and vegetables like grapefruit, tomatoes, strawberries, cantaloupe and green peppers, they can be recommended as excellent sources of ascorbic acid.

DIET AFTER ORAL SURGERY

One of the first questions the patient will ask after the removal of his teeth or any other oral surgical procedure is, "What can I eat?" A vague answer should be avoided. It is best to give a specific list of foods or beverages.

If the patient has had one of the general anesthetics like ether or an intravenous barbiturate which causes a disturbance of fat metabolism, it is best to avoid foods high in fat content for the first twelve hours or so after surgery. The patient should be given as much clear fluids as he can tolerate post nauseum. In addition to water, beverages like cola drinks, ginger ale, apple juice and orange juice as well as clear broths are best tolerated. Assuring an adequate fluid intake is most important.

In cases of oral surgery done under local anesthesia, in addition to the above mentioned beverages, sherbets, junkets, custards, gelatin and ice cream may be advised. If the patient is hungry, gruel or cereal topped with sugar and milk as well as milk, eggs or eggnogs or some type of chicken, pea or vegetable soup could be suggested.

Whichever of these dietary suggestions are adopted, they should be written on the prescription pad with the other routine postoperative instructions.

On the first or second postoperative day, when the patient is questioned about his comfort, further instructions may be given concerning the diet. The patient may continue to use liquid foods to prevent wound irritation, but this can be made adequate by using foods from the 4 Food Groups. For example, he may have the following foods in each group:

Milk group. Use milk in all forms. For extra nourishment nonfat milk solids may be added to regular milk. Add 3 tbsp. of milk solids to each 8 oz. glass of whole milk. Soft, plain ice creams are also soothing. Milk shakes and malted milks are recommended. Cream may be added to milk if desired.

Meat group. Eggs in the form of strained eggnoggs may be used in a liquid diet. They may also be used in soft or baked custards. Strained baby meats may be diluted with milk or bouillon to make soups.

Vegetable-fruit group. Citrus juices such as orange and grapefruit are highly recommended, as well as tomato juice and other fruit and vegetable juices. Puréed fruits and vegetables, such as baby foods, may be used. Strained fruits may be used with milk as a drink, and strained vegetables may be cooked with milk and butter and other seasonings as soup.

Bread-cereal group. Strained gruels.

A typical day's meals for the day or two immediately following multiple extractions might be as follows:

Breakfast
Pineapple-grapefruit juice
Strained oatmeal gruel
Coffee—with cream and sugar, if desired

Mid-morning
Orange eggnog

Noon
Strained cream of tomato soup
Custard with cream
Tea or coffee

Mid-afternoon
Chocolate milk shake

Evening
Strained pea soup
Spanish cream (or any custard pudding)
Tea or coffee

Bedtime
Cocoa

From the liquid diet the patient can change to the soft type if and when his gums allow. For example:

Milk group. Soft cheeses such as cottage cheese and cream cheese, in addition to milk and ice cream.

Meat group. Tender or ground meats, chicken, fish without bones, and cooked legumes.

Vegetable-fruit group. Cooked or canned fruits and ripe bananas. Vegetables without skins or seeds, mashed potatoes.

Bread-cereal group. Soft bread, macaroni, noodles, rice, spaghetti, cooked breakfast cereals with milk, and ready-to-eat flaked and puffed cereals such as wheat or corn flakes and puffed wheat and rice.

Even without being specifically told, the patient will gradually go to the firmer foods as the soreness in his mouth disappears. The important point to stress is that adequate diets can easily be eaten if sufficient amounts of foods from the 4 Food Groups are eaten each day.

DIET FOR A PATIENT WITH FRACTURED JAWS

Patients with jaw fractures often suffer other injuries which involve severe blood loss or even shock. For such patients one of the first treatments is the administration of whole blood. After the initial effects of the injury have subsided and the jaw fractures have been immobilized and reduced, feeding becomes a major consideration. The problem involves not only how much and what to feed but also the method of administration.

Before consideration of these problems some basic principles of the nutrient requirements of this type patient should be mentioned: (1) At least 2000 cc. of fluid should be given to maintain proper electrolytic balance. (2) Protein should be increased to compensate (a) for loss of nitrogen from injury and (b) for tissue repair. The normal requirement of a healthy man is 1 Gm. of protein per kg. of body weight. However, in the case of patients with fractured jaw from 1.5 to 2 Gms. of protein per kg. of body weight should be attained if possible. (3) Adequate calories (in most cases about 2500 calories) from the other nutrients must be provided daily to spare the protein from being used as an energy provider. (4) If elevation of temperature accompanies the injury, vitamins B complex and C requirements will be increased and, therefore, a multivitamin water-soluble capsule of B complex and C in therapeutic dosage (see Appendix IV for different types) should be prescribed.

Parenteral feeding is rarely indicated in fractured jaw cases and is only done in the event of a severe vomiting or other serious complication. In these cases one may administer 5 per cent or 10 per cent dextrose in water with added vitamins plus 5 per cent protein hydrolysate. As soon as practicable, the oral route should be used.

When a patient cannot cooperate, tube feeding is used. Henry and Barrow[3] suggest using a small caliber plastic tube (2.5 mm. or less) which is easily passed through the patient's nose down into the stomach. In the place of the usual prepared liquid feedings they use natural foods that have been liquefied. By use of a blender, foods such as meats, vegetables and fruits can be liquefied and then strained into a fine tube. The liquefied food is then forced through the tube by a mechanical pump. If a mechanical pump is not available, the foods may be forced through the tube by use of an asepto syringe.

Oral feeding is always preferable to tube feeding. As soon as the patient is able to cooperate he should be encouraged to take his liquids through a straw or bent plastic tubing. The same liquid foods which were recommended on page 395 for patients following multiple extractions may be used for the patient with a reduced and wired fractured jaw. Since the patient is likely to be on a liquid diet for several weeks, very careful attention must be given to diet adequacy. The following is a suggested total daily food plan: (1) one quart of milk or more, (2) two eggs, (3) at least one serving of strained meat or chicken, (4) four servings of fruit and vegetable juices with two of these being citrus or rich in vitamin C, (5) two or more servings of liquid gruels, and (6) additional calories added through the use of cream and sugars.

In addition to prescribing the proper diet and then serving these foods, care must be taken to see that the patient actually ingests all the prescribed foods. It must be emphasized that food is as important a medicine as an antibiotic or anodyne. He must eat everything that is prescribed for complete and quick recovery.

If the patient is unable to consume adequate amounts of food, special supplements may be added. If he cannot or does not relish fruit or vegetable juices, vitamin supplements of B complex and C in therapeutic doses should be prescribed (See Appendix IV for brand names). Protein supplements or oral fat emulsions may also be used if there are indications that the patient needs more nourishment than can be supplied through the use of ordinary foods.

Protein supplements such as Sustagen supply concentrated energy and protein in a small volume; an 8 oz. glass provides 390 calories, 23.5 Gms. of protein and some vitamins and minerals. One cup of Sustagen can be mixed with an equal amount of water and flavored with ½ tsp. of vanilla, 1 tsp. of instant coffee, ⅓ cup of orange juice or 1 tbsp. of cocoa. Another recipe for Sustagen is 1 cup of milk, 1 egg, 1 tsp. of vanilla, and 1 large scoop of ice cream. (Measure milk and vanilla into a mixing bowl. Add egg and mix, using rotary egg beater. Add Sustagen to milk and beat until mixture is smooth. Chill thoroughly and then add ice cream.) This will yield a 14 oz. glass of fluid which provides 975 calories and 52 Gms. of protein. Other protein supplements such as Meritene can be used in the same way. For the patient with a poor appetite who needs a high protein intake these are invaluable. As soon as the patient's appetite improves, he may discontinue the supplements and receive his nourishment from ordinary foods included in the liquid or soft diet.

Oral fat emulsions have been used for patients who are undernourished and need a concentrated source of calories. Slightly less than ½ cup of an oral fat emulsion supplies 400 calories. For the patient for whom eating is difficult and for whom calories are a prime concern, consideration should be given to the use of oral fat emulsions. Since fat is the most concentrated source of energy, the rationale for oral or intravenous fat emulsions is a sound one, providing the patient has no untoward reactions. Adequate fat will spare protein from being used as an energy provider.

After the wires have been removed from the jaws the patient is gradually introduced to solid foods. At first a soft diet is used, such as is described in the previous section on multiple extractions. It must be emphasized that the most difficult part of mastication is biting; therefore, foods such as sandwiches, raw apples and raw vegetables should not even be attempted until complete healing has taken place.

DIET FOR PATIENT WITH CLEFT PALATE

From birth the child with a cleft palate, with or without a cleft lip, presents feeding problems.[6] Early in life he may have to be fed with a medicine dropper or a Brecht feeder. However, it is recommended that he be fed from a bottle just as soon as possible. The sucking motions he uses in extracting milk through a nipple are necessary for development of the muscles needed for speech and for the development of all mouth tissues.

In an excellent paper by Zickefoose,[10] the result of interviews with 58 mothers of children with cleft palates, she presents some helpful suggestions for feeding cleft-palate children. Many of the suggestions come from the mothers themselves. Among the suggestions are the following:

1. Enlarging the hole in the nipple on the baby's bottle to enable him to get his milk more easily.
2. Boiling new nipples prior to use to soften them.
3. Thinning puréed foods (fruits, vegetables, meats) with milk or broth so that these foods may be fed from a bottle with a nipple with an enlarged hole. (Other mothers found that thickening puréed foods by adding crumbs helped their children to eat them better.)
4. Frequent burping aided in releasing excessive air intake.
5. Eating slowly and taking small bites helped to prevent regurgitation in the older child.
6. Using a straw helped some children to take liquids more easily.
7. Since feeding a child with a cleft palate takes longer than feeding an ordinary child, a mother needs to allow more time. Fatigue on the part of the parent may interfere with the child's receiving adequate nourishment.

The cleft-palate baby needs the same foods as any infant. In addition to his milk formula, he needs to have supplements of vitamin D and vitamin C started during the first month of life. Cereals, egg yolk, strained fruits and vegetables and puréed meats should also be fed as early as with other children. He should also be fed from a cup and spoon at the same time as other children.

As in all surgery patients, proper diet must be stressed before and after the plastic repair. This is particularly important because at the age when this surgery is usually done children's appetites are poorest.

Diet Following Repair of Cleft Palate

Immediately following repair of the cleft, a liquid diet will be provided until healing is complete. The foods to be included in a nourishing liquid diet should be adequate in protein, minerals and vitamins to promote healing. Suggestions of liquid foods that will make up an adequate diet have been outlined in the early part of this chapter.

After the cleft is repaired, the child will be able to eat all kinds of foods. As with any child, he needs adequate amounts of the 4

Food Groups daily. To repeat, these are: milk group, 4 servings; meat group, 2 servings; vegetable-fruit group, 4 servings, with one of these being a rich source of vitamin C and another a rich source of vitamin A (at least every other day); bread-cereal group, 4 servings of enriched or whole grain.

In addition to the essential foods, a child with a repaired cleft palate should be encouraged to eat foods which require him to use his tongue and his muscles of mastication. Foods should be provided that will exercise the muscles that are used in biting, chewing, swallowing, licking, sucking and blowing. Raw fruits and raw vegetables are especially recommended because they require the use of so many muscles of mastication. Sucking and blowing through a straw or sucking the juice from an orange which has had a hole cut in it will provide exercise for the lip and the tongue muscles. Licking an ice cream cone is another tongue exercise that can be suggested. Soft, cooked fruits such as apple sauce also require the use of the tongue. Careful attention to diet will aid in promoting improved speech, good dental health and improved general health for the child with a cleft palate.

REFERENCES

1. Asirvadham, M.: The bone marrow and its leucocytic response in protein deficiency. J. Infect. Dis., *83:*87, 1948.
2. Cannon, P. R.: The importance of proteins in resistance to infection. J.A.M.A., *128:*360, 1945.
3. Henry, F. A., and Barrow, J.: Tube feeding in oral surgery. J. of Oral Surg., *12:*238, 1954.
4. Koster, H., and Shapiro, A.: Serum proteins and wound healing. Arch. Surg., *41:*723, 1940.
5. Localio, S. A., Casale, W., and Hinton, J. W.: Wound healing—experimental and statistical study: experimental observations. Surg. Gynec. & Obst., *77:*243, 1943.
6. Patterson, I.: Feeding the Child with a Cleft Palate. Public Health Nursing, *43:*148, 1951.
7. Robertson, E. C., and Tisdall, F. F.: Nutrition and resistance to disease. Canad. M. A. J., *40:*282, 1939.
8. Whipple, A. O.: The critical latent or lag period in healing of wounds. Ann. Surg., *112:*481, 1940.
9. Wissler, R. W.: The effects of protein depletion and subsequent immunization upon the response of animals to pneumococcal infection; experiments with rabbits. J. Infect. Dis., *80:*250, 1947.
10. Zickefoose, M.: Feeding problems of children with cleft palates. Children, *4:*225, 1957.

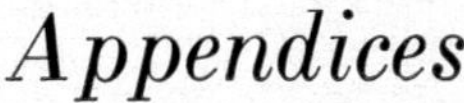

Appendices

APPENDIX I. FOOD NOMOGRAM

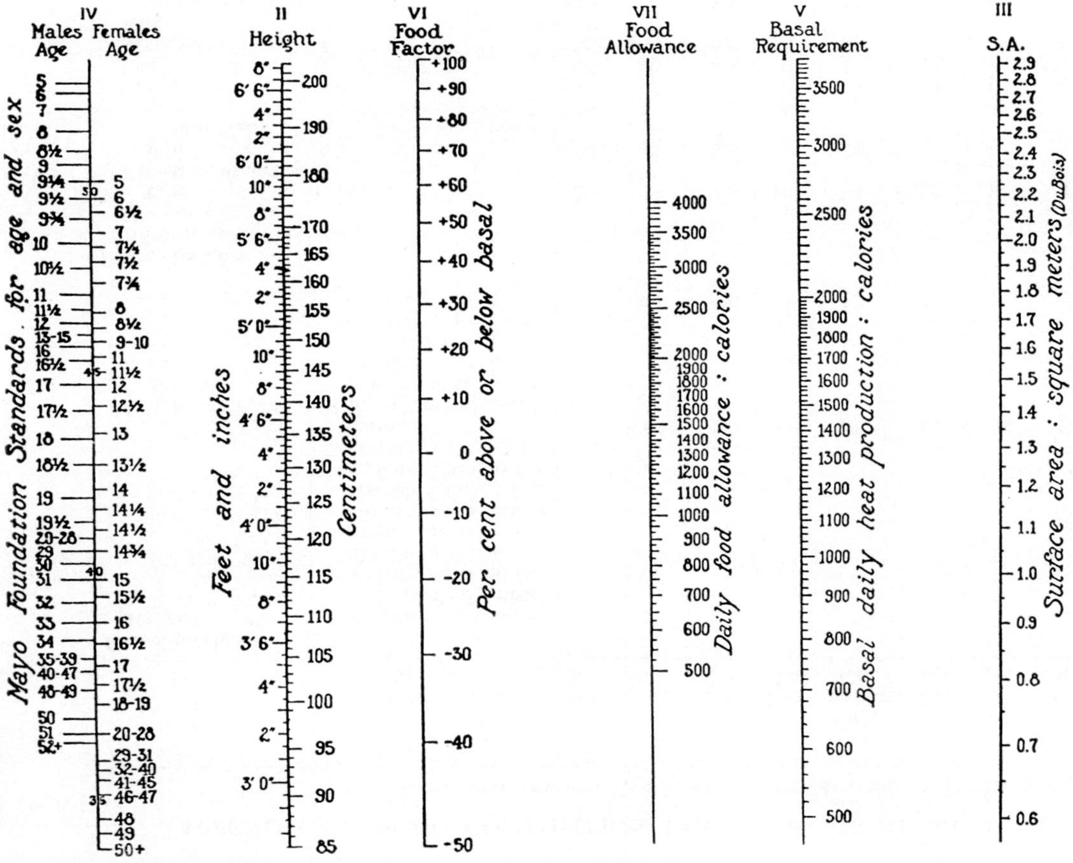

Food Nomogram

Directions: The standards for age are arranged on the basis of the common method of expressing age as of the last birthday. To determine the desired calorie allowance, proceed as follows: (1) Locate the weight on Scale I by means of a pin stuck through the eraser of a lead pencil. (2) Place the edge of the ruler against the pin and swing the other end of ruler to the patient's height on Scale II. (3) Transfer the pin to the point where the ruler crosses Scale III which gives the surface area in sq. meters (this value need not be read). (4) Holding the ruler against pin on the surface area scale, swing the left hand end of the ruler to the patient's standard for age and sex given on Scale IV. (5) Transfer the pin to where the ruler now crosses Scale V which gives the basal heat production of the patient for 24 hours and represents the calories of food required by the fasting patient when resting in bed (basal calories). The calories necessary for activity bear a percentage relationship to those demanded for the resting condition. The so-called "white collar worker" when at work will need about 50 per cent more than his basal calories. When activity is restricted, as in the hospital, the extra calories necessary will range from 10 to 30 per cent of the basal calories. Therefore (6) estimate the per cent of calories above the basal and locate this point on Scale VI. With the ruler connect this point with the point located previously on Scale V, and where the ruler now crosses Scale VII read the amount of food calories to be provided by the diet.

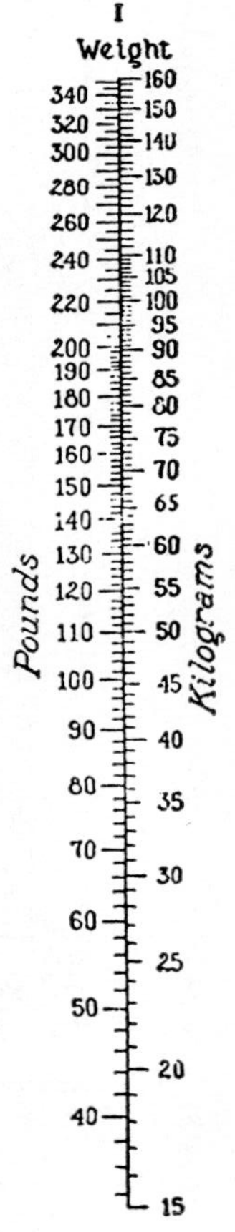

IV Males Age / Females Age — *Mayo Foundation Standards for age and sex*

II Height — *Feet and inches* / *Centimeters*

VI Food Factor — *Per cent above or below basal*

VII Food Allowance — *Daily food allowance : calories*

V Basal Requirement — *Basal daily heat production : calories*

III S.A. — *Surface area : square meters (DuBois)*

I Weight — *Pounds* / *Kilograms*

APPENDIX II. FOOD COMPOSITION TABLE FOR SHORT METHOD OF DIETARY ANALYSIS

Food Composition Table for Short Method of Dietary Analysis[1]

Food*	Approximate Measure	Wt. Gm.	Calories	Prot. Gm.	Fat Gm.	Carbohydrate Gm.	Ca Gm.	P Gm.	Fe Mg.	Vit. A I.U.	Ascorbic Acid Mg.	Thiamine Mg.	Riboflavin Mg.	Niacin Mg.
Cereal products:														
Refined	1 sl. bread (30 Gm.); ½ c. cooked cereal and cereal products (20 Gm. dry); ½-1 c. prep. cereal (20 Gm.); 3 soda crackers (20 Gm.); 1½ c. popcorn (20 Gm.); 1 griddle cake (4-in. diam.).	. .	80	2.5	1	15	.01	.02	.2	. .	. .	.02	.02	.3
Whole grain and enriched	1 sl. bread (30 Gm.); ½ c. cooked cereal (20 Gm. dry); ½-1 c. prepared cereal (20 Gm.); 2 graham crackers (20 Gm.).	. .	80	2.5	1	15	.02	.03	.6	. .	. .	.07	.04	.6
Dairy products:														
Butter, Margarine	1 tsp.	5	35	. .	4	. .	. .	. .	. .	165	. .	. .	. .	. .
Cheese, Cheddar type	1 cu. in.	30	125	7.5	10	1	.22	.15	.3	420	. .	.01	.13	. .
Cheese, cottage, skim	½ c.	100	95	19.5	1	2	.10	.19	.3	20	. .	.02	.31	.1
Cream, light	⅛ c. (for heavy cream add ½ serving butter)	30	60	1.0	6	1	.03	.02	. .	250	. .	.01	.04	. .
Custard	½ c.	130	150	7.0	7	15	.15	.16	.6	440	. .	.06	.26	.1
Egg	1 medium	50	80	6.5	6	. .	.03	.10	1.4	570	. .	.05	.14	.1
Ice cream	½ c.	80	165	3.0	10	16	.10	.08	.1	420	1	.03	.15	.1
Milk														
Buttermilk, skim	1 c.	240	85	8.5	. .	12	.30	.23	.2	. .	2	.10	.43	.2
Whole	1 c.	240	165	8.5	9	12	.28	.22	.2	385	2	.10	.41	.2

Desserts:													
Cake, plain, chocolate	1 piece cake 2½ x 2½ x 2½ (75 Gm.), for iced add 1 serving sweets; 1 waffle, 6-in. diam. (60 Gm.); 2½ doughnuts, cake type (add 1 serving fat)	. .	250	5.0	8	40	.09	.10	.4	140	. .	.02	.06	.2
Cookies, plain	2 medium	40	175	2.5	5	30	.01	.03	.4	100	. .	.02	.02	.2
Pie crust	⅙ shell, single crust	25	110	1.5	6	12	. .	.01	.4	. .	. .	.05	.04	.5
Puddings, cream fillings	½ c.	140	150	4.5	5	22	.14	.13	.1	225	. .	.04	.22	.1
Fats:	2 sl. bacon (20 Gm. raw); 1 tbsp. fat (12 Gm.); 1 tbsp. mayonnaise (15 Gm.); 1 cu. in. salt pork (15 Gm.); 2 tbsp. French dressing (30 Gm.)	. .	105	1.5	11	. .	. .	.01	.2	15	. .	.03	.02	.4
Fish:													
Cod, haddock, cooked	1 medium serving	75	55	13.5	. .	. .	.01	.15	.4	. .	1	.04	.06	1.6
Halibut, herring, tuna, whitefish, cooked	1 medium serving tuna (60 Gm.); others (75 Gm.)	60	115	17.0	5	. .	.01	.19	.8	60	. .	.04	.06	6.0
Salmon, cooked	1 medium serving	75	125	15.0	7	. .	.11	.23	.8	135	. .	.02	.12	5.6
Fruits:													
Banana	1 small	100	90	1.0	. .	22	.01	.03	.6	430	10	.04	.05	.7
Cantaloupe	½ melon, 4½-in. diam.	150	30	1.0	. .	7	.02	.02	.6	5,130	50	.07	.06	.8
Citrus	1 medium orange; ½ medium grapefruit; ½ c. juice; 1 medium large lemon	100	45	.5	. .	11	.03	.02	.4	115	45	.06	.02	.2

Food Composition Table for Short Method of Dietary Analysis[1]

Food*	Approximate Measure	Wt. Gm.	Calories	Prot. Gm.	Fat Gm.	Carbohydrate Gm.	Ca Gm.	P Gm.	Fe Mg.	Vit. A I.U.	Ascorbic Acid Mg.	Thiamine Mg.	Riboflavin Mg.	Niacin Mg.
Fruits (*Continued*)														
Yellow—fresh, canned, dried	fresh (100 Gm.); 1 medium peach, 2 to 3 apricots, 3 plums; dried (30 Gm.); for sweetened, canned, dried or fresh add ½ serving sweets	. .	70	.5	. .	17	.01	.03	.6	910	6	.01	.03	1.0
Other—dried	3 to 4 dates; 1½ to 2 small figs; dried apple; ¼ c. raisins	30	80	.5	. .	20	.03	.03	.9	15	. .	.04	.03	.3
Other—fresh and canned	½ c.	100	55	.5	. .	13	.01	.01	.4	95	4	.04	.03	.2
Gravy, white sauce	¼ c.	65	105	2.5	8	6	.07	.06	.2	225	. .	.04	.11	.2
Legumes:														
Beans, peas	½ c. cooked; dried (30 Gm.)	. .	100	6.5	. .	18	.05	.13	2.0	10	1	.19	.07	.7
Soybeans	½ c. cooked; dried (30 Gm.)	. .	105	10.5	5	4	.07	.18	2.4	35	. .	.32	.09	.7
Meat:														
Beef, lamb, veal, cooked	1 medium serving	75	240	19.0	18	. .	.01	.15	2.3	. .	. .	.07	.17	3.7
Fowl, cooked	1 medium serving	75	150	15.0	10	. .	.01	.16	1.7	. .	. .	.04	.08	5.2
Liver, cooked	1 small serving	60	125	14.0	5	6	.01	.29	4.7	32,100	19	.16	2.38	8.9
Luncheon meats, cooked	2 sl. sausage, minced ham, dried beef, luncheon roll (30 Gm.); ½ frankfurter	. .	85	6.0	7	. .	.01	.05	.9	. .	. .	.08	.08	.8
Pork, ham, cooked	1 medium serving	75	280	18.0	23	. .	.01	.16	2.2	. .	. .	.47	.17	3.5

Nuts:	1 tbsp. peanut butter; 8 to 15 walnut halves; 16 peanuts; 12 to 15 almonds; 12 pecan halves	15	90	4.0	7	3	.01	.06	.3	..	..	.04	.02	2.3
Sweets:														
Candy, sugar, syrup	1 tbsp. sugar, jelly, jam, syrup, honey; 1 serving plain Jello, plain candy (fondant or mints, 14 Gm.); 6-oz. bottle soft drink	..	55	..	..	14	..	..	..	..	..	..	..	..
Candy bar	1 2-oz. chocolate-coated bar	..	290	4.0	15	34	.06	.09	1.1	65	..	.04	.17	1.1
Molasses; sorghum	1 tbsp.	20	50	..	..	13	.04	.01	1.8	..	..	.02	.03	.6
Vegetables:														
Cabbage—cooked and sauerkraut	⅔ c.	100	25	1.5	..	5	.05	.03	.5	90	30†	.05	.05	.3
Cabbage, raw; cauliflower, cooked	1 c. cabbage (50 Gm.); ⅔ c. cauliflower (70 Gm.)	..	15	1.0	..	3	.02	.03	.5	50	22	.04	.04	.2
Corn; parsnips, cooked	½ c. corn; 1 large parsnip	100	85	2.0	1	19	.03	.07	.6	195	10‡	.07‡	.09‡	.6‡
Green and yellow:														
Asparagus cooked	⅔ c.	100	20	2.0	..	3	.02	.05	1.0	1,040	18‡	.13‡	.17‡	1.2‡
Broccoli, cooked	⅔ c.	100	30	3.0	..	5	.13	.08	1.3	3,400	74	.07	.15	.8
Carrots, cooked	⅔ c.	100	30	.5	..	7	.03	.03	.6	12,500	4‡	.05‡	.05‡	.4‡
Green beans, cooked	½ c.	100	25	1.5	..	5	.04	.02	.7	660	14‡	.07‡	.10‡	.5‡
Leafy green, cooked	⅔ c. spinach, turnip, kale, other greens	100	30	2.5	..	5	.20§	.05	2.7	10,400	33‡	.08‡	.21‡	.6‡
Peas, fresh, cooked, canned	½ c.	100	70	4.0	..	13	.02	.09	1.8	630	15‡	.25‡	.14‡	2.3‡
Sweet potato, cooked	½ large	100	140	2.0	1	31	.03	.05	.8	8,605	22‡	.10‡	.06‡	.7‡

Food Composition Table for Short Method of Dietary Analysis[1]

Food*	Approximate Measure	Wt. Gm.	Calories	Prot. Gm.	Fat Gm.	Carbohydrate Gm.	Ca Gm.	P Gm.	Fe Mg.	Vit. A I.U.	Ascorbic Acid Mg.	Thiamine Mg.	Riboflavin Mg.	Niacin Mg.
Potato, cooked	1 small (100 Gm.); for fried add 1 to 2 servings fat; for French fried (50 Gm.) add 1 to 2 servings fat	..	85	2.0	..	19	.01	.06	.7	20	14‡	.09‡	.03	1.0
Tomato, fresh, canned, or juice	½ c.; 1 small tomato (100 Gm.); for 2½ tbsp. catsup (50 Gm.) add ½ serving sweets	..	20	1.0	..	4	.01	.02	.5	1,035	18	.05	.03	.8
Other, cooked	½ c. beets, eggplant, onions, etc.	100	40	1.0	..	9	.03	.05	.6	80	8	.03	.04	.3
Other, commonly served raw	2 pieces celery; 8 sl. cucumber; ⅛ head lettuce	50	10	.5	..	2	.02	.02	.2	105	4	.02	.03	.2

[1] Leichsenring, J. M., and Wilson, E. D.: J. Am. Dietet. A. *27*:386, 1951.

* The nutritive value of food mixtures such as macaroni and cheese, Spanish rice, chow mein, creamed vegetables, soups and so on should be computed on the basis of the kind and the approximate amount of the foods in the combination.

† For sauerkraut, reduce by one half.

‡ For canned, reduce by one half.

§ Calcium may be unavailable in chard, spinach and beet greens.

Explanation of use of Appendix II on following page.

Food Composition Table for Short Method of Dietary Analysis

Explanation of Use

To illustrate the use of the food composition table, a sample day's menu from one of the homemaker's record is given below:

Breakfast

Tomato juice	1 serving
Oatmeal	1 serving
Cream (light)	2 servings
Sugar	2 tsp.
Bread, white enriched	1 sl.
Butter	1 tsp.
Milk, whole	1 c.

Lunch

Macaroni and cheese	1 serving
Head lettuce, French dressing	1 serving
Applesauce, sweetened	1 serving
Cupcake	1
Bread, whole wheat	1 sl.
Butter	1 tsp.
Milk, whole	1 c.

Midafternoon

Chocolate bar	1

Dinner

Liver	1 small serving
Potato, baked	1 small
Butter	2 tsp.
Green beans, buttered	1 serving
Celery	2 pieces
Bread, white enriched	1 sl.
Butter	1 tsp.
Chocolate pie	1 serving
Milk, whole	1 c.

This day's menu may be summarized as follows in preparing to calculate the nutritive value from the figures in the table:

Foods	Servings
Cereals:	
Refined	1
Whole grain or enriched	4
Dairy products:	
Butter	5½
Cheese, Cheddar	1
Cream, light	2
Milk, whole	3¼
Desserts:	
Cake, plain	⅔
Pie crust	1
Pudding	1
Fruit: other, fresh or canned	1
Meat: liver	1
Sweets	1
Candy bar	1
Vegetables:	
Green beans	1
Potato	1
Tomato	1
Other, raw	1

APPENDIX III. FOODS AND MIXED DISHES CLASSIFIED ACCORDING TO FOOD GROUPS AND AMOUNTS COMMONLY CONSIDERED AS ONE SERVING

(Unless specified each serving = 1 unit of the food group)

Foods and Mixed Dishes	*Amount Commonly Considered as One Serving*	*Food Group*
apple	1 med. size, 3–4 oz.	veg.-fruit
apple juice	½ cup	veg.-fruit
apricots	3–4 oz., 2–3 med.	veg.-fruit
asparagus	½ cup (4 oz.)	veg.-fruit
avocado	½ cup (4 oz.)	veg.-fruit
bacon	2 slices	fat
bananas	1 med.	veg.-fruit
beans (dry)	½ cup, cooked	meat
beans (fresh) green or wax	½ cup, cooked (4 oz.)	veg.-fruit
beef	2–3 oz., cooked hamburger	meat
beet greens	½ cup (4 oz.)	veg.-fruit
beets	½ cup (4 oz.)	veg.-fruit
berries	½ cup (4 oz.)	veg.-fruit
biscuits (baking powder)	1 medium, 2″ in diameter	bread-cereal
blanc mange	½ cup	milk (½) sugar—3 tsp.
bread, corn	1 piece—2″ square	bread-cereal
bread, all varieties	1 slice (1 oz.)	bread-cereal
broccoli	½ cup (4 oz.)	veg.-fruit
brussel sprouts	½ cup (4 oz.)	veg.-fruit
butter	1 tsp.	fat
buttermilk	1 cup	milk
cabbage	½ cup (4 oz.)	veg.-fruit
cantaloupe	¼ medium melon	veg.-fruit
carrots	½ cup (4 oz.)	veg.-fruit
cauliflower	½ cup (4 oz.)	veg.-fruit
cereals, cooked (oatmeal, corn meal, Cream of Wheat, etc.)	½ cup (1 oz.)	bread-cereal
cereals, ready-to-eat, flaked or puffed	¾ cup–1 cup (1 oz.)	bread-cereal
celery	½ cup (4 oz.)	veg.-fruit
chard	½ cup (4 oz.)	veg.-fruit
cheese, cheddar, American, Swiss	1 oz.	milk
cheese, cream	2 tbsp.	fat
cheese, soft type, cottage	½ cup	milk (⅓)
cheese bits	½ cup (10 to 20 crackers)	bread-cereal
cherries	3–4 oz., 15 large	veg.-fruit
chicken	½ breast or 1 leg and thigh (4 oz.)	meat
chickory	½ cup (4 oz.)	veg.-fruit
clams	3–4 oz., cooked (½) cup	meat
cocoa, made with milk	1 cup	milk
collards	½ cup (4 oz.)	veg.-fruit
corn	½ cup (4 oz.) 1 ear—5 inches	veg.-fruit

Foods and Mixed Dishes	*Amount Commonly Considered as One Serving*	*Food Group*
crackers, round, thin	6 crackers	bread-cereal
saltines	3 crackers	bread-cereal
graham	3 crackers	bread-cereal
oyster	24 crackers	bread-cereal
cress	½ cup (4 oz.)	veg.-fruit
cucumbers	½ cup (4 oz.)	veg.-fruit
custard pudding (½ cup)	½ cup	milk (½) sugar—3 tsp.
dandelion greens	½ cup (4 oz.)	veg.-fruit
duck	2–3 oz., cooked	meat
egg, in any form	2	meat
eggplant	½ cup (4 oz.)	veg.-fruit
English muffins	1 muffin	bread-cereal
escarole	½ cup (4 oz.)	veg.-fruit
figs (fresh)	3 small	veg.-fruit
fish—cod, haddock, bass, mackerel, flounder, halibut	3–4 oz., cooked	meat
fish chowder	1⅓ cup	meat (½) milk veg.-fruit (½)
grapefruit	½ medium	veg.-fruit
grapes	3–4 oz., 22 Tokay 60 green, seedless	veg.-fruit
greens, all kinds cooked	½ cup	veg.-fruit
grits	½ cup (1 oz.)	bread-cereal
guava	3 oz.	veg.-fruit
heart	2–3 oz., cooked	meat
ice cream	½ cup	milk (¼)
kale	½ cup (4 oz.)	veg.-fruit
kidney	2–3 oz., cooked	meat
lamb	2 rib chops, ½ inch thick	meat
lentils, dried	½ cup, cooked	meat
lettuce	½ cup (4 oz.)	veg.-fruit
liver	2–3 oz., cooked	meat
lobster	2–3 oz., cooked	meat
macaroni	½ cup	bread-cereal
macaroni and cheese	1 cup (8 oz.)	bread-cereal milk
mango	3–4 oz.	veg.-fruit
margarine	1 tsp.	fat
mayonnaise	1 tbsp.	fat
meat loaf	3–4 oz.	meat bread-cereal (¼)
meat stew	1 cup (8 oz.)	veg.-fruit meat
meat, lean,—beef, lamb, pork, veal	3–4 oz.	meat
melons, honeydew	¼ melon; ½ cup diced	veg.-fruit
milk (fresh, diluted, evaporated, reconstructed or dried)	½ cup	milk

Foods and Mixed Dishes	*Amount Commonly Considered as One Serving*	*Food Group*
muffins	1 med.	bread-cereal
mushrooms	½ cup	veg.-fruit
nectarines	1 medium	veg.-fruit
noodles	½ cup	bread-cereal
nuts	2 tbsp., ½ oz.	meat (¼)
okra	½ cup (4 oz.)	veg.-fruit
olives	10–12	fat
onions	½ cup (4 oz.)	veg.-fruit
oranges	1 medium, 3–4 oz.	veg.-fruit
oysters	6–8 medium	meat
pancakes	1, 4 inch pancake	bread-cereal
papaya	3–4 oz. (½ cup)	veg.-fruit
parsnips	½ cup (4 oz.)	veg.-fruit
peaches	1 medium, 3–4 oz.	veg.-fruit
peanut butter	2 tbsp.	meat (½)
pears	1 medium, 3–4 oz.	veg.-fruit
peas, fresh or canned	½ cup, cooked	veg.-fruit
peas, dried	½ cup, cooked	meat
peppers	½ cup (4 oz.)	veg.-fruit
pies, cream—1 crust (custard, squash)	⅙ of a pie	bread-cereal (½) milk (½) sugar, 2 tbsp.
pies, fruit—2 crusts (apple, berry, peach, cherry, etc.)	⅙ of a pie	bread-cereal veg.-fruit sugar, 2 tbsp.
pies, lemon meringue 1 crust	⅙ of a pie	bread-cereal (½) sugar, 3 tbsp.
pineapple	3–4 oz., ½ cup diced	veg.-fruit
plums	½ cup (1 medium)	veg.-fruit
popcorn	¾–1 cup	bread-cereal
popovers	1 popover	bread-cereal
pork	1 chop, 1 inch thick	meat
potato chips	8–10 pieces	bread-cereal
potatoes	1 med. size, 3–4 oz.	veg.-fruit
pretzel sticks	½ cup (10 to 20 crackers)	bread-cereal
prunes	4 medium	veg.-fruit
rabbit	2–3 oz., cooked	meat
radishes	½ cup (4 oz.)	veg.-fruit
rice	½ cup	bread-cereal
rolls, plain	1 roll, medium, Parker House or Cloverleaf	bread-cereal
rutabaga	½ cup (4 oz.)	veg.-fruit
Ry-Krisp	4 crackers	bread-cereal
salmon	2–3 oz., cooked	meat
sandwiches	2 slices bread	bread-cereal (2)
	Filling:	
	2 oz. meat, fish, chicken, egg or peanut butter	meat (½)
	1 slice cheese	milk
	lettuce, tomato	veg.-fruit

Foods and Mixed Dishes	*Amount Commonly Considered as One Serving*	*Food Group*
sardines	2–3 oz.	meat
sauerkraut	½ cup	veg.-fruit
sausage (bologna, frankforts, liverwurst, etc.)	2–3 oz., 3 slices 1 large or 2 small frankforts	meat
shredded wheat	¾–1 cup, 1 oz.	bread-cereal
shrimp	2–3 oz., cooked	meat
soup, vegetable	1 cup	veg.-fruit
soup, cream of tomato, asparagus, corn	1 cup	milk (½)
soup, clear, chicken or beef bouillon	1 cup	meat (½)
soup, noodle, rice or barley	1 cup	bread-cereal (½)
spaghetti	½ cup	bread-cereal
spaghetti (Italian style) with meat sauce	1 cup spaghetti ½ cup meat sauce	bread-cereal (2) meat, (½)
spinach	½ cup (4 oz.)	veg.-fruit
squash	½ cup (4 oz.)	veg.-fruit
strawberries	3–4 oz., 1 cup	veg.-fruit
swordfish	2–3 oz., cooked	meat
tangerines	3–4 oz., 1 medium	veg.-fruit
tapioca pudding	½ cup	milk (½) sugar, 3 tsp.
tomatoes	1 med. size, 3–4 oz.	veg.-fruit
tortillas	1 medium	bread-cereal
tuna	2–3 oz., cooked	meat
turkey	2–3 oz., cooked	meat
turnips	½ cup (4 oz.)	veg.-fruit
turnip greens	½ cup (4 oz.)	veg.-fruit
veal	2–3 oz., cooked	meat
venison	2–3 oz., cooked	meat
waffles	½ medium	bread-cereal
watermelon	1/16 of a melon, ½ cup diced	veg.-fruit
white sauce, for creamed chicken, meat, fish, or vegetables	½ cup	milk (½)
yams	1 medium	veg.-fruit
yoghurt	1 cup	milk

APPENDIX IV. SOME REPRESENTATIVE VITAMIN PREPARATIONS FROM A FEW DIFFERENT DRUG HOUSES

	Product	Mfg.	B_1 mg.	B_2 mg.	Niac. mg.	Pant. mg.	B_6 mg.	C mg.	A units	D units	B_{12} mcg.	Folacin mg.	Misc.
Vitamins B complex and C in Maintenance Doses	B-compules with Vitamin C	Abbott	3	3	20	3	0.1	30					Liver fraction 330 mg.
	Betacebrin Syrup	Lilly (in pints)	1	1	8			40					Yeast 250 mg. per 5 cc.
	Beta-Cevalin Comp.	Lilly	5	5	25	12.5	2.5	75			1		Liver 455 mg.
	Cebefortis Tab.	Upjohn	5	5	50	25	1.5	150			2	0.5	
	Novo-Basic	E. R. Squibb & Sons	5	5	50	10	1	150			2	15	
	Totabex Caps	C. D. Smith	3	2	15	2	0.25	30					
	Vitikon Syrup	Upjohn (in 4 & 12 oz.) per teaspoon	2	3	30			100					
Vitamins B complex and C in Therapeutic Doses	Allbee with Vitamin C	A. H. Robins Co., Inc.	15	10	50	10		250					
	A.S.F. Caps	Roerig	10	10	100	20	2	300			4	1.5	Menadione (Kanalogue) 2 mg.
	Convalets Filmtabs	Abbott	10	10	100	20	2	300			4	1.5	

Vitamins B complex and C in Therapeutic Doses	Novogran	E. R. Squibb & Sons	10	10	100	20	2	300			4	1.5	Menadione (Kanalogue) 2 mg.
	Panalins-T	Mead Johnson	10	10	100	20	2	300			4	1.5	
	Probec-Tabs (formerly Stuart Therapeutic B complex, C)	Stuart	10	10	150	10	5	150			5 mcg. 50% USP crystalline 50% B_{12} concentrate		
	Provite B with C	Ives-Cameron	25	12.5	100	5	1.5	100			2		
	Stress Caps	Lederle	10	10	100	20	2	300			4	1.5	Menadione (Kanalogue) 2 mg.
	Surgimin-T	Walker	10	10	100	20	2	300			4	1.5	
	Thera-combex Kaps	Parke, Davis	25	15	100	10	1	150			5	2.5	
	Vio-Bec Caps	Rowell	25	25	100	40	10	250					
Vitamins A, D, B Complex and C in Maintenance Doses	Mixed Vitamin Caps	Mead-Johnson	3	4	25			100	10,000	1,000			
	Multi-Vi Caps	White	1.5	2	10			37.5	5,000	500			
	Pan-Concemin	Merrell	3	2	20	2	1	50	5,000	800			
	Unicaps	Upjohn	2.5	2.5	20	5	0.5	50	5,000	500	2	0.25	
	Vi-Zo-8	Pitman-Moore	1.5	2	5	1		30	5,000	800			E-6.2 mg.

	Product	Mfg.	B_1 mg.	B_2 mg.	Niac. mg.	Pant. mg.	B_6 mg.	C mg.	A units	D units	B_{12} mcg.	Folacin mg.	Misc.
Vitamins A, D, B Complex and C in Maintenance Doses	Paladac Multi-V	Parke, Davis (3 therapeutic doses per 4 cc.)	3	3	20	5	1	50	5,000	1,000	5		
	Procebrin Multi-Vitamin Drops	Lilly (no therapeutic doses) contains per 0.6 cc.	2	1	16	3	1	120	6,000	1,600			
Vitamins A, D, B Complex and C in Therapeutic Doses	Alin-Diem Caps	McNiel	5	10	50			150	25,000	1,000			
	Bio Formula	Walker	25	10	150			150	25,000	2,500			
	Magnicaps	Plessner	10	5	150			150	25,000	1,000			
	Theragran (also liquid, same contents)	E. R. Squibb & Sons	10	10	150			150	25,000	1,000			
	Therapeutic Formula E	Ives-Cameron	10	10	150			150	25,000	1,000			E-3.4 mg.
	Thera-Vita	Warner	10	10	100	10	1	150	12,500	1,250			

There are many other preparations listed in Edwin P. Jordan, ed.: Modern Drug Encyclopedia and Therapeutic Index. 7th ed. New York, Drug Publications, Inc., 1958.

APPENDIX V. EQUIVALENT WEIGHTS AND MEASURES

Equivalent Weights and Measures

Comparative Values of Weight and Volume of Water

1 liter	=	1 kilo.	= 2.2 lbs.
1 fluid ounce	=	30 Gm.	= 1.04 ozs.
1 pint	=	473 Gm.	= 1.04 lbs.
1 quart	=	.946 kilo.	= 2.1 lbs.

Table of Common Measures and Metric Equivalents

1 tsp.	=	5 cc.	
1 tbsp.	=	14 cc.	(approx. 15 Gm.)
1 cup	=	225 cc.	(approx. 240 Gm.)

(*See* Table of Measures and Approximate Weights, p. 407)

Comparative Temperatures

Boiling water, sea level	100	212
Body temperature	37	98.6
Tropical temperature	30	89
Room temperature, average	20	70
Freezing	0	32

Table of Measures and Approximate Weights

3 teaspoons	1 tbsp.
16 tablespoons	1 cup
½ cup	1 gill
2 cups	1 pt.
4 cups	1 qt.
2 pints	1 qt.
4 quarts	1 gal.
1 tablespoon butter	½ oz.
*1 tablespoon liquid	½ oz.
1 tablespoon flour	¼ oz.
1 tablespoon sugar	⅜ oz.
*1 cup liquid	8 ozs.
1 cup flour	4½ ozs.
1 cup butter	8 ozs.
1 cup sugar	10 ozs.

* Water or milk.

Equivalent Weights and Measures

Weight Equivalents

	Milligram	Gram	Kilogram	Grain	Ounce	Pound
1 microgram (mcg.)	.001	.000001				
1 milligram (mg.)	1.	.001		.0154		
1 gram (Gm.)	1,000.	1.	.001	15.4	.035	.0022
1 kilogram (Kg.)	1,000,000.	1,000.	1.	15,400.	35.2	2.2
1 grain (gr.)	64.8	.065		1.		
1 ounce (oz.)		28.3		437.5	1.	.063
1 pound (lb.)		453.6	.454		16.0	1.

Volume Equivalents

	Cubic Millimeter	Cubic Centimeter	Liter	Fluid Ounce	Pint	Quart
1 cubic millimeter (cu. mm.)	1.	.001				
1 cubic centimeter (cc.)	1,000.	1.	.001			
1 liter (L.)	1,000,000.	1,000.	1.	33.8	2.1	1.05
1 fluid ounce		30. (29.57)	.03	1.		
1 pint (pt.)		473.	.473	16.	1.	
1 quart (qt.)		946.	.946	32.	2.	1.

Linear Equivalents

	Millimeter	Centimeter	Meter	Inch	Foot	Yard
1 millimeter (mm.)	1.	.1	.001	.039	.00325	.0011
1 centimeter (cm.)	10.	1.		.39	.0325	.011
1 meter (M.)	1,000.	100.	1.	39.37	3.25	1.08
1 inch (in.)	25.4	2.54	.025	1.	.083	.028
1 foot (ft.)	304.8	30.48	.305	12.	1.	.33
1 yard (yd.)	914.4	91.44	.914	36.	3.	1.

As given in Cooper, L. F., Barber, E. M., Mitchell, H. S., and Rymbergen, H. J.: Nutrition in Health and Disease. Philadelphia, J. B. Lippincott Company.

APPENDIX VI. AVERAGE HEIGHT AND WEIGHT TABLES FOR CHILDREN

Height-Weight Tables for Girls *

Juvenile and Adolescent Ages

Height in Inches	5 Yrs	6 Yrs	7 Yrs	8 Yrs	9 Yrs	10 Yrs	11 Yrs	12 Yrs	13 Yrs	14 Yrs	15 Yrs	16 Yrs	17 Yrs	18 Yrs
38	33	33												
39	34	34												
40	36	36	36											
41	37	37	37											
42	39	39	39											
43	41	41	41	41										
44	42	42	42	42										
45	45	45	45	45	45									
46	47	47	47	48	48									
47	49	50	50	50	50	50								
48		52	52	52	52	53	53							
49			54	55	55	56	56							
50			56	57	58	59	61	62						
51			59	60	61	61	63	65						
52			63	64	64	64	65	67						
53			66	67	67	68	68	69	71					
54				69	70	70	71	71	73					
55				72	74	74	74	75	77	78				
56					76	78	78	79	81	83				
57					80	82	82	82	84	88	92			
58						84	86	86	88	93	96	101		
59						87	90	90	92	96	100	103	104	
60						91	95	95	97	101	105	108	109	111
61							99	100	101	105	108	112	113	116
62							104	105	106	109	113	115	117	118
63								110	110	112	116	117	119	120
64								114	115	117	119	120	122	123
65								118	120	121	122	123	125	126
66									124	124	125	128	129	130
67									128	130	131	133	133	135
68									131	133	135	136	138	138
69										135	137	138	140	142
70										136	138	140	142	144
71										138	140	142	144	145

* Prepared by Bird T. Baldwin, Ph.D., and Thomas D. Wood, M.D. Published originally by American Child Health Association.

Height-Weight Tables for Boys *

Juvenile and Adolescent Ages

Height in Inches	5 Yrs	6 Yrs	7 Yrs	8 Yrs	9 Yrs	10 Yrs	11 Yrs	12 Yrs	13 Yrs	14 Yrs	15 Yrs	16 Yrs	17 Yrs	18 Yrs	19 Yrs
38	34	34													
39	35	35													
40	36	36													
41	38	38	38												
42	39	39	39	39											
43	41	41	41	41											
44	44	44	44	44											
45	46	46	46	46	46										
46	47	48	48	48	48										
47	49	50	50	50	50	50									
48		52	53	53	53	53									
49		55	55	55	55	55	55								
50		57	58	58	58	58	58	58							
51			61	61	61	61	61	61							
52			63	64	64	64	64	64	64						
53			66	67	67	67	67	68	68						
54				70	70	70	70	71	71	72					
55				72	72	73	73	74	74	74					
56				75	76	77	77	77	78	78	80				
57					79	80	81	81	82	83	83				
58					83	84	84	85	85	86	87				
59						87	88	89	89	90	90	90			
60						91	92	92	93	94	95	96			
61							95	96	97	99	100	103	106		
62							100	101	102	103	104	107	111	116	
63							105	106	107	108	110	113	118	123	127
64								109	111	113	115	117	121	126	130
65								114	117	118	120	122	127	131	134
66									119	122	125	128	132	136	139
67									124	128	130	134	136	139	142
68										134	134	137	141	143	147
69										137	139	143	146	149	152
70										143	144	145	148	151	155
71										148	150	151	152	154	159
72											153	155	156	158	163
73											157	160	162	164	167
74											160	164	168	170	171

* Prepared by Bird T. Baldwin, Ph.D., and Thomas D. Wood, M.D. Published originally by American Child Health Association.

APPENDIX VII. AVERAGE HEIGHT AND WEIGHT TABLE FOR ADULTS

Ideal Weights for Men *

(Ages Twenty-five and Over)

Height (With Shoes)		Weight in Pounds (As Ordinarily Dressed)		
Feet:	*Inches:*	Small Frame	Medium Frame	Large Frame
5	2	116–25	124–33	131–42
5	3	119–28	127–36	133–44
5	4	122–32	130–40	137–49
5	5	126–36	134–44	141–53
5	6	129–39	137–47	145–57
5	7	133–43	141–51	149–62
5	8	136–47	145–56	153–66
5	9	140–51	149–60	157–70
5	10	144–55	153–64	161–75
5	11	148–59	157–68	165–80
6	0	152–64	161–73	169–85
6	1	157–69	166–78	174–90
6	2	163–75	171–84	179–96
6	3	168–80	176–89	184–202

Ideal Weights for Women *

(Ages Twenty-five and Over)

Height (With Shoes)		Weight in Pounds (As Ordinarily Dressed)		
Feet:	*Inches:*	Small Frame	Medium Frame	Large Frame
4	11	104–11	110–18	117–27
5	0	105–13	112–20	119–29
5	1	107–15	114–22	121–31
5	2	110–18	117–25	124–35
5	3	113–21	120–28	127–38
5	4	116–25	124–32	131–42
5	5	119–28	127–35	133–45
5	6	123–32	130–40	138–50
5	7	126–36	134–44	142–54
5	8	129–39	137–47	145–58
5	9	133–43	141–51	149–62
5	10	136–47	145–55	152–66
5	11	139–50	148–58	155–69

* Figures from Metropolitan Life Insurance Company, Statistical Bureau, 1943.

APPENDIX VIII. COMPOSITION OF FOOD EXCHANGES

Composition of Food Exchanges

List	*Food*	*Measures*	*Gm.*	*C*	*P*	*F*	*Cal.*
1	Milk Exchanges	½ pint	240	12	8	10	170
2a	Vegetable Exchanges	as desired	...	..	..	..	...
2b	Vegetable Exchanges	½ cup	100	7	2	..	36
3	Fruit Exchanges	varies	...	10	..	..	40
4	Bread Exchanges	varies	...	15	2	..	68
5	Meat Exchanges	1 oz.	30	..	7	5	73
6	Fat Exchanges	1 tsp.	5	..	..	5	45

APPENDIX IX. LISTS OF FOOD EXCHANGES, ARRANGED BY FOOD TYPE

LIST 1. MILK EXCHANGES

Carb.—12 gm., Protein—8 gm., Fat—10 gm., Calories 170

	Meas.	*Gm.*
*Milk, whole	1 cup	240
Milk, evaporated	½ cup	120
*Milk, powdered	¼ cup	35
*Buttermilk	1 cup	240

* Add 2 fat exchanges if fat free.

LIST 2. VEGETABLE EXCHANGES

A.—These vegetables may be used as desired in ordinary amounts. Carbohydrate and Calories negligible

Asparagus
Broccoli
Brussels Sprouts
Cabbage
Cauliflower
Celery
Chicory
Cucumbers
Escarole
Eggplant

Lettuce
Mushrooms
Okra
Pepper
Radishes
Rhubarb
Sauerkraut
String Beans, young
Summer Squash
Tomatoes

"GREENS"

Beet
Chard
Collard
Dandelion
Kale
Mustard
Spinach
Turnip

B.—Vegetables: 1 Serving equals ½ cup equals 100 grams. Carb.—7 gm., Protein—2 gm., Calories—36

Beets
Carrots
Onions

Peas, green
Pumpkin
Rutabaga

Squash, winter
Turnips

LIST 3. FRUIT EXCHANGES
Carbohydrate—10 gm., Calories—40

	Meas.	*Gm.*
Apple	1 sm. (2″ diam.)	80
Applesauce	½ cup	100
Apricots, fresh	2 medium	100
Apricots, dried	4 halves	20
Banana	½ small	50
Berries: Straw., Rasp., Black	1 cup	150
Blueberries	⅔ cup	100
Cantaloupe	¼ (6″ diam.)	200
Cherries	10 large	75
Dates	2	15
Figs, fresh	2 large	50
Figs, dried	1 small	15
Grapefruit	½ small	125
Grapefruit Juice	½ cup	100
Grapes	12	75
Grape Juice	¼ cup	60
Honeydew Melon	⅛ (7″ diam.)	150
Mango	½ small	70
Orange	1 small	125
Orange Juice	½ cup	100
Papaya	⅓ medium	100
Peach	1 medium	100
Pear	1 small	100
Pineapple	½ cup	80
Pineapple Juice	⅓ cup	80
Plums	2 medium	100
Prunes, dried	2 medium	25
Raisins	2 tbsp.	15
Tangerine	1 large	100
Watermelon	1 cup	175

LIST 4. BREAD EXCHANGES

Carbohydrate—15 gm., Protein—2 gm., Calories—68

	Meas.	*Gm.*
Bread	1 slice	25
Biscuit, Roll	1 (2″ diam.)	35
Muffin	1 (2″ diam.)	35
Cornbread	1 (1½″ cube)	35
Flour	2½ tbsp.	20
Cereal, cooked	½ cup	100
Cereal, dry (flake & puffed)	¾ cup	20
Rice, Grits, cooked	½ cup	100
Spaghetti, Noodles, etc., cooked	½ cup	100
Crackers, graham (2½″ sq.)	2	20
Oyster	20 (½ cup)	20
Saltines (2″ sq.)	5	20
Soda (2½″ sq.)	3	20
Round, thin (1½″ diam.)	6–8	20
Vegetables		
Beans & Peas, dried, cooked (lima, navy, split peas, cowpeas, etc.)	½ cup	90
Baked Beans, no pork	¼ cup	50
Corn	⅓ cup	80
Parsnips	⅔ cup	125
Potatoes, white, baked, boiled	1 (2″ diam.)	100
Potatoes, white, mashed	½ cup	100
Potatoes, sweet, or Yams	¼ cup	50
Sponge Cake, plain	1 (1½″ cube)	25
Ice Cream (Omit 2 fat exchanges)	½ cup	70

LIST 5. MEAT EXCHANGES

Protein—7 gm., Fat—5 gm., Calories—73

	Meas.	*Gm.*
Meat & Poultry (med. fat) (beef, lamb, pork, liver, chicken, etc.)	1 oz.	30
Cold Cuts (4½″ sq., ⅛″ thick)	1 slice	45
Frankfurter	1 (8–9/lb.)	50
Fish: Cod, Mackerel, etc	1 oz.	30
Salmon, Tuna, Crab	¼ cup	30
Oysters, Shrimp, Clams	5 small	45
Sardines	3 medium	30
Cheese, cheddar, American	1 oz.	30
Cottage	¼ cup	45
Egg	1	50
Peanut Butter*	2 tbsp.	30

* Limit use or adjust carbohydrate.

LIST 6. FAT EXCHANGES
Fat—5 gm., Calories—45

	Meas.	*Gm.*
Butter or Margarine	1 tsp.	5
Bacon, crisp	1 slice	10
Cream, light, 20%	2 tbsp.	30
Cream, heavy, 40%	1 tbsp.	15
Cream Cheese	1 tbsp.	15
French Dressing	1 tbsp.	15
Mayonnaise	1 tsp.	5
Oil or Cooking Fat	1 tsp.	5
Nuts	6 small	10
Olives	5 small	50
Avocado	⅛ (4″ diam.)	25

Index

Page numbers in *italic* type indicate illustrations.

Sample Forms

For the convenience of the reader there are reproduced on the following pages blank forms similar to Tables 21, 22, 24, and 27 in Chapter XV, and Table 33 in Chapter XVII. These can be used as models from which additional copies may be made.

DIET EVALUATION SUMMARY

FOOD GROUPS	1st Day	2nd Day	3rd Day	4th Day	5th Day	Ave. per Day	Recommended Amounts Child	Adol.	Adults	Difference
MILK GROUP							3-4 serv.	4 or more serv.	2 serv.	
MEAT GROUP							2 or more servings			
VEGETABLE-FRUIT GROUP Total No. Serv. (Including those rich in Vitamin C & Vitamin A							4 or more servings (Including --- - 1 serving -1 serving every other day -)			
BREAD-CEREAL GROUP Enriched or Whole grain							4 or more serv.			

SWEETS INTAKE

FORM	WHEN EATEN	1st Day	2nd Day	3rd Day	4th Day	5th Day	Total No. Exposures
Sugar in solution	During meal						
	End of meal						
	Between meals						
Retentive sweets	During meal						
	End of meal						
	Between meals						
Solid sweets	During meal						
	End of meal						
	Between meals						
						Grand total	

DIET EVALUATION SUMMARY

FOOD GROUPS	1st Day	2nd Day	3rd Day	4th Day	5th Day	Ave. per Day	Recommended Amounts Child	Adol.	Adults	Difference
MILK GROUP							3-4 serv.	4 or more serv.	2 serv.	
MEAT GROUP							2 or more servings			
VEGETABLE-FRUIT GROUP Total No. Serv. (Including those rich in Vitamin C & Vitamin A							4 or more servings (Including --- - 1 serving -1 serving every other day -)			
BREAD-CEREAL GROUP Enriched or Whole grain							4 or more serv.			

SWEETS INTAKE

FORM	WHEN EATEN	1st Day	2nd Day	3rd Day	4th Day	5th Day	Total No. Exposures
Sugar in solution	During meal						
	End of meal						
	Between meals						
Retentive sweets	During meal						
	End of meal						
	Between meals						
Solid sweets	During meal						
	End of meal						
	Between meals						
						Grand total	

FOOD INTAKE CHART WITH SPECIAL CONSIDERATION TO PHYSICAL FORM OF FOOD

FOOD GROUPS	PHYSICAL FORM	1st Day	2nd Day	3	4	5	Average Per Day	Recommended Intake	Diff.
I MILK	Liquid Soft							2 Serv.	
	Hard								
II MEAT	Soft Chopped							2 Serv.	
	Solid								
III VEGETABLE FRUIT	Juices, Processed							4 Serv.	
	Raw or Slightly cooked								
IV BREAD-CEREAL	Soft, cooked							4 Serv.	
	Dry, crusty, Toasted								

FOOD INTAKE CHART WITH SPECIAL CONSIDERATION TO PHYSICAL FORM OF FOOD

FOOD GROUPS	PHYSICAL FORM	1st Day	2nd Day	3	4	5	Average Per Day	Recommended Intake	Diff.
I MILK	Liquid Soft							2 Serv.	
	Hard								
II MEAT	Soft Chopped							2 Serv.	
	Solid								
III VEGETABLE FRUIT	Juices, Processed							4 Serv.	
	Raw or Slightly cooked								
IV BREAD-CEREAL	Soft, cooked							4 Serv.	
	Dry, crusty, Toasted								

FIRST DAY			SECOND DAY			THIRD DAY		
Food:	Quantity:	Prepared:	Food:	Quantity:	Prepared:	Food:	Quantity	Prepared.
BREAKFAST:			BREAKFAST:			BREAKFAST:		
10:00 A.M.			10:00 A.M.			10:00 A.M.		
LUNCH:			LUNCH:			LUNCH:		
3:00 P.M.			3:00 P.M.			3:00 P.M.		
DINNER:			DINNER:			DINNER:		
EXTRAS:			EXTRAS:			EXTRAS:		

FOURTH DAY

Food: Quantity: Prepared:

BREAKFAST:

10:00 A.M.

LUNCH:

3:00 P.M.

DINNER:

EXTRAS:

FIFTH DAY

Food: Quantity: Prepared:

BREAKFAST:

10:00 A.M.

LUNCH:

3:00 P.M.

DINNER:

EXTRAS:

FOOD INTAKE DIARY

Of:

FOR THE FIVE DAYS (include one WEEKEND DAY or a HOLIDAY)

INSTRUCTIONS

1. Record every type of food consumed, solid or liquid, at mealtime, between meals, at the soda fountain, while watching television. Record also, candies, Lifesavers, gum, cough drops or syrups.
2. For each meal, list the food, preparation, (fried, boiled, etc.) and amount in household measures (1 t., 1 T., 1 cup (8 oz.), 1 4 oz. glass, no. of pieces).
3. For fruits and vegetables, record whether raw, fresh, frozen or canned.
4. Record amount of sugar or sugar products and cream or milk added to cereal, beverages or other foods.
5. Record foods in the order in which they are eaten.
6. Particular information on extras is most important to us. Do not leave out the smallest detail.

FIRST DAY			SECOND DAY			THIRD DAY		
Food:	Quantity:	Prepared:	Food:	Quantity:	Prepared:	Food:	Quantity	Prepared.
BREAKFAST:			BREAKFAST:			BREAKFAST:		
10:00 A.M.			10:00 A.M.			10:00 A.M.		
LUNCH:			LUNCH:			LUNCH:		
3:00 P.M.			3:00 P.M.			3:00 P.M.		
DINNER:			DINNER:			DINNER:		
EXTRAS:			EXTRAS:			EXTRAS:		

FOURTH DAY

Food: Quantity: Prepared:

BREAKFAST:

10:00 A.M.

LUNCH:

3:00 P.M.

DINNER:

EXTRAS:

FIFTH DAY

Food: Quantity: Prepared:

BREAKFAST:

10:00 A.M.

LUNCH:

3:00 P.M.

DINNER:

EXTRAS:

FOOD INTAKE DIARY

Of:

FOR THE FIVE DAYS (include one WEEKEND DAY or a HOLIDAY)

INSTRUCTIONS

1. Record every type of food consumed, solid or liquid, at mealtime, between meals, at the soda fountain, while watching television. Record also, candies, Lifesavers, gum, cough drops or syrups.
2. For each meal, list the food, preparation, (fried, boiled, etc.) and amount in household measures (1 t., 1 T., 1 cup (8 oz.), 1 4 oz. glass, no. of pieces).
3. For fruits and vegetables, record whether raw, fresh, frozen or canned.
4. Record amount of sugar or sugar products and cream or milk added to cereal, beverages or other foods.
5. Record foods in the order in which they are eaten.
6. Particular information on extras is most important to us. Do not leave out the smallest detail.

DIET "PRESCRIPTION" FOR CONTROL OF RAMPANT CARIES

I. Total Sweets Intake ________ per week   Recommended Substitutes:

II. Number of Detergent Foods Used ________ per week   Improve by Increasing:

III. a) DIET

FOOD GROUPS	Actual Intake	Recommended Intake	Improve by + Increase	- Decrease
MILK GROUP				
MEAT GROUP				
VEGETABLE-FRUIT GROUP				
BREAD-CEREAL GROUP				

b) MEAL PLAN

Recommended Typical Meal Plan	Patient's Typical Meal Plan	Recommended Improvements
Breakfast		
Meat or Milk - 1 serv. or more		
Bread-Cereal - 2 serv. or more		
Vegetable-Fruit - 1 serv.		
Lunch		
Bread-Cereal - 2 serv. or more		
Meat - 1 serv. or more		
Vegetable-Fruit - 2 serv. or more		
Milk - 1 serv.		
Dinner		
Meat - 1 serv. or more		
Vegetable-Fruit - 2 serv. or more		
Bread-Cereal - 1 serv. or more		
Milk - 1 serv.		

c) MENU PLAN *

BREAKFAST	LUNCH	DINNER

* Use Exchange List of Foods as a guide for selection of foods to include and avoid in designing menus to suit individual taste.

DIET "PRESCRIPTION" FOR CONTROL OF RAMPANT CARIES

I. Total Sweets Intake________ per week — Recommended Substitutes:

II. Number of Detergent Foods Used ________ per week — Improve by Increasing:

III. a) DIET

FOOD GROUPS	Actual Intake	Recommended Intake	Improve by + Increase	- Decrease
MILK GROUP				
MEAT GROUP				
VEGETABLE-FRUIT GROUP				
BREAD-CEREAL GROUP				

b) MEAL PLAN

Recommended Typical Meal Plan	Patient's Typical Meal Plan	Recommended Improvements
Breakfast		
Meat or Milk - 1 serv. or more		
Bread-Cereal - 2 serv. or more		
Vegetable-Fruit - 1 serv.		
Lunch		
Bread-Cereal - 2 serv. or more		
Meat - 1 serv. or more		
Vegetable-Fruit - 2 serv. or more		
Milk - 1 serv.		
Dinner		
Meat - 1 serv. or more		
Vegetable-Fruit - 2 serv. or more		
Bread-Cereal - 1 serv. or more		
Milk - 1 serv.		

c) MENU PLAN *

BREAKFAST	LUNCH	DINNER

* Use Exchange List of Foods as a guide for selection of foods to include and avoid in designing menus to suit individual taste.